Lecture Notes of the Institute for Computer Sciences, Social Informatics and Telecommunications Engineering   159

More information about this series at http://www.springer.com/series/8197

Vladimir Atanasovski · Alberto Leon-Garcia (Eds.)

Future Access Enablers for Ubiquitous and Intelligent Infrastructures

First International Conference, FABULOUS 2015
Ohrid, Republic of Macedonia, September 23–25, 2015
Revised Selected Papers

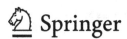 Springer

Editors
Vladimir Atanasovski
Ss. Cyril and Methodius University
  in Skopje
Skopje
Macedonia

Alberto Leon-Garcia
University of Toronto
Toronto
Canada

ISSN 1867-8211 ISSN 1867-822X (electronic)
Lecture Notes of the Institute for Computer Sciences, Social Informatics
and Telecommunications Engineering
ISBN 978-3-319-27071-5 ISBN 978-3-319-27072-2 (eBook)
DOI 10.1007/978-3-319-27072-2

Library of Congress Control Number: 2015955868

Springer Cham Heidelberg New York Dordrecht London

Printed on acid-free paper

Springer International Publishing AG Switzerland is part of Springer Science+Business Media
(www.springer.com)

Preface

The world of smart environments enabled by broadband and pervasive communications is changing toward ubiquitous interconnected digital surroundings that offer increasing opportunities for novel access and core technologies, novel applications and services, and novel communications solutions. This volume constitutes the refereed proceedings of the First EAI International Conference on Future Access Enablers of Ubiquitous and Intelligent Infrastructures (FABULOUS 2015), held in Ohrid, Macedonia, in September 2015. The submitted papers were carefully reviewed before being selected for presentation and inclusion in this volume. The papers cover the broad areas of future wireless networks, ambient and assisted living, smart infrastructures, and security and they reflect the fast developing and vibrant penetration of IoT technologies in diverse areas of human lives. They aim to consolidate the main results achieved in this area.

November 2015   Liljana Gavrilovska

Organization

FABULOUS 2015 was organized by the EAI in cooperation with ICST.

Steering Committee

Imrich Chlamtac	Create-Net, Italy
Liljana Gavrilovska	Ss. Cyril and Methodius University in Skopje, Macedonia
Alberto Leon-Garcia	University of Toronto, Canada

Organizing Committee

General Co-chairs

Imrich Chlamtac	Create-Net, Italy
Liljana Gavrilovska	Ss. Cyril and Methodius University in Skopje, Macedonia

TPC Chair

Alberto Leon-Garcia	University of Toronto, Canada

Publication Chair

Vladimir Atanasovski	Ss. Cyril and Methodius University in Skopje, Macedonia

Workshops Chair

Aleksandar Risteski	Ss. Cyril and Methodius University in Skopje, Macedonia

Publicity and Social Media Co-chairs

Marina Petrova	RWTH Aachen, Germany
Mile Stankovski	Ss. Cyril and Methodius University in Skopje, Macedonia
Dimitar Trajanov	Ss. Cyril and Methodius University in Skopje, Macedonia

Web Chair

Valentin Rakovic	Ss. Cyril and Methodius University in Skopje, Macedonia

Sponsorship Chair

Miroslav Jovanovic	Makedonski Telekom, Macedonia

Demo Chair

Pero Latkoski	Ss. Cyril and Methodius University in Skopje, Macedonia

Technical Program Committee

Aguayo-Torres Mari Carmen	Universidad de Malaga, Spain
Akyildiz Ian	Georgia Tech, GA, USA
Atanasovski Vladimir	Ss. Cyril and Methodius University in Skopje, Macedonia
Bader Carlos Faouzi	Supelec, France
van de Beek Jaap	Luleå University of Technology, Sweden
Bhargava Vijay	University of British Columbia, Canada
Chen Lei	Sam Houston State University, USA
Chomu Konstantin	Ss. Cyril and Methodius University in Skopje, Macedonia
Correia M. Luis	IST, T.U. Lisbon, Portugal
Da Silva Luiz	Trinity College Dublin, Ireland
Di Benedetto Maria-Gabriella	University of Rome La Sapienza, Italy
Denkovski Daniel	Ss. Cyril and Methodius University in Skopje, Macedonia
Fratu Octavian	University Politehnica of Bucharest, Romania
Giorgetti Andrea	University of Bologna, Italy
Koucheryavy Yevgeni	Tampere University of Technology, Finland
Kyriazakos Sofoklis	Aalborg University, Denmark
Latkoski Pero	Ss. Cyril and Methodius University in Skopje, Macedonia
Lazaridis Pavlos	Alexander Technological Educational Institute of Thessaloniki, Greece
Milutinovic Veljko	University of Belgrade, Serbia
Mohorcic Mihael	Jozef Stefan Institute, Slovenia
de Nardis Luca	University of Rome La Sapienza, Italy
Neskovic Aleksandar	University of Belgrade, Serbia
Popovski Petar	Aalborg University, Denmark
Poulkov Vladimir	Technical University of Sofia, Bulgaria
Rakovic Valentin	Ss. Cyril and Methodius University in Skopje, Macedonia
Sayrac Berna	Orange, France
Schwefel Hans-Peter	FTW, Vienna, Austria
Shuminoski Tomislav	Ss. Cyril and Methodius University in Skopje, Macedonia
Stankovski Mile	Ss. Cyril and Methodius University in Skopje, Macedonia
Tafazolli Rahim	University of Surrey, UK
Trajkovic Vladimir	Ss. Cyril and Methodius University in Skopje, Macedonia
Trobec Roman	Jozef Stefan Institute, Slovenia

Contents

X   Contents

Special Session on Cyberspace Security

Demo Session: Student Innovation Corner

Regular Session

Special Session on Software-Defined Infrastructures and Smart Applications

SAVI Testbed Architecture and Federation

Thomas Lin, Byungchul Park, Hadi Bannazadeh,
and Alberto Leon-Garcia[⊠]

Department of Electrical and Computer Engineering, University of Toronto,
Toronto, ON M5S 3G4, Canada
{t.lin,byungchul.park,hadi.bannazadeh,alberto.leongarcia}@utoronto.ca

Abstract. The flexibility of cloud computing has afforded users the ability to develop and deploy fully customizable cloud-based applications and services. Thus far, this flexibility has primarily been constrained to the likes of x86 servers and storage devices. The SAVI application platform testbed was developed to realize the hypothesis that all physical infrastructure resources can be virtualized. Key to this work is a novel control and management framework based on Software-Defined Infrastructure (SDI), a concept which provides a unified programmable interface over heterogeneous infrastructures. In this paper, we present the architecture of the Canadian SAVI national testbed based on the SDI framework. The design of an autonomous SAVI node will be described and the multi-node deployment that comprise the national testbed will be discussed. In addition, the orchestration of applications across the multi-node testbed will be described. Lastly, we will report on the progress of our recent efforts to federate the SAVI testbed with the American GENI national testbed.

Keywords: Cloud computing · Cloud federation · SDI · Testbed

1 Introduction

Continual advances in the information and communication technology fields over the past decade have resulted in increased performance of commodity off-the-shelf CPUs, higher speed Ethernet technologies, and higher capacity storage devices, all at ever lowering costs. In turn, cloud computing has become increasingly affordable and available, transforming the way people and businesses create, host, and deliver new services and applications. In anticipating that cloud-based platforms will form the basis of future applications and services with lifecycles ranging from a few hours to multiple months, or even years, the Smart Applications on Virtual Infrastructure (SAVI) project[1] was launched to investigate the design of future application enablement platforms upon which applications and services can be flexibly deployed, maintained, and retired, all on a fully virtualized infrastructure. SAVI is an NSERC (Natural Sciences and Engineering Research Council of Canada) strategic research network comprised of a partnership between industry, academia, and research networks.

---

[1] http://www.savinetwork.ca.

© Institute for Computer Sciences, Social Informatics and Telecommunications Engineering 2015
V. Atanasovski, L.-G. Alberto (Eds.): Fabulous 2015, LNICST 159, pp. 3–10, 2015.
DOI: 10.1007/978-3-319-27072-2_1

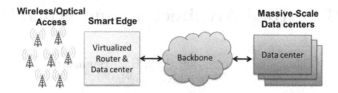

Fig. 1. Conceptual view of multi-tier cloud.

SAVI believes that the flexibilities and economies of scale seen today with cloud-based computing and storage resources can be further extended to other types of resources. Thus, key to the development of the SAVI application platform testbed was the inclusion of heterogeneous resources in the form of alternative computing resources (e.g. programmable hardware, network processors, GPUs, etc.) and network devices that are programmable via software-defined networking (SDN) techniques. This assortment of heterogeneous resource types in a cloud setting enables users to create novel applications on-the-fly without having to purchase physical hardware. SAVI also views future cloud application platforms as comprising multiple tiers, with smaller clouds at the edge closer to the users for providing localized services (e.g. smart grid alarms, transportation safety applications, monitoring in remote health) at reduced access latencies. We use the term "Smart Edge" to describe these heterogeneous clouds at the network edge. This led SAVI to develop its testbed in a multi-tiered fashion, as seen in Fig. 1, comprising of two main tiers and an access tier. The main tiers involve core datacentres, which are massive in scale and may be located in regions with inexpensive or renewable energy, as well as smaller Smart Edge datacentres strategically located closer to the end-users. The access tier is seen as enabling users to access the applications platform through devices that connect to a high-bandwidth, integrated wireless/optical access network. The application platform thus provides direct network connectivity (i.e. not over the public internet) to the applications and services of interest.

In this paper, we present the SAVI testbed architecture based on the concept of software-defined infrastructure (SDI), and we explore how to orchestrate applications across the multi-node national deployment. We include a brief report summarizing the work to date on federating the SAVI and GENI testbeds. The paper is organized as follows. Section 2 will present the SDI architecture for performing converged control and management of networking and heterogeneous cloud resources. In Sect. 3, we first introduce the architectural design of a single SAVI node, followed by a discussion of the multi-node national deployment that constitute the SAVI testbed. Our efforts to date at federating with the GENI[2] testbed in the United States are briefly summarized in Sect. 4, and we conclude in Sect. 5.

---

[2] https://www.geni.net/.

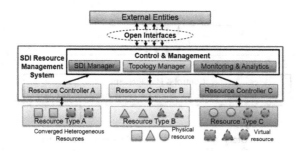

Fig. 2. Software-defined infrastructure.

2   SAVI SDI Architecture

We investigate the hypothesis that all physical resources can be virtualized and managed using Infrastructure-as-a-Service (IaaS) and Platform-as-a-Service (PaaS) principles and we arrive at the Software-Defined Infrastructure (SDI) architecture [1] to realize the hypothesis. SDI is a concept which provides an abstraction for unified control and management over an underlying set of heterogeneous resources. The abstraction exposes a set of open interfaces (i.e. APIs) to external users and entities, upon which infrastructure control applications may be built in a programmatic fashion. Figure 2 depicts the high level architectural overview of the SDI resource management system (RMS). There are three control and management components essential to the SDI RMS: the SDI manager, the topology manager, and the monitoring and analytics (M&A) system.

The SDI manager, responsible for the decision making and execution of control and management tasks, coordinates with the topology manager as well as the monitoring and analytics system. In order for an SDI manager to control and manage all the resource types that exist in a given infrastructure (e.g. x86 servers, FPGAs, GPUs, sensors, network switches, access points, etc.), we associate each resource type with a specialized resource controller capable of interfacing with that type. The resource controllers essentially act as proxies for the control and management components, and are responsible for performing the necessary tasks to virtualize the resources under their control. New resource types can be added into the testbed by simply finding an appropriate controller and interfacing it with the SDI manager.

The topology manager keeps a record of all the resources in the infrastructure, both physical and virtual, and tracks their relationships with one another. Like the SDI manager, the topology manager leverages the various resource controllers in order to accomplish its task. It provides information regarding the current state and configuration of each resource type, thus enabling external entities as well as the SDI manager to perform infrastructure-state-aware management.

Lastly, the M&A system [2] is responsible for collecting, storing, and analyzing data from the entire infrastructure. It is able to monitor and collect data from both the physical resources as well as the virtual resources. If given access, it is also able to collect data regarding applications running within virtual machines.

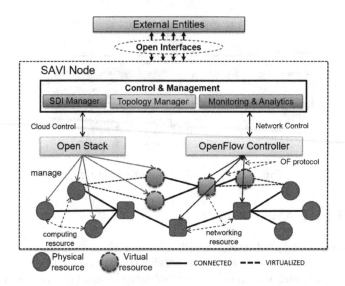

Fig. 3. Design of SAVI node based on SDI.

The collected raw data can be queried directly or fed into an analytics framework whereupon the SDI manager or other external entities can query the results and use them to inform crucial control and management decisions.

3   SAVI National Infrastructure

The infrastructure of the SAVI national testbed is comprised of multiple nodes deployed over several university campuses. The current deployment spans seven universities containing one core datacentre interconnected with seven smaller smart edge datacentres located closer to the end-users. The interconnection between nodes utilizes a dedicated layer 2 optical fibre network.

3.1   SAVI Node Design

Figure 3 shows the design of a SAVI node based on the SDI architecture to manage both cloud and networking resources. It contains the three major SDI RMS components (SDI manager, topology manager, and M&A), as well as two resource controllers realized using OpenStack and an OpenFlow controller [3]. The SDI manager controls and manages virtual computing resources using Open-Stack as the computing resource controller. For heterogeneous resources, we have extended OpenStack to support the virtualization of unconventional resources within our testbed (e.g. FPGAs, GPUs, etc.) by adding new device drivers. For networking resources, an OpenFlow controller is utilized. The OpenFlow controller receives all network events from the OpenFlow-enabled switches and conveys them to the SDI manager. The SDI manager performs all management

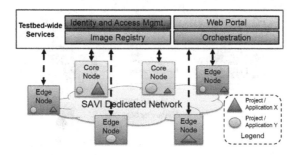

Fig. 4. Muti-node design of SAVI tesbed deployment.

functions based on data provided by the OpenStack and OpenFlow controllers, as well as the topology manager and M&A components. This data allows the SDI manager to conduct infrastructure-state-aware resource management such as fault tolerance, path optimization, resource scheduling and network-aware VM replacement. It determines appropriate actions for controlling computing and networking resources and applies the actions to resources through the Open-Stack and OpenFlow controllers.

3.2   SAVI Multi-node Deployment

The multi-node design of the SAVI testbed is depicted in Fig. 4. With the exception of a few testbed-wide services, each node essentially operates autonomously. Each node contains the necessary hardware and software for virtualizing the compute, network, and storage resources local to that node, as well as all the control and management functionalities. However, there are a few essential services that every node shares; these testbed-wide services include: 1. the identity and access management (IAM) service; 2. the image registry service; 3. the SAVI web portal; and 4. the orchestration service.

The IAM service is responsible for storing the credentials for all the users of the testbed, their associations with various projects, as well as a catalog of all the services throughout the testbed. The catalog is crucial as it offers clients and users a centralized lookup service to discover the endpoint URLs (point of contact for open APIs) of any service given the ID of an autonomous node. Users can thus provision resources spread across various nodes that are associated with the same project identification. A logically centralized image registry is also crucial as it allows users to use the same image irrespective of location. Finally, both the web portal and the orchestration services offers a testbed-wide view for users to deploy multi-node applications and services.

3.3   Testbed-Wide Orchestration

The SAVI testbed provides a centralized orchestration service with an end-to-end view of the entire infrastructure, thus providing the ability to deploy platform-wide applications and services. We leverage the OpenStack orchestration service,

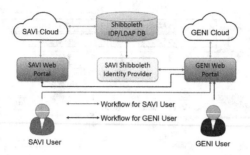

Fig. 5. Authentication workflow of federated SAVI-GENI cloud.

Heat, to manage the lifecycle of multi-node resource deployments. Multi-node deployments enables users to create, update, and retire complex applications that can fully leverage the multi-tiered aspect of the SAVI testbed. The virtual infrastructure for these multi-node applications and services can be fully described in text-based "templates", which can be deployed by the orchestration service in a single action. Changes to the application infrastructure merely requires changing the template and pushing it to the orchestration service. For example, envision a scenario in which a video-on-demand service is deployed such that the content servers are located in the Core, with caches and virtualized transcoders located at the smart edges to provide clients with low-latency access to the content in a multitude of different video formats. Updates to the service can be triggered either manually through the orchestration service, or automatically, by tying the testbed's monitoring service directly to the orchestration service. Thus, virtualized resources such as the transcoders and caches, can be automatically scaled in and out depending on the current load on the system.

4   Federation with GENI

Cloud federation involves the interconnection of multiple cloud environments for the enablement of cross-cloud applications. Cloud federation offers substantial benefits for both the cloud provider and the users [4]. It enables cloud providers to expand their geographic spheres and accommodates abrupt resource demands by leveraging the resources of federated clouds. In addition, users can utilize heterogeneous resources that may not be available in a certain cloud environment, as well as deploy applications and services spanning a wider geographical reach.

GENI [5] is a National Science Foundation (NSF) funded nationwide cloud infrastructure located in the United States. It is a collaborative and exploratory environment for academia and industry to do experimental research in computer networking and distributed systems, and to accelerate the transition of this research into products and services.

The SAVI teams at the University of Victoria and the University of Toronto are currently working in close collaboration with the GENI project office to federate the two testbeds. In this section, we present a brief summary of this effort on behalf of all researchers involved; further details regarding this work will be presented in the future. This work involves different levels: 1. federated authentication and user-base; and 2. providing common APIs for both SAVI and GENI. Currently, we have achieved the first goal and have developed a command line Common Interface tool to interface with both GENI and SAVI.

Figure 5 describes the authentication workflow of the federated SAVI-GENI cloud. For a SAVI user to access the GENI cloud, the user first visits the GENI portal which redirects them to the SAVI Shibboleth[3] Identity Provider (SSIDP). The SSIDP verifies the users SAVI credentials against an LDAP database containing the credentials of all SAVI users. If authenticated, the SSIDP redirects and logs the user into the GENI portal. Once in the GENI Portal, the user can request resources using the web interface or through the downloadable command line Common Interface tool. For a GENI user to access the SAVI cloud, the user selects "SAVI access" from within the GENI portal, which posts a user certificate to the SAVI IAM. If authenticated, the SAVI IAM issues the user a set of SAVI credentials. The user may then request resources through the SAVI web portal or through the Common Interface tool.

To provide an example of SAVI-GENI federation, we have presented tutorial sessions in three different conferences (GEC23, Tridentcom 2015, and SAVI Workshop 2015) showcasing the ability for users to create a slice spanning the SAVI and GENI testbeds, and jointly orchestrating the actions of VMs across both cloud infrastructures. The federation of SAVI with GENI provides a powerful testbed and application platform for experimenters and developers alike.

We would like to acknowledge Sudhakar Ganti, Sushil Bhojwani, Riz Panjwani, and Rick McGeer from the University of Victoria, as well as Tom Mitchell, Niky Riga, and Vicraj Thomas from the GENI office, for all their contributions towards this work.

5 Conclusion

In this paper we introduced the architecture for the multi-node SAVI national testbed, a cloud-based applications platform which features a novel control and management framework based on software-defined infrastructure. The SDI management system facilitates the realization of converged control over a fully virtualized platform featuring heterogeneous resources. Together, the open APIs atop the SDI management system, the testbed orchestration system, the variety of available resources at the smart edges, and the federation with GENI, now affords users the ability and opportunity to provision novel applications and services anytime with a wide geographical reach.

---

[3] https://shibboleth.net/.

References

1. Kang, J.M., Bannazadeh, H., Rahimi, H., Lin, T., Faraji, M., Leon-Garcia, A.: Software-defined infrastructure and the future central office. In: International Conference on Communications (ICC), pp. 225–229 (2013)
2. Lin, J., Ravichandiran, R., Bannazadeh, H., Leon-Garcia, A.: Monitoring and measurement in software-defined infrastructure. In: IFIP/IEEE International Symposium on Integrated Network Management (IM), pp. 742–745 (2015)
3. McKeown, N., Anderson, T., Balakrishnan, H., Parulkar, G., Peterson, L., Rexford, J., Shenker, S., Turner, J.: OpenFlow: enabling innovation in campus networks. SIGCOMM Comput. Commun. Rev. **38**(2), 69–74 (2008)
4. Goiri, I., Guitart, J., Torres, J.: Characterizing cloud federation for enhancing providers' profit. In: IEEE International Conference on Cloud Computing, pp. 123–130 (2010)
5. GENI design principles. GENI planning group, IEEE Computer, vol. 39(9), pp. 102–105 (2006). doi:10.1109/MC.2006.307

VNF Service Chaining on SAVI SDI

Pouya Yasrebi[1,2](✉), Spandan Bemby[1,2], Hadi Bannazadeh[1,2],
and Alberto Leon-Garcia[1,2]

[1] University of Toronto, Toronto, ON, Canada
{pouya.yasrebi,spandan.bemby,hadi.bannazadeh,
alberto.leongarcia}@utoronto.ca
[2] University of Toronto - St. George Campus, 40 St George St,
Toronto, ON M5S 2E4, Canada

Abstract. Managing computational resources and networking elements over today's heterogeneous infrastructure has become very challenging. A need for virtualizing network functions has emerged to reduce infrastructure operating costs. In this paper we consider using software-defined infrastructure (SDI) resource management system (RMS) to achieve service chaining of virtualized network functions (VNFs). SDI allows for the integrated control and management of heterogenous resources. In an SDI environment, the end user has access to interfaces that allow programmatic management of the resources. The user can define their own service graph (SG), which determines the path that traffic must take through various VNFs. The ability to dynamically realize the SG is what is referred to by service chaining. Use cases of service chaining include adding a firewall in front of web server and multicasting. Furthermore, we tested the firewall use case in two scenarios to verify validity of our service chaining implementation.

Keywords: Software defined infrastructure · Network function virtualization · Virtualized network function · Software defined networking · OpenFlow · Smart application on virtual infrastructure

1 Introduction

Application infrastructures consist of two primary components: computing and networking. Due to recent advances in computing and networking technologies, these infrastructures are experiencing two notable changes. First, computing is shifting towards the cloud because of reduced costs through shared resources. Second, traditional networking is being replaced by software-defined networking (SDN) due to its greater flexibility and reduced management cost. Typically, compute and networking resources were controlled and managed separately. However, in [2], Kang et al. presented the software-defined infrastructure (SDI) architecture for a resource management system (RMS) that allows for integrated management of networking and compute resources.

The SDI [6] RMS manages resources in a hierarchical fashion, whereby individual resources are controlled by the corresponding resource controller.

© Institute for Computer Sciences, Social Informatics and Telecommunications Engineering 2015
V. Atanasovski, L.-G. Alberto (Eds.): Fabulous 2015, LNICST 159, pp. 11–17, 2015.
DOI: 10.1007/978-3-319-27072-2_2

These resource controllers are managed by a centralized entity, an SDI manager, which allows for integrated management of heterogeneous resources, such as networking, computing, and other unconventional resources like FPGAs and wireless access. The SDI manager also exposes interfaces that allow applications to programmatically manage their resources while having access to topology information and monitoring data. These SDI interfaces also facilitate functions such as orchestration and service chaining.

The SDI RMS is responsible for coordinating all interactions with resources, including the deployment of applications. Deployment consists of various parts including, resource allocation, configuration, and satisfying quality of service (QoS) SLAs. The SDI RMS delegates the allocation and configuration of resources to an orchestration system built upon OpenStack. Orchestration refers to the management, i.e. the creation, deletion, and modification, of a lifecycle of a cloud application or service. The orchestration engine abstracts various functions, and facilitates the management of resource lifecycles.

An application deployment consists of various pluggable modules, such as network functions (NF) that must be connected together. These pluggable functions are also referred to as virtual network functions (VNF). NFV supplies modules, that traditionally were provided to consumers as priority boxes, as processes in virtual machines (VM). In general, an application may want to specify a service graph (SG), that defines traffics order of traversal through a set of VNFs [3]. An SG includes a set of Service Level Agreements (SLA) that the infrastructure must fulfill. To satisfy these SLAs, the VNFs must be connected virtually, i.e. service chained. Chaining refers to the modification in configuration of network components such as switches, to direct packets through the set of intended modules.

This paper is organized as follows. Section 2 describes how we perform service chaining in an SDI environment. Section 3 describes what orchestration is and how we leverage an orchestration engine to facilitate service chaining. Section 4 considers our experiments with service chaining and their evaluation. Finally, the conclusion is presented in Sect. 5.

2   Service Chaining in SAVI

In this section we provide a more concrete definition of service chaining. We then consider the features provided by the SDI RMS, and how these can facilitate service chaining.

An application deployment consists of services that the end-user interacts with, e.g. a web server, and other NFs, i.e. transparent components like a load balancer. NFV refers to the virtualization of arbitrary NFs, such as deep packet inspection (DPI) firewalls, load balancers, etc. Individual NFs can be composed into a SG, that specifies a list of services and the order of traversal. For instance, consider a web application (app) deployment. This app may consist of a firewall that filters the traffic and a load balancer that distributes the load across horizontally scaled web servers. The SG is an abstract object that corresponds to a set of SLAs. The realization of a SG is service chaining. Service chaining consists of two parts: creating the VNFs specified in the SG, and chaining them together. These can be done through the orchestration engine and the SDI manager, respectively. Specifically, the SDI manager has state information of the infrastructure and can direct the resource controllers to execute certain operations (See Fig. 1). These combined, allow the SDI manager to perform functions such as fault tolerance and dynamic installation of network flows.

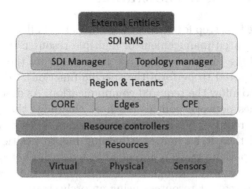

Fig. 1. SDI overall architecture

To facilitate service chaining, the SDI manager exposes many primitive functions, such as: tapping and blocking. Tapping refers to sending a copy of the incoming traffic to a host that was not the intended destination. Blocking concerns dropping packets according to system requirements in switches.

As an example of chaining, lets consider a WordPress deployment consisting of two VMs- one running a web server and the other running a database. It is desirable to allow the application to dynamically change their SG. For instance, the application may want to insert an inline deep packet inspection (DPI) VNF in front of the web server. The applications requirement can be satisfied using service chaining. Now lets consider how service chaining in the web server example could be realized. First, the application would request the SDI manager to perform service chaining by inserting a DPI VNF in front of the web server. The SDI manager would direct the network controller to install special high-priority flows in the switches of the underlying infrastructure to ensure all traffic headed for the web server goes to the DPI VNF. In this case we would have to configure the DPI unit to forward the traffic to the web server. Alternatively, we could use tapping so that the traffic is sent to the web server and mirrored to the DPI VNF [9]. Since resource controllers can be directed to execute commands at any time, service chaining can be performed on a live system without service disruption.

Multicasting is another example of an application that can leverage VNF chaining. Lets consider the sequences of events when deploying a multicasting application. First, the orchestration engine creates casting modules such as virtualized transceivers and load balancers. Migrating the chained casting modules could reduce total bandwidth usage by reconstructing a more efficient multicast tree. In [10], Zhang et al. demonstrated cost reductions in deployments of multicast trees with a newly proposed routing algorithm that used dynamic chaining of VNFs.

3   Integration with Orchestration

Orchestration is the first step for service chaining. The challenge in service chaining consists of integrated management of multiple resource types such as computing and networking resources. First, we have to create the VNFs (these are typically VMs configured to perform the specific function). Second, we need to connect the nodes to allow the required communication. As described above, the SDI manager applies network policies (such as chaining) that ensure that the traffic traverses the required VNF(s). In our previous DPI example, first a DPI unit is created and then it is chained. Chaining has to position the firewall in such a way that all packets that are intended to reach the web server have to be redirected from the gateway through the firewall and to the web server.

Applications can request resources using an orchestration service on an SDI environment. For our experiments we utilized the Heat Orchestration project [4] from OpenStack. Heat facilitates the management of the creation, modification, and deletion of cloud infrastructure resources over the applications life cycle. Applications specify what resources they need and how they should be configured in descriptive template files. The orchestration engine then parses these templates to provision and configure the required resources. The applications can also modify and delete resources by providing new or modified templates to the orchestration engine. Therefore, the orchestration service allows management of complex topologies without increasing the cost of managing that complexity. Furthermore, template files for Heat are compatible with Amazon Web Services (AWS) CloudFormation (another orchestration service).

4   Implementation and Evaluations

We have conducted our service chaining experiments on the SAVI testbed to prove our concepts. The SAVI TB is an experimental platform intended to allow investigation into future application infrastructures. The SAVI TB is based on the SDI resource management architecture [1,5].

We conducted the following experiment to demonstrate dynamic service chaining. Our experiment consisted of a WordPress deployment and a DPI unit that were subsequently chained. We initiated two attacks to a web server and then attempted to block the attacks via a network intrusion detection and prevention system (NIDPS) that blocks the attackers in the same IDS. For both tests, the initial setups consisted of a web server (WS) running WordPress, and a database (DB) running MySQL. Both WS and DB were created using a Heat orchestration template on the SAVI TB. The WS and DB were configured to allow the WordPress contents to be stored on the DB. This version of WordPress was a generic template representing a typical blogging web site over the Internet. Hence, it did not have any advanced filtering techniques embedded in itself.

We used a web user interface (Web UI) to allow users to request to chain the NIDPS between the client (potential attacker) and the web server. This web UI allows a user to conveniently login with credentials and select their SAVI node and project [5]. After login, the user could observe and select intended VMs for chaining operation and apply the modifications on the fly. The web UI sends the users request to the SDI manager to apply a network policy that steers the web traffic destined for the WordPress web server through the DPI.

Hence, to block the attack we utilized the NIDPS between attacker and the WordPress. Snort [8] is a highly active open source project that has been widely employed as a DPI. It incorporates groups of learned network policies to judge the validity of a packet or a group of packets passing through it. In addition, Snort was configured to act as a NIDPS. Merely, creating a DPI does not block the attack; we needed to chain it between the attacker and the WS. We tested our chaining and orchestration processes on the following two attack scenarios. The goal in both are to provide access for normal users and block attackers from overloading or corrupting the web server.

4.1 URL Injection Attack

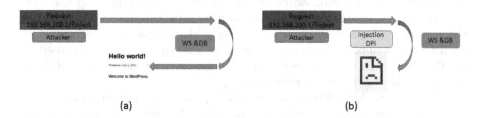

Fig. 2. URL injection attack

We first wanted to verify that attack would affect the web server without presence of a firewall. A normal user will insert correct address of the web server to the address bar, but an attacker would attempt to inject an extra text in the URL aiming to obtain or corrupt information on the Database (URL injection). Therefore, we initiated a sample URL injection attack on the web server (as seen in Fig. 2 part a), that passed an invalid argument to the WS. Specifically, we made malicious HTTP GET request by attaching a text at the end of the URL. Despite the malicious URL, the webpage still loaded, meaning the attack was successful. URL injection [7]could represent a general variety of access control or virus injection problems. To prevent such attacks we used the web UI to chain the firewall between the WS and the gateway. Afterward the same attack was initiated. This time the DPI detected the attack and the web page didn't load. Hence the service chaining was successful (as seen in Fig. 2 part b).

4.2   DOS Attack

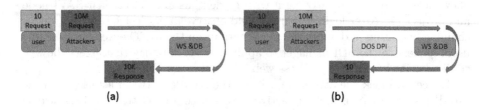

Fig. 3. DOS attack.

Our second test scenario was the detection and blockage of Denial of Service (DoS) attack. As upgraded networking and computing provide users with more bandwidth and processing, compromised users can more efficiently send high bandwidth (tens of Mbps) of requests to overload an attack target. This attack can be identified by deep inspection (i.e. using Snort) of packet headers that are being sent to a WS to identify malicious users. Specifically, malicious users send more than a threshold of requests that a web server could handle in a period of time. In [9] the network switch leading to the WS was tapped by the IDS. The IDS was processing the data and malicious attackers were reported to the SDI manager. The SDI manager subsequently blocked the malicious traffic at the ingress switch of the network. However, in this paper, where IDS is used as NIDPS, there is no longer a need to use SDI for blocking the attacker as Snort detects and blocks the attack right away.

We tested the WS without the firewall in place and initiated a DoS attack from multiple users. The attack made the web server slower and in some cases even inaccessible (as seen in Fig. 3 part a). Afterward by modifying the proper inputs to the web UI, a new DPI was placed in the middle of WS and the gateway. The new DPI was able to block the attackers from reaching the WS and protected the system against this DoS attack. Therefore the normal users were still able to access the WS even after the attack was initiated (as seen in Fig. 3 part b).

5   Conclusion

The SDI RMS allows converged management of networking and computing resources. These features, among other things allow us to easily perform service chaining. Service chaining consists of provisioning the required NFs and chaining them together. The SDI RMS exposes functions that allow us to apply converged network and computing policies. Furthermore, we leverage the orchestration engine to provision and configure the VNFs. Using the orchestration service greatly reduces the complexity and effort in managing resource lifecycles. Service chaining and orchestration have eased development of complex architectures for hyper-dynamic applications. Therefore, employing instant placement modification of VNFs and dynamic application of network policies on SAVI testbed has brought SDI closer than ever to a promising autonomic platform.

References

1. Kang, J.-M., Lin, T., Bannazadeh, H., Leon-Garcia, A.: Software-defined infrastructure and the savi testbed. In: 9th International Conference on Testbeds and Research Infrastructures for the Development of Networks and Communities (TRIDENTCOM 2014), Guangzhou, People's Republic of China (2014)
2. Kang, J.-M., Bannazadeh, H., Leon-Garcia, A.: Savi testbed: control and management of converged virtual ict resources. In: 2013 IFIP/IEEE International Symposium on Integrated Network Management (IM 2013), pp. 664–667, May 2013
3. Keeney, J., van der Meer, S., Fallon, L.: Towards real-time management of virtualized telecommunication networks. In: 2014 10th International Conference on Network and Service Management (CNSM), pp. 388–393, November 2014
4. Kumar, R., Gupta, N., Charu, S., Jain, K., Jangir, S.K.: Open source solution for cloud computing platform using openstack. Int. J. Comput. Sci. Mob. Comput. **3**(5), 89–98 (2014)
5. Lin, T., Park, B., Bannazadeh, H., Leon-Garcia, A.: Savi testbed architecture and federation. In: 1st EAI International Conference on Future Access Enablers of Ubiquitous and Intelligent Infrastructures (Fabulous), September 2015
6. Lin, T., Kang, J.-M., Bannazadeh, H., Leon-Garcia, A.: Enabling sdn applications on software-defined infrastructure. In: Network Operations and Management Symposium (NOMS). IEEE, pp. 1–7, May 2014
7. Mookhey, K., Burghate, N.: Detection of sql injection and cross-site scripting attacks. Symantec SecurityFocus (2004)
8. Roesch, M., et al.: Snort: lightweight intrusion detection for networks. In: LISA 1999, pp. 229–238 (1999)
9. Yasrebi, P., Monfared, S., Bannazadeh, H., Leon-Garcia, A.: Security function virtualization in software defined infrastructure. In: 2015 IFIP/IEEE International Symposium on Integrated Network Management (IM), pp. 778–781, May 2015
10. Zhang, S., Zhang, Q., Bannazadeh, H., Leon-Garcia, A.: Routing algorithms for network function virtualization enabled multicast topology on sdn. IEEE Trans. Netw. Serv. Manage. **PP**(99), 1 (2015)

SAVI vCPE and Internet of Things

Jieyu Lin, Hadi Bannazadeh$^{(\boxtimes)}$, Petros Spachos, and Alberto Leon-Garcia

Department of Electrical and Computer Engineering, University of Toronto,
Toronto, ON M5S 3G4, Canada
{jieyu.lin,hadi.bannazadeh,petros.spachos,alberto.leongarcia}@utoronto.ca

Abstract. As cloud computing technologies continue to develop and evolve, cloud infrastructure has become heterogeneous and multi-tiered. A new demand in cloud computing is to provide cloud functionalities at the customer premise to support customer needs. This demand is addressed in this paper by providing virtual Customers Premise Edge (vCPE) as a third tier of the SAVI Testbed, which is a platform established for experimentation of future applications. A smart room monitoring use case is used to demonstrate the functionalities and efficiency of the vCPE in the SAVI Testbed.

Keywords: vCPE · Internet of Things · SDI · Cloud computing · Wireless sensor network

1 Introduction

With the continuous development of cloud computing and Internet of Things (IoT) technologies, cloud computing infrastructure has become heterogeneous and multi-tiered. The traditional cloud computing infrastructure contains only data centers that reside geographically far away from users. These data centers contains large numbers of compute, network and storage resources. However, deploying applications on top of traditional data centers can introduce high communication latency due to the physical distance. To address this issue and improve content delivery for applications, cloud infrastructure has become multi-tiered, where the first tier is the traditional cloud data centers, and the second and third tiers are smaller but fast and agile data centers/computing devices that are geographically closer to user.

In the Smart Application and Virtual Infrastructure (SAVI) project, we envision the cloud to have a three-tiers infrastructure. Tier 1 has core data centers that are traditional data centers discussed above. Tier 2 has Smart Edges that are agile data centers residing closer to end users. In addition to the traditional compute, network and storage resources, Smart Edges also provide other heterogeneous resources such as programmable hardware (FPGA), GPUs, Software Defined Radio (SDR), and wireless access point. The Smart Edge is mainly to deliver quality applications that require high responsiveness and have requirements that can only be satisfied with a heterogeneous data center close to the end users. Examples applications could be content-delivery systems, smart city management systems, emergency response systems and utility management systems.

© Institute for Computer Sciences, Social Informatics and Telecommunications Engineering 2015
V. Atanasovski, L.-G. Alberto (Eds.): Fabulous 2015, LNICST 159, pp. 18–25, 2015.
DOI: 10.1007/978-3-319-27072-2_3

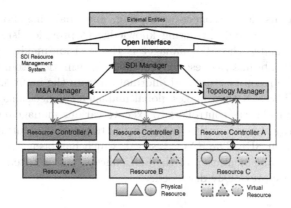

Fig. 1. SDI architecture

Smart Edges are connected to the Core data centers through backbone networks. Finally Tier 3 has sensors and virtual Customer Premise Edge (vCPE). Sensors continuously monitor the physical world. These sensors includes mobile sensors such as smartphones, car sensors and sensor that are installed statically such as temperature, light, carbon-dioxide sensors inside buildings. vCPE extends cloud management and functionalities to the the customers premise to support various demands from customers.

1.1   Software Defined Infrastructure (SDI)

The cloud infrastructure necessarily contains converged heterogeneous resources. Heterogeneous resources enable more functionalities, flexibilities, and performance. However, they also create more demands on the management system. In order to make informed decisions in a heterogeneous cloud environment, it is important to the have a global view of the all the resources and management in an integrated fashion. Existing control and management systems mostly use separate controllers for different types of resources, which introduces high management and maintenance overhead. To address this limitation, we have proposed Software Defined Infrastructure (SDI). [3] SDI provides integrated management of heterogeneous resources in a logically centralized view. It offers flexibility and intelligence for infrastructure management.

Figure 1 shows the high level architecture of the SDI Resource Management System (RMS). In a virtualized, heterogeneous infrastructure, we have different types of physical and virtual resources. In this architecture, type-specific resource controller directly control each type of resource. On top of all the type-specific controllers, we have our SDI modules (i.e. SDI manager, M&A Manager, Topology Manager) that acts as a top-level manager which obtains a global view of the all the resources and conduct integrated management of all types of resources.

The topology manager is responsible for discovering the relationship and interconnections between different resources. The monitoring and analytics manager is responsible for collecting, storing, and analysing monitoring data from all the resources and extracting knowledge to provide visibility into the infrastructure. Finally, the SDI manager is the decision-making point in this architecture. SDI obtains the resource topology information from the topology manager, and the resource state and information from the monitoring and analytic manager. The SDI then makes global management decisions and communicates with the resources controllers to execute various management functions.

The SAVI project was launched with the goal to investigate future application platforms based on SDI. The SAVI Testbed, which has been operational since July 2013, is an implementation of the SDI concept and is based on the three-tiered architecture previously discussed.

2   SAVI vCPE

The Smart Edge envisioned in SAVI primarily focuses on small to mid-size heterogeneous data centers capable of providing virtualized resources to many applications that can serve a large number of end users, either in a city, a small town or even a large sport stadium that justifies investment for such an infrastructure.

A natural extension to a SAVI Smart Edge is a system that can host applications that need to serve only a small number of users in a very close proximity. These end users can be residents of a house or employees at a small office or a remote branch of a large enterprise. In such environments, there may be times when there is a need to have a small set of virtualized resources that can be flexibly programmed to address a specific application. Primarily, there are applications such as smart home management that not only need a small amount of resources to serve (for instances) as a local at-home compute node, but also be able to continue operation independently in the event of network disruptions and disconnections from resources deployed at a larger Smart Edge or remote cloud.

One might debate why there needs to be a virtualized set of resources in such environments. The answer lies in the fact that virtual resources are much easier to manage through their life-cycle and provide lower costs compared to purpose-built boxes that are made specifically for a single application and cannot be readily reprogrammed to address another set of requirements by another application. This in fact fits quite well with the Network Function Virtualization (NFV) paradigm that has received a lot of attention recently. To utilize advancements with NFV functions we would require virtualized resources closer to a few end users for some of these applications.

Therefore, we introduce the SAVI Smart virtualized Customer Premise Edge (SvCPE) to address requirements of such applications. By introducing SvCPE, we introduce a new third-tier in SAVI application-delivery platform. Target applications and common use cases for SvCPE could be any or a combination of the following services:

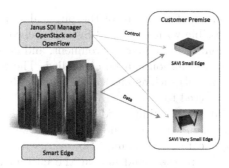

Fig. 2. vCPE in SAVI testbed

- A collection point for Internet of Things devices
- Smart Home and Office Sensor Management
- Smart Home and Office Power Management
- Security Enforcement Point
- Web Acceleration and Service Delivery Point including common NFVs such as Proxy, Firewall, IDS/IPS and VPN services.

In the rest of this section we describe the SvCPE design in more detail focusing on two types of SvCPE: The Small SvCPE and Very Small SvCPE.

2.1 Small SAVI vCPE

A Small SAVI vCPE (SvCPE) is a node with computing and networking capabilities managed by a Smart Edge but located in the customer premise. The SvCPE supports compute and networking virtualization and can host multiple applications deployed simultaneously on it. The SvCPE is connected to the SAVI Smart Edge with VPN technology. Therefore, it is seen as an extension of SAVI Smart Edge Resources and has all the capabilities provided from the virtualized system in SAVI, such as tenant isolation. Since it is controlled by the SAVI Smart Edge SDI Manager, the SvCPE can leverage advanced features of the SAVI SDI, for example, NFV service chaining and live migration of virtual resources. Figure 2 shows the relation of the SvCPE to the SAVI Smart Edge via its Data and Management logical links connections.

There are many use cases for a Small Smart Edge.

1. Network and Web functionalities such as routing, DHCP, firewall, proxy servers can be deployed on the SvCPE. When equipped with WiFi access point capability, the SvCPE can directly offer WiFi service to on-premise users. As it can be easily programmed using SAVI SDI, the applications deployed can be customized based on the specific requirements of each location.
2. SvCPE is SDN capable and therefore an application can have a fine-grained control on how networking traffic is steered at each particular node. This is very handy when deploying virtualized security applications such as Deep Packet Inspection as described in [6].

3. Monitoring and control of the state of the physical world at the customer premise is made possible with the Small SvCPE. Sensors can be connected to the SvCPE to monitor an indoor environment, and devices such as indoor lights, temperature, ventilation can be controlled. The SvCPE enables IoT wireless network protocols such as ZigBee and Bluetooth, and wireless sensor network can be connected to as well.
4. Application availability can be improved with the SvCPE. When applications are deployed on the cloud, network interruption between the cloud and the user can reduce application availability. However, with SvCPE, application can be deployed both in the cloud and at the customers site, so network disruption will have less impact on the availability of the application. For instance, changes made by users can be updated to the cloud when the network is restored.

The location of the SvCPE in the customer premise changes the environment and requirements for physical size and shape comparing to computing rack servers in a cloud. In particular, the computing power needed at a site is limited. Based on this concerns, we selected a mini-PC such as Gigabyte Brix (shown in top-right of Fig. 2) as the Small SvCPE in a proof-of-concept implementation. Gigabyte Brix comes with an Intel CPU, supports up to 16 GB of RAM and an mSATA connection to a SSD. Its relatively small physical size allows it be located in any convenient location in the customers site. This mini-PC can host up to two VMs each with one virtual CPU and it also has in-built Wifi, Bluetooth and three USB connections to external storage if needed. In next section, we will describe how we used this SvCPE to deliver a Smart Home Monitoring system.

2.2 VSvCPE: A Very Small vCPE

The Very Small vCPE is a lightweight node that is used mainly to support advanced SDN and network functionalities, but not compute and storage virtualization. The VSvCPE operates on top of low-cost hardware and is often used for situations where a larger number of nodes are needed to support high quality application delivery.

Most of the use cases discussed in the SvCPE section are applicable for the Very Small node as well, but without virtual computing and storage support. For instance the VSvCPE could be used as a smart on-premise router to provide features such as advanced traffic steering that is required for NFV service chaining, traffic tapping, blocking. These services can be delivered in coordination with resources and NFVs deployed on the SAVI Smart Edge or remote cloud.

For a proof-of-concept, we selected two types of hardware for the Very Small VSvCPE: NetGate APU kit, and Raspberry Pi 2. The NetGate APU kit (shown in Fig. 2) is a development board that has an AMD APU on-board and multiple Ethernet ports. A Linux system (often OpenWRT) can be installed on the system for network related tasks or light-weight computing tasks. The Raspberry Pi 2 is a ARM based development board which is very small in size. It uses an SD card for storage and it has on board memory. Raspberry Pi 2 has one onboard Ethernet port and two USBs which can also be used for WiFi adaptor or extra Ethernet adaptors. A Debian-based Linux system can also be installed on the Raspberry Pi 2, so providing network and performing computing task is relatively simple.

3 Use Case

There are many use cases that can be supported by the vCPE as we have discussed in the previous section. Due to space limitation, we will focus on one use case in this paper: smart room monitoring using sensors connected to vCPE. This use-case has been implemented using SvCPE and here we provide a brief report on this system.

3.1 Smart Room Monitoring

As new buildings are becoming more energy efficiency and airtight, Indoor Air Quality (IAQ) has become an important health and safety factor for indoor environment. However, many indoor environments have limited or no detection mechanisms for health and safety purposes. For this use case, we are demonstrating a real-time wireless ad-hoc sensor network system that supports carbon dioxide monitoring in a complex indoor environment. The system is deployed on the SAVI Testbed vCPE and is connected to our monitoring and analytics manager, called MonArch [2], for data storage and analysis.

Sensor Node   Relay Node   Control Room

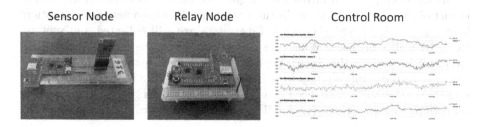

Fig. 3. System framework of the wireless indoor monitoring system

In the following, we will present the architecture of the indoor monitoring system. Then we describe how the indoor monitoring system is deployed on top of the vCPE and discuss about the benefit of this approach.

System Architecture. The system framework of the wireless indoor monitoring system is shown in Fig. 3. This system framework consists of three units:

Sensor Nodes[5]: Each sensor node consists of a carbon dioxide sensor and radio module. Multiples of these nodes are put together to form a wireless sensor network. The data generated in the sensors is passed to the radio module for formatting and transmitting towards to destination.

Relay Nodes: A wireless ad-hoc network that is responsible for forwarding any received packet toward the destination by following an opportunistic routing protocol and cognitive networking techniques [4]. This network supports dynamic join/leave of sensor and relay nodes.

Control Room: The destination of sensor data where data aggregation and network maintenance take place.

MonArch is a monitoring and analytics system in the SAVI Testbed. The indoor monitoring system takes care of the wireless sensor network and MonArch is responsible for collection, storing and analyzing monitoring data.

Deployment on SAVI vCPE. To deploy the indoor monitoring system on the vCPE, we connect the destination node of the wireless sensor network to the vCPE machine. Then we run the control room software and the MonArch Super Agent in the vCPE so that data are aggregated and sent to the Smart Edge node for storage.

One of the features of the vCPE is to provide uninterrupted service even when there is a network disruption between itself and data centers. This feature is provided for this use case as well. To achieve uninterrupted service, an Apache Kafka [1] instance is deployed locally on the vCPE. Sensor data are collected by the MonArch Super agent and submitted to the local Kafka instance. Then on the Smart Edge size, the sensor data are aggregated into the top level Kafka which is part of the MonArch system. In this case, when there is a network disruption between the vCPE and the Smart Edge, data are still collected and sent to the local Kafka instance. When the network recovers, the queued monitoring data will be sent to the Smart Edge and aggregated to the top level Kafka. As a result, there will no data lost. If the monitoring data stored in the Smart Edge are continuously visualized in a GUI, the sensor data generated during the networking disconnection period will be shown when the connection restores.

4   Conclusion

In this paper, we discussed about the three-tiered architecture of the SAVI Testbed and how vCPE is design and implemented as the third tier in the architecture. The features of vCPE is demonstrated through the smart room monitoring use case. In summary, vCPE in the SAVI Testbed can provide cloud management and functionalities to the customer premise to enable new types of applications.

References

1. Kreps, J., Narkhede, N., Rao, J., et al.: Kafka: A distributed messaging system for log processing. In: Proceedings of the NetDB, pp. 1–7 (2011)
2. Lin, J., Ravichandiran, R., Bannazadeh, H., Leon-Garcia, A.: Monitoring and measurement in software-defined infrastructure. In: 2015 IFIP/IEEE International Symposium on Integrated Network Management (IM), pp. 742–745. IEEE (2015)
3. Lin, T., Park, B., Bannazadeh, H., Leon-Garcia, A.: Savi testbed architecture and federation. In: 1st EAI International Conference on Future Access Enablers of Ubiquitous and Intelligent Infrastructures (Fabulous), September 2015
4. Spachos, P., Hantzinakos, D.: Scalable dynamic routing protocol for cognitive radio sensor networks. Sens. J. IEEE **14**, 2257–2266 (2014)
5. Spachos, P., Song, L., Hatzinakos, D.: Prototypes of opportunistic wireless sensor networks supporting indoor air quality monitoring. In: 2013 IEEE Consumer Communications and Networking Conference (CCNC), pp. 851–852. IEEE (2013)
6. Yasrebi, P., Bembey, S., Bannazadeh, H., Leon-Garcia, A.: Virtual network function service chaining on SAVI SDI. In: 1st EAI International Conference on Future Access Enablers of Ubiquitous and Intelligent Infrastructures (Fabulous), September 2015

Application Platform for Smart Transportation

Ali Tizghadam[⊠] and Alberto Leon-Garcia

Department of Electrical and Computer Engineering,
University of Toronto, Toronto, Canada
{ali.tizghadam,alberto.leongarcia}@utoronto.ca

Abstract. This paper presents CVST, an open scalable platform for smart transportation application development. CVST resources can be elastically scaled up/down, or scaled out to robustly adjust to the varying demands on CVST portal. CVST provides APIs to access all live and historical transportation data as well as analytics and algorithmic engines that are provisioned within the platform. Third party application developers and researchers can create their own space in the CVST cloud environment and build their applications.

Keywords: Transportation · ITS · Smart applications · Connected vehicles

1 Introduction

Connected Vehicles and Smart Transportation (CVST) project [1] is a Canadian Government-University-Industry partnership to build a flexible and open platform in support of smart transportation applications. CVST platform consists of four major components:

- **Resource Management Platform:** Integrates advanced wireless and sensor communications with mobile computing techniques in a cloud-based environment. The required resources for smart transportation applications are created and managed in this layer which is supported by another major research initiative (SAVI) in Canada led by University of Toronto [2].
- **Data Dissemination Platform:** Collects transportation data streams from a diverse set of sources / sensors including road camera, loop detectors, mobile traffic sensors, social media sources, public transit, and other private data. Using underlying resources, the CVST data management platform can scale to accommodate new data sources seamlessly. The CVST data management platform anonymizes the data (if required), unifies the format of different data types, cleanses the data and publishes it on a frontend portal.
- **Analytics (Business Intelligence) Platform:** Offers a wide range of statistics and business intelligence (knowledge) by exploiting advanced data mining methods on real-time and historical transportation data.
- **Application Platform:** Enables development of third party applications by offering access to raw and processed data in the CVST platform along with

© Institute for Computer Sciences, Social Informatics and Telecommunications Engineering 2015
V. Atanasovski, L.-G. Alberto (Eds.): Fabulous 2015, LNICST 159, pp. 26–32, 2015.
DOI: 10.1007/978-3-319-27072-2_4

access to other installed applications / algorithms. The following list identifies a subset of applications that can be developed on the CVST platform: real-time dashboards, real-time monitoring of traffic patterns and demand, optimization of traffic flows in a region, personal route assistance, short-term and long-term modeling of mobility patterns in a region, automatic traffic signal control.

The focus of this paper is on second and third layers of the CVST Platform, i.e. the data dissemination layer and the analytics block. In the reminder of this paper we discuss general architecture of the CVST platform and its constituting blocks, with a focus on data ingestion, dissemination and analytics.

2   CVST Platform Architecture

Figure 1 denotes the major building blocks of the CVST platform including data ingestion through collectors, data dissemination layer, analytics and algorithmic engines,application programming interfaces (APIs), and end-user portal.

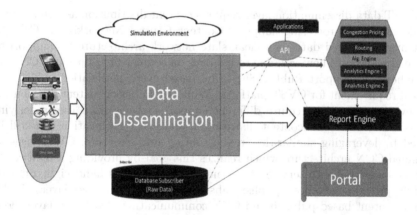

Fig. 1. High-level diagram of CVST platform including data collectors, data dissemination block, analytics engines, application programming interfaces, simulation engines, front-end portal, and database.

2.1   Data Ingestion and Data Collectors

The CVST platform collects a rich set of data from a variety of transportation data sources including but not limited to highway traffic sensors, road cameras, road incidents, road closures, twitter traffic reports,public transportation (bus location information, bike station data), border delay time, and loop detector per lane data.

2.2   Data Dissemination Layer

This layer is at the heart of all data communication processes within the CVST platform. Figure 2 shows different blocks of the data dissemination layer.

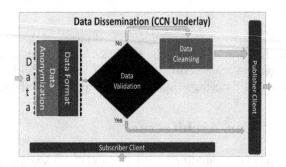

Fig. 2. Components of "Data Dissemination" layer in CVST platform

CVST data dissemination layer requires content distribution as well as event notification and processing support. Content Centric Networking (CCN) [3], built around named data, is a clean-slate network architecture for supporting future applications; however, due to its focus on content distribution, CCN does not inherently support Publish-Subscribe based event notification, which is a critical requirement for CVST platform. While semantics of content distribution and event notification require different support systems from the underlying network infrastructure, content distribution and event notification can still be united by leveraging similarities in the routing infrastructure. CVST uses an extended-CCN architecture which realizes this goal by providing a lightweight content based pub-sub service at the network layer. This lightweight pub-sub module provides advanced publish-subscribe services at higher layers. Lightweight content based pub-sub and CCN communication at network layer along with advanced publish-subscribe together are presented as data collection and dissemination fabric in CVST platform.

Storing data in the data dissemination layer follows a publish-subscribe paradigm. The Central database of CVST platform is in fact a subscriber within the pub-sub block that subscribes to all new data update events for all existing data types supported by CVST platform. This way all data entering to CVST platform will be recorded for future analysis.

For privacy-sensitive data types the CVST platform uses an anonymization service and the published data for subscriber is in fact this anonymized data. Data anonymization service should be able to anonymize different types of data including camera feeds and mobile records each of which has different requirements; therefore, anonymization service requires separate algorithms per specific data type.

The CVST data dissemination layer also performs data validation checks on input data before being published, the data will be checked for integrity and missing data parts, in case on observing anomalies, the system tries to cleanse the data and then it will publish in on data dissemination platform.

2.3   Algorithmic and Analytic Engines

The published data in CVST data dissemination layer, gets delivered by appropriate subscription to the analytics layer where a number of different instances of Hadoop and Spark clusters are installed. Hadoop clusters are used primarily for batch processing of complex analytics tasks that do not need to be performed fast. In contrast Spark is used for fast in memory-processing. Figure 3 shows building blocks of an Spark cluster that is used within CVST platform to analyze bus location data within GTA (Greater Toronto Area).

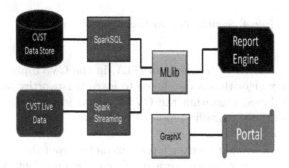

Fig. 3. High-level diagram of Spark Cluster within CVST platform for in-, memory analytics.

The "Spark Streaming" block of the spark cluster retrieves live CVST data by subscribing to the target published data and / or through APIs, while "Spark-SQL" queries historical data from CVST data warehouse. The data will be delivered to "MLLib", a library of different algorithms for data mining and machine learning, the data will be processed then and the results will be delivered to the front-end portal after being visualized by another integrated library for graph visualization (GraphX).

Algorithms - Twitter Data. The CVST platform uses a number of data mining algorithms for different purposes on various CVST data. For instance, some data types require pre-processing in order to be admitted to the data dissemination layer of the CVST platform; therefore, admission control algorithms have been developed for the CVST portal. One prime example of data types requiring admission control is Twitter data.

Incidents are among the most important causes of traffic jam in large cities; therefore, it is required to have accurate incident reports. CVST looks for Twitter traffic data that is published related to GTA road incidents. There are many

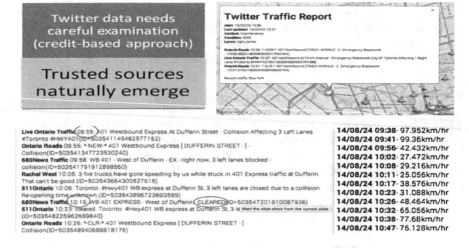

Fig. 4. Sample Twitter traffic report (incident)

unreliable tweets related to incidents in GTA, in the CVST platform a credit-based evolutionary algorithm is developed to learn trustworthy sources of data. Using this credit-based algorithm the CVST portal identifies some important trustable data sources for traffic reports throughout GTA and visualizes their data on CVST portal.

Figure 4 shows a sample Twitter report extracted from the CVST historical data. As one can observe, there are a number of independent twitter sources that have reported the same incident including "680News Traffic" (680News is a radio station in GTA), "Live Ontario Traffic", and "Ontario Roads". As Fig. 4 shows, the tweets have reported the starting time of the incident as well as the termination time.

Video Analytics. Currently, in the Greater Toronto Area, digital cameras are used to monitor the traffic; however, they require live human operator supervision. CVST platform proposes a module to use digital video streams from traffic cameras across GTA to extract traffic information and to use this information to predict future conditions. Traffic information include, mean speed of vehicles, traffic density and traffic flow information in numerical terms.

The video analytics engine of CVST platform (Fig. 5 has two main blocks, extraction of traffic information from video stream and prediction of future traffic conditions. There are several alternative approaches to extract information from video streams for traffic surveillance. Currently, CVST video analytics module makes use of Haar Cascade Classifiers within OpenCV project [4] to detect vehicles, and takes advantage of particle filters to track the vehicle through subsequent frames. In order to extract useful traffic information from the video feeds, algorithm parameters need to be calibrated appropriately depending on the camera position. Only after these steps have been completed, we can calculate traffic flow parameters.

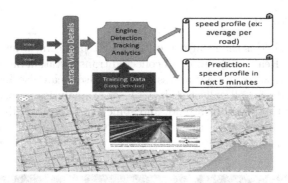

Fig. 5. Video and image analytics within CVST platform

Another block of video analytics module is short-term traffic prediction. There are different approaches to estimate road traffic given the view of the road, in this research we used a machine learning method, where the forecasting module uses a set of highway traffic data (extracted form existing loop detectors along GTA highways) as training dataset and combined with the information extracted from video feeds provides short-term traffic prediction on roads with video feeds.

Other Analytics. The analytics modules explained are examples of different analytics blocks that are developed in CVST platform. Other analytics components of the platform could be directly explored via the portal [1]. For example, there is a comprehensive set of detailed reports that can be generated about buses and bike stations within GTA, a user can configure the desired report, such as bus frequency or average travel time for a specific route and particular time frame, using CVST portal and the portal will visualize the requested report.

2.4 Application Programming Interfaces

A major promise of CVST project is to offer an open platform to encourage smart transportation applications. As the first step towards realizing an open smart platform CVST offers APIs for all data types maintained within the platform as well as remote procedure calls to the algorithms and analytics functions created in the platform for various transportation purposes. In addition to the typical pull-based APIs (REST), the CVST platform offers a push-based API using subscription feature of data dissemination layer. To elaborate, consider a subscriber who is interested in incidents that are taking place in a specific highway between two pre-determined intersections. The pub-sub system will check the publishers data and if it finds a match for this subscription it will forward the data to the user who has subscribed. This means that when the data is ready, it will be pushed to the end user.

2.5   CVST Portal

The CVST portal [1] is the front-end of the CVST platform, where all visualization takes place. Real-time view of all collected transportation data is illustrated in the portal and users can get access to them. Users can also browse through the historical data for all collected data. A set of analytics reports can also be generated using the portal front-end, and some short-term trends of data types can be observed by selecting the target data. One example of such embedded trending graphs is shown in Fig. 6.

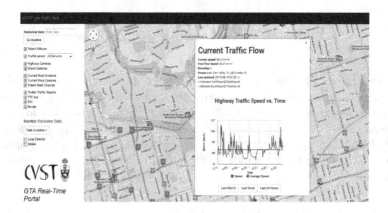

Fig. 6. CVST Portal - embedded trended history of highway traffic data

3   Conclusion

This paper presented a summary of the CVST platform which is an effort to create an open, scalable and flexible platform to create smart transportation applications. CVST offers a wide range of transportation data along with associated analytics, as well as open API-based access to the CVST data and algorithms. Moreover, the CVST platform offers developer accounts for researchers who are willing to contribute their algorithms to the CVST platform. Current focus of CVST platform is to extend the capabilities of the publish-subscribe block and to offer customized subscription for end users through mobile phones.

References

1. (for CVST portal: portal.cvst.ca). www.cvst.ca
2. www.savinetwork.ca
3. Jacobson V., Smetters D. K., Thornton J. D., Plass M., Briggs N., Braynard R.: Networking named content. In: Proceedings of ACM CoNEXT, New York, NY (2009)
4. www.opencv.org

Special Session on Recent Advances in IoT Communications

Mission Critical IoT Communication in 5G

Qi Zhang[1](✉) and Frank H.P. Fitzek[2]

[1] Qi Zhang Department of Engineering, Aarhus University,
8200 Aarhus, Denmark
qz@eng.au.dk
[2] 5G Lab Germany, Technische Universitt Dresden,
01062 Dresden, Germany
frank.fitzek@tu-dresden.de

Abstract. 5G is envisioned to support unprecedented diverse applications and services with extremely heterogeneous performance requirements, i.e., mission critical IoT communication, massive machine-type communication and Gigabit mobile connectivity. This imposes enormous challenges to fulfil the key performance requirements, in particular, mission critical IoT communication, which calls for a dramatic paradigm change in 5G. This paper presents vision and challenges of mission critical IoT scenarios and the enabling technologies in 5G. Several research opportunities are given as example for inspiration purpose.

Keywords: IoT · Tactile internet · 5G · SDN · NFV · fog/edge computing

1 Vision and Challenges of Mission Critical IoT

Internet of Things (IoT) represents a vision in which the Internet as an open global platform will extend into the physical realm by embedding sensors and actuators into physical objects such as appliances, machines, medical devices, and vehicles and letting them communicate, compute and coordinate. IoT is able to provide machines, people and business real-time access the state of things and control, which has a great potential to enable a wide range of innovative applications and services [1,2]. Cisco estimated in 2011 that the number of smart objects will rise to 50 billion by 2020 [3] and increased that number up to 500 billion devices [4] in 2014. McKinsey report [5] shows that the IoT has the potential to create economic impact of $2.7–$6.2 trillion annually by 2025.

Despite the fact that IoT has an enormous potential to bring innovations to new business and our daily life, IoT is facing a long list of unsolved technical challenges related to heterogeneous devices, limited spectrum, hardware miniaturization, energy harvesting, privacy and security, etc. [1]. One of the most crucial challenges is the communication for mission critical applications. Here the meaning of *mission critical* is not limited to the conventional definition of "risk to life" but also covering the risks to interrupt public services, disturb public order, jeopardize enterprise operation and cause significant loss in business and assets. The typical mission critical IoT use cases, just to name a few,

© Institute for Computer Sciences, Social Informatics and Telecommunications Engineering 2015
V. Atanasovski, L.-G. Alberto (Eds.): Fabulous 2015, LNICST 159, pp. 35–41, 2015.
DOI: 10.1007/978-3-319-27072-2_5

include the communication between vehicle and the transportation infrastructure and the cooperation among vehicles in smart transportation, remote surgery in healthcare, robotics cooperation or remotely maneuver in public safety agent or industrial process automation and control, and many others.

To enable mission critical IoT applications it requires an extra care in the design from hardware of smart objects, software, cyber physical system (CPS), to communication infrastructure and network architecture. However, the state-of-the-art IoT solutions evolved from the traditional embedded wireless sensor and actuator networks and M2M communication in LTE, fall far short of the stringent requirements for mission critical applications. This paper will focus on how to provide mission critical communication with ultra-low latency, ultra-high reliability, and security to smart objects and CPSs in 5G by leveraging a number of key enabling technologies in the air interface and network architecture.

2   Classification of IoT

IoT has a wide range of applications and use cases, with heterogeneous communication performance requirements. There exists different ways to categorize IoT applications. It can be basically classified as *monitoring-based* and *control-oriented* or mission-critical and non-mission-critical which are differentiated in the requirements on reliability, availability and end-to-end latency. Figure 1 illustrates the basic performance requirements of the different categories in terms of latency, reliability and availability.

	Monitoring-based	Control-oriented
Mission-critical	Low latency Carrier grade reliability Approx. 100% Availability	Ultra-low latency Carrier grade reliability Approx. 100% Availability
Non Mission-critical	Moderate latency Moderate reliability High availability	Ultra-low latency Moderate reliability High availability

Fig. 1. The matrix of IoT classification and the performance requirements.

The primary purpose of *monitoring-based* IoT applications is to periodically collect sensor data of the smart objects and transmit it, often in small packets, to the cloud. For example, goods periodically report its location and other context data, e.g., vibration and temperature, to the cloud for object tracking or a windmill periodically reports the velocity of wind and power generation to the cloud for electricity generation prediction. Such applications mainly focus on collecting sensor data via smart objects and providing remote monitoring and various big data analytics services. The sensor data can also occasionally trigger certain actuators, for instance, when the power usage of a household reported by a smart meter exceeds the peak power limit, the demand response server will schedule the smart appliances through home energy management gateway, or when the ECG sensor data shows a symptom of heart attack or severe mental stress, it can trigger the smartphone to call for caregiver or launch a stress intervention. The majority of *monitoring-based* IoT applications are not mission-critical and the main challenge regarding communication in 5G is to provide massive machine-type communication (MTC), even up to 10^7 links/km^2, with ultra-low energy consumption, long life time and low signalling overhead.

The primary objective of *control-oriented* IoT applications is to steer and control remotely, which uses the sensor data to control the actuators in real-time. Taking driverless car as an example, it captures sensor data, e.g., text/images of the road signs and communicates with the cars in its proximity, to control the steering wheel, adapt the speed and avoid collisions. Industrial robot is another good case in point and is remotely maneuvered in hazardous environment for industrial process automation and control. The *control-oriented* IoT applications rely on mission critical communication (also referred to mission-critical machine-type communications). Depending on the concrete application, the performance requirements in terms of latency, reliability, and availability can vary. For example, in the driverless car scenario, round-trip latency is one of the crucial metrics to avoid collisions, which depends on the relative speed between vehicles and a vehicle to the obstacles. A simple calculation can show that for a vehicle with 120 km/h, 1 ms round-trip latency corresponds to 3 cm between a vehicle and a static obstacle or 6 cm between two moving vehicles. Reliability of 99.9999 % shall be guaranteed to ensure maximum 31.5 s downtime per year.

2.1   Mission Critical IoT and Tactile Internet

The Tactile Internet coined by Professor Fettweis can enable precise haptic interaction not only machine-to-machine but also human-to-machine relying on 1 ms round-trip latency combining with high availability, reliability and security [6]. The Tactile Internet covers the application fields of health care, traffic, education, robotics, manufacturing, sports, games, etc. The common character of the Tactile Internet is to steer and/or control of a physical or virtual object remotely using tactile input and also audio and/or visual feedback with imperceptible latency [6]. The scope of the Tactile Internet is partially overlapped with mission critical IoT, in particularly, in the fields of traffic, robotics, manufacturing, health care, and utility. The Tactile Internet and mission critical IoT share similar requirements in terms of communication. However, the Tactile Internet can be additionally applied in virtual reality and augmented reality for training physical movements for sports or training operating machines for education purpose. The reliability and security requirements in education and sports application fields are not as stringent as the ones in other fields, i.e., they are not mission critical according to the definition in Sect. 1. For some mission critical monitoring based IoT applications, the end-to-end latency constraint is not as low as 1 ms but reliability and availability are more crucial, for example, the applications of catastrophe monitoring of tsunamis and earthquake. The relation between mission critical communication for IoT and the Tactile Internet is illustrated in Fig. 2. It is clear that to tackle the challenges of mission critical communication in 5G will benefit mission critical IoT applications as well as Tactile Internet applications.

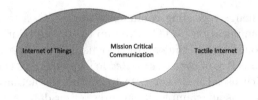

Fig. 2. Mission-critical communication for IoT and Tactile Internet.

3   Mission Critical IoT Communications in 5G

Mission critical IoT communication is one of the main goals in 5G. A number of initiatives in the industrial and academic communities and standardization bodies are working on this. For example, EU project METIS [8] and 5GNOW [9] aim to lay the foundation of 5G on ultra-reliable communication to enable mission-critical M2M applications. The Alcatel-Lucent collaboration with 5G Lab Germany at TU Dresden will initially focus on leveraging multiple device-to-radio connections to enhance reliability for mission-critical communication. The researchers in the leading companies, Ericsson Research, Huawei research institutions, Intel Strategic Research Alliance, etc. have been active in investigating the feasibility requirements and have proposed enabling solutions for mission-critical communication in 5G.

3.1   Possible Enabling Technologies

The key performance requirements of mission critical IoT communication have an important impact on the design choices of each component in the communication link and the optimization across the entire protocol stack. Taking 1 ms end-to-end latency as an example, the latency at different components can be distributed as follows: about 300 μs for processing on the devices including the sensors at the transmitter and the actuators at the receiver, 100 μs for air interface in one way, 500 μs for network processing including the base station and control/steer server [7]. It is intuitive to resort to the methods such as shortening the frame size, using instant-access resource allocation to avoid the medium-access latency, and moving the network processing function to the edge of the network closer to the devices. For example, to fulfil 100 μs air interface, the transmission time interval (TTI) has to be shortened to 100 μs maximum as TTI is the inherent lower bound of the PHY latency. And an enormous processing and storage capacity will be accumulated in the proximity of the smart objects through virtualized network functions and fog/edge computing. In the following, we will briefly present the enabling technologies in software-defined air interface and network architecture.

Air Interface. 5G needs to design a new air interface not only to deal with heterogeneous traffic types, e.g., massive sporadic machine-type traffic, real-time mobile traffic, but also to achieve ultra-low latency and ultra-reliable mission critical communication. To address the requirements and challenges, several designs of 5G air interface have been proposed. 5GNOW [10] has proposed to use non-orthogonal asynchronous waveforms in the new physical layer to replace the synchronism and orthogonality in OFDM. Among the superior waveform alternatives, e.g., universal filtered multi-carrier (UFMC), filtered bank multi-carrier (FBMC), filtered-OFDM (F-OFDM), and generalized frequency-division multiplexing (GFDM), in particular, GFDM could be an enabler for ultra-low latency due to its flexibilty and block structure. A GFDM frame can be designed to fulfil 100 μs time constraint together with a flexible capability of non-continuous subcarrier allocation or non-proportional subcarrier spacing to improve throughput [10]. Moreover, the GFDM block structure has an advantage in using special sequences with impulse self-correlation properties as preamble of the GFDM frame to efficiently initiate communication procedure, which can enable fast detection of a new communication process in random access. A software defined air interface has been proposed in [11] to offer flexibility to diverse application scenarios. Among the building blocks of the new air interface, sparse code multiple access (SCMA) has been adopted as another waveform in the air interface. SCMA is not only able to tolerate overloaded signal superposition[1], which is favorable for massive connectivity; but also an enabler for grant-free multiple access using blind detection technique [12,13]. Grant-free multiple access effectively eliminates the signaling and latency in the request-grant dynamic scheduling schemes. Additionally, other technologies like massive MIMO increasing network capacity and coverage, and advanced error control coding, promise benefits contributing to realize carrier grade reliability and improve availability.

Network Architecture. The extremely diverse and heterogeneous (even virtual contradictory) use cases requires 5G to offer a wide range of connectivity, which urges a dramatic change in network architecture as well. Moreover, different mission critical IoT use cases have differentiated requirements for connectivity in terms of latency, reliability and others. One of the keys to address these challenges is to enable higher-degree flexibility in the network by the concept of *network slices*. Each slice can be customized to match requirements of specific use case to optimize the network resource utilization. *Network slides* leverage the software-defined networking (SDN), network function virtualization (NFV) and cloud technologies to provide an abstraction of the physical network infrastructure realizing network-wide programmability and separate hardware from software making the network functions independent from a specific location and node. For instance, a "plastic" architecture for 5G based on the advances of SDN is proposed in [14], consisting of three levels of control, i.e., device, edge and orchestration controllers. The network functions can be implemented "centralized" or "distributed at the edge" depending on the performance requirements of the supported services, and the logical network elements can be dynamically instantiated in the cloud infrastructure. This architecture promises

---

[1] The number of multiplexed users is more than the length of the multiplexed codewords, i.e., the number of orthogonal resources.

to significantly reduce the latency by exploiting SDN to implement the network functions in an optimal location and eliminating the forwarding path latency with pro-active configuration [14]. The device and edge controllers might be feasible to implement the concept of "Neural Bearer" from [16] beyond the state-of-art D2D and MANET, which is envisioned to enable several carrier grade communications simultaneously through different radio interfaces with multiple transceivers.

A similar promising enabling technology, fog/edge computing, is a highly virtualized platform at the edge of the network, providing compute, storage and networking services between smart objects and traditional cloud computing data center with salient characteristics of low latency, location awareness, wide-spread geographical distribution, and support for mobility, real-time interaction and many others [15]. Fog/edge computing integrated with SDN and NFV can significantly reduce the latency in network processing to meet the objective of 500 μs limit. Additionally, distributed intelligence in fog/edge network will provide multiple connections increasing diversity whilst NFV will facilitate the resource coordination among multi-RAT (radio access technology) thanks to its fast instantiation of network functions capability, thereby; ultra-reliable, always available and dependable connectivity can be realized.

4   Research Opportunities and Conclusion

It is an exciting era to witness the rapid development of IoT and the converging visions of 5G. It is clear that to address the challenges in 5G, especially, mission critical IoT communication, it calls for a complete design paradigm change. Here we have no intention to give a complete list of research opportunities in this regards, but merely briefly present several examples.

To further enhance reliability, advanced error control coding scheme can be applied, e.g., polar codes concatenated with cyclic redundancy codes is promising to outperform turbo or LDPC codes according to the simulation results in the literature. It is particularly interesting to find a simple encoder and faster decoding algorithm for polar codes with short block size, which is necessary to minimize the end-to-end latency. Retransmission scheme might not be a viable solution for carrier grade reliability, additionally due to the latency constraints.

To fully leverage the benefits of fog/edge computing, a better integration of SDN and NFV with fog/edge networking should be studied considering the dynamic nature of the components of the fog. Especially the combination of SDN and NFV is leading to a fusion of transport and storage.

Additionally, network coding (NC) probably is an efficient technique to tackle or ease the challenges of data storage and networking in fog network and improve the processing speed, by reducing the impact due to the dependency of computation performance and data locality. It is viable to combine NC with multi-RATs to ensure faster and reliable data delivery over multiple connections simultaneously and avoid the complicate RATs selection problem. NC encoded packets can enhance the security and reliability in distributed storage in fog computing. NC is going well together with SDN and NFV concepts and relies only on one code for storage and transportation. Furthermore NC can decrease latency using new mechanisms like sliding window and re-coding [17].

It is also worth investigating ultra-lean methods for graceful degradation, e.g., joint source-channel coding and partial packet recovery, to improve reliability and availability. Joint optimization of sampling at a device with transmission scheme leveraging the sensor data model could be a feasible approach to shorten the device processing latency whilst enhance reliability and availability.

References

1. Miorandi, D., et al.: Internet of things: vision, applications and research challenges. J. Ad Hoc Netw. **10**(7), 1497–1516 (2012)
2. Atzori, L., et al.: The internet of things: a survey. Comput. Netw. **54**(15), 2787–2805 (2010)
3. Evans, D.: The internet of things: how the next evolution of the internet is changing everything. In: Cisco Internet Business Solutions Group (IBSG)
4. Chamber, J.: Beyond the hype: internet of things shows up strong at mobile world congress, PC World (2014)
5. Manyika, J., et al.: Disruptive Technologies: Advances that will Transform Life, Business, and the Global Economy. McKinsey Global Institute, San Francisco (2013)
6. Fettweis, G.P.: The tactile internet: applications and challenges. IEEE Veh. Technol. Mag. **9**(1), 64–70 (2014)
7. Fettweis, G.P., et al.: The tacile Internet, ITU-T Technology Watch Report, August 2014
8. METIS 2020: Mobile and wireless communications Enablers for the Twenty-twenty Information Society. https://www.metis2020.com
9. 5GNOW 5th Generation Non-Orthogonal Waveforms for Asynchronous Signalling. http://www.5gnow.eu/
10. Wunder, G., et al.: 5GNOW: non-orthogonal, asynchronous waveforms for future mobile applications. IEEE Commun. Mag. **52**(2), 97–105 (2014)
11. 5G: New Air Interface and Radio Access Virtualization. Huawei white paper, April 2015
12. Au, K., et al.: Uplink contention based SCMA for 5G radio access. In: IEEE Globecom Workshop on Emerging Technologies for 5G Wireless Cellular Network, pp. 900–905 (2014)
13. Bayesteh, A., et al.: Blind detection of SCMA for uplink grant-free multiple-access. In: 2014 11th International Symposium on Wireless Communications Systems (ISWCS), pp. 853–857, 26–29 August 2014
14. Trivisonno, R., et al.: SDN-based 5G mobile networks: architecture, functions, procedures and backward compatibility. Trans. Emerg. Telecommun. Technol. **26**(1), 82–92 (2015)
15. Bonomi, F., et al.: Fog computing and its role in the internet of things. In: Proceedings of the First Edition of the MCC Workshop on Mobile Cloud Computing, MCC 2012, pp. 13–16, Helsinki, Finland (2012)
16. Soldani, D., Manzalini, A.: A 5G infrastructure for anything-as-a-service. J. Telecommun. Syst. Manag. 3:114 (2014). http://www.omicsgroup.org/journals/a-g-infrastructure-for-anythingasaservice-2167-0919-114.php?aid=33681, doi:10.4172/2167-0919.1000114
17. Szab, D., et al.: Towards the tactile internet: decreasing communication latency with network coding and software defined networking. In: European Wireless Conference (2015)

A Stochastic Geometry Framework
for Full-Duplex Machine Type Communications

Andrea Munari[(⊠)], Petri Mähönen, and Marina Petrova

Institute for Networked Systems, RWTH Aachen University,
Kackertstraße 9, 52072 Aachen, Germany
{amu,pma,mpe}@inets.rwth-aachen.de

Abstract. This paper focuses on the role played by in-band full-duplex
in asynchronous random access networks. With an eye on 5G, we tackle
a scenario characterised by a large population of uncoordinated users
exchanging sporadic traffic in the form of short data packets. In this context, we introduce an analytical framework based on stochastic geometry
that captures the tradeoffs induced by the presence of some full-duplex
links. Via closed-form expressions, we study the behaviour of the system as a function of the packet length, and derive the optimal fraction
of full-duplex communications that shall be performed to maximise the
network throughput. The role of imperfect self-interference cancellation
is accurately accounted for, drawing interesting insights on the benefits,
the design tradeoffs and the challenges to be solved when applying full
duplex to machine type communications.

Keywords: Full-Duplex · Stochastic geometry · Aloha · M2M communications

1 Introduction

Machine type communications (MTC) have earned a central role in the design
of the 5G paradigm, thanks to the flourishing sprout of applications that see a
massive number of terminals exchange information in a sporadic fashion. From
this standpoint, the traditional quest to provide higher data rates to connections
in a centralised system has been flanked by the need to optimise throughput at
a network level for short packet transfers among uncoordinated terminals. While
the issue has partially been tackled by advanced random access schemes [1], the
support of ever growing populations of users calls for further improvements in
spectrum utilisation.

Along this perspective, in-band full-duplex communications are emerging as
an interesting solution. Following this approach, terminals can send and receive
at the same time over the same frequency band, potentially doubling the capacity of a link. The key challenge to enable such operations is clearly represented
by the need for a node to cancel the self-interference it generates when transmitting, which is several order of magnitudes larger than the power of any useful

© Institute for Computer Sciences, Social Informatics and Telecommunications Engineering 2015
V. Atanasovski, L.-G. Alberto (Eds.): Fabulous 2015, LNICST 159, pp. 42–50, 2015.
DOI: 10.1007/978-3-319-27072-2_6

signal coming from surrounding terminals. Relevant advances have been made recently in this direction, and several works have proven the feasibility of full-duplex connections with relatively simple hardware and software defined radios, complemented by the design of MAC protocols for ad hoc networks, see, e.g., [2,3] and references therein. Nevertheless, the potential of this paradigm from a network-wide perspective is not yet fully understood. A first relevant step in this direction was taken in [4], where stochastic geometry tools were used to analyse slotted random access. This contribution highlighted the key tradeoff that characterises full-duplex systems, where the increase in spatial reuse enabled by simultaneous bidirectional communications is beset by the additional interference generated by concurrent transmissions, and showed how the capacity doubling achievable at a single link does not scale in larger topologies. Starting from this ground, recent studies have proposed the application of full-duplex to 5G MTC [5], focusing on the impact of some bidirectional device-to-device links in a cellular scenario.

On the other hand, the fundamental question of whether full-duplex can represent a valid game-changer for the performance of large-scale MTC networks still remains open. In this paper we tackle the issue focusing on a more complex yet realistic scenario in which nodes lack any form of coordination. This maps not only to a random access to the shared medium, but also to completely asynchronous transmissions, bringing the additional challenge of a time-varying interference. By means of a stochastic geometry framework, we derive closed form expressions that clarify the role of packet length on the effectiveness of full-duplex, and that capture the optimal fraction of transmissions that shall operate in bidirectional mode. Moreover, the impact of imperfect self-interference cancellation is discussed, deriving interesting design hints that offer a deeper understanding of the applicability of the paradigm to MTC as well as pointing out the key challenges to be addressed.

2   System Model and Preliminaries

For our analysis we will focus on an infinite population of users spread over the plane, that share a common medium in an uncoordinated fashion to exchange data packets. The communication parameters, common to all terminals, are set so that every transmission lasts D seconds. The network is organised in node pairs or *clusters*, and each user only establishing one-hop links with its companion, located at distance r. Clusters can be operated either in *half-duplex* or *full-duplex* mode. In the former case, one terminal transmits packets according to the underlying medium access strategy, while the other simply acts as receiver and does not generate traffic. As to the latter mode, instead, both nodes access the channel simultaneously, leveraging full-duplex capabilities to send and receive data at the same time. In order to cover a broad range of network configurations, we assume that a fraction q of clusters resort to full-duplex operations, whereas the remaining perform half-duplex access. Medium contention is performed asynchronously via random access, following a simple unslotted Aloha protocol. No feedback nor specific retransmission policies are considered. Instead, we assume users to always have traffic for their intended destination, so that a (possibly bidirectional) packet exchange within a pair is established following random backoff periods.

In order to capture analytically the behaviour of the system, we model transmissions in the network via a homogeneous time-space Poisson point process (PPP) $\Psi = \{\mathbf{x}_i, T_i\}$ of intensity λ. Following this approach, the number of links (both half- and full-duplex) established in a region of area A over T seconds is described as a Poisson r.v., with parameter λAT. Within the considered PPP, $\mathbf{x}_i$ represents the position of the transmitter for half-duplex clusters, or the position of one of the nodes for full-duplex pairs. In the latter case, the companion node is located at $\mathbf{x}_i + \mathbf{w}_i$, where $\mathbf{w}_i$ is randomly and independently distributed over a circle of radius r centered at $\mathbf{x}_i$. On the other hand, T_i identifies the start time of the transmission performed by the cluster. The hybrid nature of links in the network is accounted for by having each pair independently decide whether to establish a half- or a full-duplex connection with probability $1 - q$ and q, respectively. By virtue of the properties of thinning for PPPs, the original process can then be written as $\Psi = \Psi_{hd} \cup \Psi_{fd}$, where Ψ_{hd} and Ψ_{fd} are two independent space-time PPPs of intensity $(1 - q)\lambda$ and $q\lambda$. From this standpoint, it is relevant to stress that we do not focus on a spatial process describing the distribution of nodes and track the evolution of their medium access over time, e.g., by means of a renewal process. Conversely, Ψ jointly captures position and transmission time of a cluster, modelling the network as a population of node pairs that are born at a random time and a random location and occupy the channel for a predefined time D before disappearing. This approach embeds some aspects of the medium access strategy, e.g., the backoff distribution, resorting to the sole parameter λ, yet will yield a compact mathematical formulation capable of identifying some key tradeoffs and has been shown to offer a very accurate estimation of the performance of unslotted systems [6]. Moreover, from a practical angle not only can the space-time process under consideration easily be mapped to mobile topologies, but also to the MTC-relevant scenario of very large populations of terminals generating sporadic traffic.

Wireless links are affected by path loss with exponent $\alpha > 2$ and Rayleigh fading, so that the incoming power at location $\mathbf{y}$ for a packet originated at $\mathbf{x}$ is given by $P L(\mathbf{x}, \mathbf{y})\zeta$, where P is the transmission power common to all users, $L(\mathbf{x}, \mathbf{y}) = k\|\mathbf{x} - \mathbf{y}\|^{-\alpha}$, k is a constant accounting for propagation factors set to one in the following, and ζ is an exponential random variable with unit mean and pdf $f_\zeta(a) = e^{-a}, a \geq 0$. Given the interference-limited nature of the networks under consideration, we disregard thermal noise and evaluate the performance of the system based on the signal-to-interference ratio (SIR). From this standpoint, the asynchronous medium access of interest leads to a time-varying interference $I(t)$ even within the duration of a packet. In an effort to account for this aspect while preserving the mathematical tractability of the problem, we model decoding of a data unit at a receiver considering the average interference it experiences, defined as:

$$\bar{I} = \frac{1}{D} \int_{T_i}^{T_i+D} I(t)dt \tag{1}$$

By virtue of the homogeneity of the PPP under consideration, we can compute without loss of generality $I(t)$ for a node located at the origin of the plane. To this aim, let $\Psi_{hd}^{(a)}(t) = \{(\mathbf{x}_j, T_j) \in \Psi_{hd} \,|\, t \in [T_j, T_j + D]\}$ and $\Psi_{fd}^{(a)}(t) = \{(\mathbf{x}_j, T_j) \in \Psi_{fd} \,|\, t \in [T_j, T_j + D]\}$ be the half- and full-duplex clusters active at time t. Then, simplifying the notation via the auxiliary variables $\ell_j = L(\mathbf{x}_j, \mathbf{0})$ and $\ell'_j = L(\mathbf{x}_j + \mathbf{w}_j, \mathbf{0})$, the interference contribution perceived at the receiver from the two sets can be written respectively in the form

$$I_{hd}(t) = \sum_{(\mathbf{x}_j, T_j) \in \Psi_{hd}^{(a)}(t)} P\ell_j \zeta_j, \quad I_{fd}(t) = \sum_{(\mathbf{x}_j, T_j) \in \Psi_{fd}^{(a)}(t)} P\left(\ell_j \zeta_j + \ell'_j \zeta'_j\right) \tag{2}$$

where $I(t) = I_{hd}(t) + I_{fd}(t)$ and all the fading coefficients are statistically independent. We then define the average signal to interference ratio experienced at a half- and a full-duplex receiver as $\overline{\mathsf{SIR}}_{hd} = PL(r)\zeta/\bar{I}$, and $\overline{\mathsf{SIR}}_{fd} = PL(r)\zeta/(\bar{I}+S)$, where, with a slight abuse of notation, $L(r) = r^{-\alpha}$ is the path loss for a link of distance r and S represents the remaining self-interference contribution that hampers reception at a transmitting terminal. Buttressed by experimental results [3], we assume a linear dependence of S to the emitted power, i.e., $S = P(1 - \eta)$. This hypothesis leads to an average SIR which is independent of P, helping to identify broadly applicable tradeoffs. Accordingly, in the remainder of our discussion we will refer to the case of unit transmission power without loss of generality.

A threshold model is assumed for decoding, with a packet being retrieved as soon as the average SIR experienced at its receiver is above θ. In the case of a half-duplex link, letting $\bar{I}_{hd}$ and $\bar{I}_{fd}$ be the average of the quantities (2) as per (1), the success probability can be expressed as $p_s^{(hd)} = \Pr\{\zeta \geq \theta(\bar{I}_{hd} + \bar{I}_{fd})/L(r)\}$, which eventually leads to

$$p_s^{(hd)} = \mathbb{E}\left[e^{-\frac{\theta}{L(r)}\bar{I}_{hd}}\right] \mathbb{E}\left[e^{-\frac{\theta}{L(r)}\bar{I}_{fd}}\right] = \mathcal{L}_{\bar{I}_{hd}}\left(\theta/L(r)\right) \cdot \mathcal{L}_{\bar{I}_{fd}}\left(\theta/L(r)\right). \tag{3}$$

Here, the first equality starts from the exponential distribution of ζ and leverages the law of total probability over the two independent processes Ψ_{hd} and Ψ_{fd} generating the interference contributions. In turn, the second step simply employs the definition of Laplace transform of a random variable x, $\mathcal{L}_x(s) \triangleq \mathbb{E}[e^{-sx}]$. Following a similar approach, it is straightforward to also derive the success probability for a full-duplex link as $p_s^{(fd)} = \beta \cdot p_s^{(hd)}$, where $\beta = e^{-(1-\eta)\theta/L(r)}$ accounts for imperfect self-interference cancellation.

In order to complement our analysis, the performance of the system is also evaluated in terms of the throughput density τ, defined as the average number of information bits per second successfully exchanged in the network per unit area. Assuming a common information bitrate of R bit/s, a successful packet contributes with RD bits to the throughput, leading to

$$\tau = \lambda DR\left[(1-q)p_s^{(hd)} + 2q\,p_s^{(fd)}\right], \tag{4}$$

where the first addend accounts for the fraction of half-duplex clusters delivering at most one data unit, while simple combinatorial calculations lead to the second addend, reporting the average number of packets exchanged within an active full-duplex pair.

3 Performance of Asynchronous Full-Duplex Networks

The framework introduced in Sect. 2 highlighted how the system performance can be characterised as soon as the Laplace transforms of the average interference generated at a receiver by half- and full-duplex links are evaluated. An elegant calculation of the former was derived in [6]. Due to space constraints, we refer the interested reader to the original work of Blaszczyszyn et al. for the details. Instead, we only report here a slightly modified version of their outcome, obtained via simple mathematical manipulations which lead to

$$\mathcal{L}_{\bar{I}_{hd}}\big(\theta/L(r)\big) = \exp\big(-4\lambda(1-q)\,D\,\Omega_{hd}\big), \tag{5}$$

where

$$\Omega_{hd} = \frac{\pi}{2}\,\theta^{2/\alpha}\,r^2\Gamma\left(1+\frac{2}{\alpha}\right)\Gamma\left(1-\frac{2}{\alpha}\right)\frac{\alpha}{\alpha+2} \tag{6}$$

and $\Gamma(x) = \int_0^\infty x^{t-1}e^{-x}\,dt$ is the complete Gamma function. The result in (5) is particularly insightful, as it isolates the role of two key performance drivers. On the one hand, an exponential dependence of the success probability on the duration D of the active links is prompted, stressing the intrinsic weakness of longer transmissions to interference. On the other hand, the factor Ω_{hd} summarises the impact of system parameters as r, θ and α, embedding the structure of the interference generated by half-duplex clusters.

Let us now focus instead on the contribution of full-duplex pairs. As a preliminary step it is useful to reshape (1), leveraging the indicator function $\mathbb{1}(\cdot)$ to express $\bar{I}_{fd}$ through a summation over the whole Ψ_{fd} as

$$\bar{I}_{fd} = \sum_{(\mathbf{x}_i,T_i)\in\Psi_{fd}} (\ell_i\,\zeta_i + \ell'_i\,\zeta'_i)\int_0^D \frac{\mathbb{1}(T_i \le t \le T_i + D)}{D}\,dt. \tag{7}$$

Simple calculations allow to evaluate the integral in (7) as $(D-|T_i|)^+/D \triangleq f(T_i)$, with $a^+ = \max\{a,0\}$, $a \in \mathbb{R}$. Taking the lead from this result, we can then elaborate on the Laplace transform $\mathcal{L}_{\bar{I}_{fd}}(s)$, $s \in \mathbb{R}$:

$$\mathcal{L}_{\bar{I}_{fd}}(s) = \mathbb{E}\left[\prod_{\Psi_{fd}} e^{-s(\ell_i\zeta_i+\ell'_i\zeta'_i)f(T_i)}\right] \overset{(a)}{=} \mathbb{E}\left[\prod_{\Psi_{fd}} \frac{1}{1+s\ell_i f(T_i)}\frac{1}{1+s\ell'_i f(T_i)}\right]$$

$$\overset{(b)}{=} \exp\left(-\lambda q \int_{\mathbb{R}^2} d\mathbf{x}\int_{\mathbb{R}} dT\left(1-\int_{\mathbb{R}^2}\frac{1}{1+s\ell_i f(T)}\frac{1}{1+s\ell'_i f(T)}g(\mathbf{w}_i)d\mathbf{w}_i\right)\right). \tag{8}$$

Here, equality (a) follows from taking the expectation over the fading coefficients and relying on their independence, while the second step first averages over the spatial distribution of the companion node of $\mathbf{x}_i$ (generically expressed as $g(\mathbf{w})$ over $\mathbb{R}^2$) and then resorts to Campbell's theorem for the homogeneous PPP Ψ_{fd} of intensity λq. The general expression in (8) can be specified for the case of interest, taking advantage of the simple structure of $f(T)$ to carry out the integration over time and recalling that $\mathbf{w}_i$ is uniformly distributed over a circle of radius r centred at $\mathbf{x}_i$. Simple yet tedious calculations eventually lead to the sought result for the Laplace transform of the interference contribution of full-duplex clusters:

$$\mathcal{L}_{\bar{I}_{fd}}\big(\theta/L(r)\big) = \exp\big(-4\lambda q\, D\, \Omega_{fd}\big), \qquad (9)$$

where we define the ancillary function

$$\Omega_{fd} = \int_0^\infty u\left(\pi - \int_0^\pi \frac{\ln\left(\frac{1+\theta r^\alpha u^{-\alpha}}{1+\theta r^\alpha (u^2+r^2+2ru\cos\varphi)^{-\frac{\alpha}{2}}}\right)}{\theta r^\alpha\left(u^{-\alpha} - (u^2+r^2+2ru\cos\varphi)^{-\frac{\alpha}{2}}\right)}\, d\varphi\right) du. \qquad (10)$$

The presented result is remarkable, as we can once more isolate the effect of the key design parameters q and D from the factor Ω_{fd}. The latter, in turn, is not affected by the fraction of full-duplex clusters in the network nor by the duration of the transmissions, but rather only characterises the interference contribution that each full-duplex link produces. Moreover, leaning on (5) and (9), a compact and insightful expression for the throughput of the rather generic network under consideration is eventually obtained, in the form

$$\tau = \lambda D\big(1 + q\,(2\beta - 1)\big)\cdot\exp\big(-4\lambda D\big[(1-q)\Omega_{hd} + q\Omega_{fd}\big]\big). \qquad (11)$$

Based on this, let us start our discussion assuming ideal self-interference cancellation ($\eta = 1$), and focus on the two extreme scenarios $q = 0$ and $q = 1$, corresponding to a purely half-duplex and a purely full-duplex network. Unless otherwise specified, we refer to a system with parameters $\lambda = 0.05$, $r = 1$, $\alpha = 4$, $R = 1$ and $\theta = 2$. The throughput density achievable in the two cases when varying the packet length D is reported in Fig. 1a, together with results obtained via Monte Carlo simulations of the described time-space PPP that validate the framework. The plot clearly highlights how, for short data units, full-duplex capabilities indeed boost performance, thanks to the higher degree of spatial reuse they enable. On the other hand, when longer packets are considered, the detrimental effect of the additional interference generated by having two concurrent transmissions per cluster kicks in, leading to a steep decrease in the achievable throughput and eventually making a simple half-duplex setting more convenient. The tradeoff between additional interference and spatial reuse when varying the packet length raises then the natural question of what is the optimal fraction q^* of clusters that shall be allowed to operate in full-duplex. The answer to this can be derived from the expression of the throughput in (11),

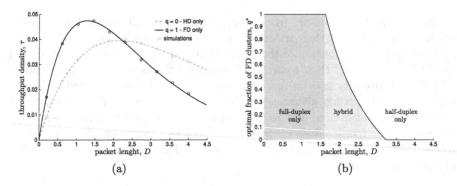

Fig. 1. (a) Network throughput density vs packet length for a purely half-duplex and a purely full-duplex; (b) Fraction of full-duplex clusters to maximise network throughput vs. packet length. Perfect self-interference cancellation is assumed.

differentiating it with respect to q. Simple calculations lead to three optimal operating regions: for $D \in [0, D_1)$, $q^* = 1$; for $D \in [D_1, D_2]$, $q^* = \delta - 1/(2\beta - 1)$; and for $D > D_2$, $q^* = 0$, where $D_1 = \delta(1 - 1/(2\beta))$, $D_2 = (2\beta - 1)\delta$, and $\delta = (4\lambda(\Omega_{fd} - \Omega_{hd}))^{-1}$. The result is reported graphically in Fig. 1b, assuming again ideal cancellation (i.e., $\beta = 1$). It is apparent that for sufficiently short packets it is indeed convenient to let as many clusters as possible (ideally, all of them) operate in full-duplex mode. Conversely, when data units are longer than the threshold D_2, even full-duplex capable nodes shall only establish half-duplex links. Remarkably, a closed form expression is available also to characterise the optimal q in the intermediate region as a function of the ancillary functions Ω. The plot offers thus an insightful design hint, prompting full-duplex as a promising solution to support the increasing throughput demand of MTC networks, which typically exhibit short and sporadic information exchanges.

Along the same line of reasoning, the simple dependence of τ on D allows to derive the duration D^* of data links that shall be set to maximise performance in a network with a fraction q of full-duplex clusters. From the analysis, $D^* = [4\lambda((1-q)\Omega_{hd} + q\Omega_{fd})]^{-1}$ follows. Not only can this result be useful to tune the communications parameters in a deployed network, but it also addresses the question on whether the doubling of the throughput approached by full duplex at a link level can be achieved when more articulated topologies are considered. To this aim, let us consider the ratio χ of the peak throughput when $q = 1$ to the same quantity for $q = 0$. Plugging the value of D^* into (11), we readily get $\chi = 2\beta \, \Omega_{hd}/\Omega_{fd}$. This expression is independent of λ, showing how the maximum gain brought by spatial reuse is intrinsically limited by the nature of the interference generated by full-duplex links. Moreover, χ is conveniently expressed as two times a correction factor which is lower than one even under the assumption of ideal self-interference cancellation, confirming and quantifying how full-duplex can in fact not double the network capacity in uncoordinated systems. For the special case $\alpha = 4$ under consideration, it is furthermore possible

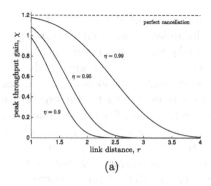
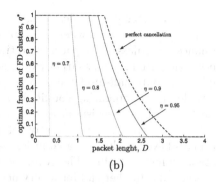

(a)   (b)

Fig. 2. (a) Peak throughput gain achievable by a purely full-duplex network over a solely half-duplex one vs link distance; (b) Optimal fraction of full-duplex clusters to maximise network throughput vs. packet length. Imperfect self-interference cancellation is considered.

to write Ω_{fd} in the form $c\,r^2$, where c is a real constant.[1] Under ideal interference cancellation, then, χ is also independent of the link distance r, and evaluates to ~ 1.2 with the assumed θ. Conversely, recalling that $\beta = \exp\left(-\left(1-\eta\right)\theta r^\alpha\right)$, a residual level of self-interference induces a dramatic degradation of the throughput gain offered by full-duplex with the link distance. This aspect is highlighted in Fig. 2a, which reports χ as a function of r, and shows how already small losses in η fundamentally limit the throughput of the full-duplex network. Even more interestingly, poorer interference cancellation levels (e.g., $\eta \leq 0.9$ in our case) eventually lead to a condition in which a purely half-duplex network outperforms its full-duplex counterpart regardless of the proximity of the communicating nodes. This offers two relevant design take-aways. In the first place, not only shall full-duplex links be employed when short data units have to be exchanged, but also, they shall carefully be triggered when source and addressee are sufficiently close to each other - a condition often met in MTC links. Secondly, the potential improvement in terms of capacity shall not distract from the importance of achieving levels of self-interference cancellation even stronger than what desirable from an isolated-link viewpoint. In the quest for low-cost terminals, this may in fact constitute a crucial challenge.

As a final remark, the presented framework also allows to understand the role played by η on the fraction of clusters that shall be operated in full-duplex mode, leaning on the optimal regions derived earlier as a function of D. The behaviour of the system is reported in Fig. 2b, where the dashed line reproduces for completeness the regions under ideal cancellation already discussed by Fig. 1b. Lower values of η progressively limit the convenience of a solely full-duplex

---

[1] The result is obtained by applying the inequality $1 - 1/x \leq \ln(x) \leq x - 1$, $x > 0$ to upper and lower bound the numerator of the inner integrand, as well by upper bonding the cosine terms as 1. The resulting rational function can easily be integrated, leading to the dependence on r^2. Further details are omitted due to space constraints.

system to shorter communications, eventually reaching a point, for $\beta = 1/2$, i.e., $\eta = 1 - \ln(2)r^{-\alpha}/\theta$, where a simpler half-duplex network offers better performance regardless of the packet duration. Furthermore, the presence of residual self-interference induces sharper transitions between the regions where only full-duplex and only half-duplex are to be preferred. Such a trend is in general not desirable, as the operating condition of most interest is exactly the one where both kind of links coexist. From this standpoint, in fact, fractional values of q can be interpreted as representative of both a network where only some of the terminals have full-duplex capabilities and of topologies in which node pairs generate asymmetric traffic. The two conditions are clearly very relevant to MTC scenarios, and further call for a very accurate cancellation of self-interference.

4   Conclusions

This paper has introduced a stochastic geometry framework that captures the performance of an asynchronous Aloha network where part of the nodes operate in full-duplex mode. Closed form expressions have been presented for the success probability and the system throughput, identifying the key tradeoffs in the system. In particular, three operating regions have been identified, showing how for short enough packets as many communications as possible shall be performed in full-duplex mode, while for packets longer than a certain threshold solely relying on half-duplex is convenient. The impact of imperfect cancellation has been discussed, and relevant insights for the applicability of full-duplex to machine type communications have been discussed.

References

1. Paolini, E., Stefanovic, C., Liva, G., Popovski, P.: Coded random access: applying codes on graphs to design random access protocols. IEEE Commun. Mag. (2015, to appear)
2. Sabharwal, A., Schniter, P., Guo, D., Bliss, D.W., Rangarajan, S., Wichman, R.: In-band full-duplex wireless: challenges and opportunities. IEEE J. Sel. Areas Commun. 32(9), 1637–1652 (2014)
3. Bharadia, D., McMilin, E., Katti, S.: Full duplex radios. In: Proceedings of ACM SIGCOMM, Hong Kong, China, 12–16 August 2013
4. Tong, Z., Haenggi, M.: Throughput Analysis for Full-Duplex Wireless Networks with Imperfect Self-interference Cancellation (2015). http://arxiv.org/abs/1502.07404
5. Ali, S., Rajatheva, N., Latva-aho, M.: Full duplex device-to-device communication in cellular networks. In: Proceedings of EuCNC, Bologna, Italy (2014)
6. Blaszczyszyn, B., Muehlethaler, P.: Stochastic analysis of non-slotted aloha in wireless ad hoc networks. In: Proceedings of IEEE INFOCOM, San Diego, CA, USA (2010)

Long-Range IoT Technologies: The Dawn of LoRa™

Lorenzo Vangelista[1,2]([✉]), Andrea Zanella[2], and Michele Zorzi[1,2]

[1] Patavina Technologies s.r.l., Padova, Italy
info@patavinatech.com
http://www.patavinatech.com/en/
[2] Department of Information Engineering, University of Padova,
Via Gradenigo 6/B, Padova, Italy
{vangelista,zanella,zorzi}@dei.unipd.it

Abstract. The last years have seen the widespread diffusion of novel Low Power Wide Area Network (LPWAN) technologies, which are gaining momentum and commercial interest as enabling technologies for the Internet of Things. In this paper we discuss some of the most interesting LPWAN solutions, focusing in particular on LoRa™, one of the last born and most promising technologies for the wide-area IoT.

Keywords: Internet of Things · 5G · Low-power wide area

1 Introduction

Although the general requirements of the next generation of communication systems, generally referred to as *5G*, are still being debated by industrial and academic experts,[1] fairly broad consensus has been reached upon a few key requirements: besides the inevitable increase in the bit rates and energy efficiency of the whole system, 5G shall seamlessly integrate Internet of Things (IoT) services, without degrading the traditional services. However, how to practically realize such an integration is still an open question.

The problem is that, up to now, the term IoT has been broadly used to indicate a number of different technologies (and research disciplines) that are somehow intended to enable the Internet to reach out into the real world of physical objects. Among the most popular technologies that are commonly associated with IoT, we can mention the radio frequency identifiers (RFID), short-range wireless communication technologies (NFC, Bluetooth, ZigBee), and ad hoc and wireless sensor networks (WSNs) [1–3]. Most of these technologies are characterized by short-range, low-power communication capabilities, which limit their application to scenarios with limited coverage areas, such as rooms or small buildings. Also in this case, multihop communication is often required to guarantee proper coverage while limiting the cost of deployment.

---

[1] http://networld2020.eu/expert-group/.

© Institute for Computer Sciences, Social Informatics and Telecommunications Engineering 2015
V. Atanasovski, L.-G. Alberto (Eds.): Fabulous 2015, LNICST 159, pp. 51–58, 2015.
DOI: 10.1007/978-3-319-27072-2_7

In the last years, however, the multi-hop paradigm for the IoT has been challenged by the idea that the only valuable and practical solution to provide ubiquitous coverage for IoT devices is to exploit the current and upcoming cellular technologies [4–6]. Cellular networks have indeed a world-wide established footprint and are able to deal with the challenge of ubiquitous and transparent coverage, thus potentially enabling the *place-&-play* functional model, according to which IoT nodes just need to be placed in the desired locations to become operational and get connected to the rest of the world [7]. On the other hand, cellular networks were not originally conceived and designed for providing machine-type services to a massive number of devices. Differently from traditional broadband services, IoT communication is expected to generate, in most cases, sporadic transmissions of short packets. At the same time, the potentially huge number of IoT devices that shall gain connectivity through a single Base Station will raise a number of issues related to the signalling and control traffic, which may become the bottleneck of the system [7]. All these aspects make current cellular network technologies unsuitable to fully support the envisioned IoT scenarios, while a number of research challenges still need to be addressed before the upcoming 5G cellular networks may natively support IoT connectivity.

In the meantime, the IoT market has been witnessing the rapid spread of new commercial technologies, based on another networking paradigm referred to as *Low Power Wide Area Network* (LPWAN). These technologies fall in between short-range multi-hop technologies and proper broadband cellular systems. Similarly to the cellular networks, LPWAN technologies are characterized by long-range links (in the orders of kilometres) and have *star network topologies*, with the peripheral nodes connected directly to a concentrator that, as for short-range multi-hop WSNs, acts as *gateway* towards the IP-world. Furthermore, their architecture allows for *wide area coverage*, which can extend to a whole nation, while sometime permitting the roaming of the peripheral nodes between networks in different countries. Last but not least, the robust modulations used by these technologies make them suitable to connect end-devices located in harsh environments (e.g., water meters placed underground or in basements), where cellular technologies may fail.

In the rest of this paper, we first provide a broad overview of the most interesting LPWAN technologies. Then, we focus our attention on the last born in the LPWAN family, namely LoRa[TM], whose specific features and market perspectives are particularly attractive in the context of IoT services. We conclude the paper with some final remarks.

2   LPWAN Technologies for Ubiquitous IoT Connectivity

Conversely to the general trend that pushes the new generations of wireless technologies towards higher and higher frequency bands, LPWAN solutions mainly operate in the band from 863 MHz to 870 MHz in Europe (so-called SDR860), according to the regulations in [8], and in the ISM band from 902 MHz to 928 MHz in the USA. Depending on the type of modulation adopted, the technologies can be broadly divided in two categories:

- Ultra Narrow Band (UNB): using narrowband channels with a bandwidth of the order of 25 kHz;
- Wideband: using a larger bandwidth (125 kHz or 250 kHz) and employing some form of spread spectrum multiple access techniques to accomodate multiple users in one channel.

In the following we discuss in greater detail some of the LPWAN products that have been gaining momentum in the last years, deferring to Sect. 3 the description of the LoRa^TM technology.

SIGFOX^TM. The first LPWAN technology proposed in the IoT market has been SIGFOX^TM [9], which was founded in 2009, and has been growing very fast since then. Its current coverage includes France, UK and Spain. The SIGFOX^TM network employs a UNB modulation, while the network layer protocols are the "secret sauce" of the SIGFOX^TM network and, as such, there exists basically no publicly available documentation. The first releases of the technology only supported uni-directional communication, i.e., from the device towards the aggregator; however bi-directional communication is now supported. Each base station can handle up to a million connected objects, with a coverage area of 30–50 km in rural areas and 3–10 km in urban areas.

Weightless^TM. A more open approach has been taken by Weightless^TM, which is an open standard backed by Neul, a UK company recently acquired by Huawei. Weightless^TM is actually a set of three standards [10], which are developed under the umbrella of the non-profit global standards organisation *Weightless SIG*. The standards are: *Weightless-N*, which supports a star network architecture and operates in sub-GHz spectrum using UNB technology, with an excellent range of several kilometres even in challenging urban environments; *Weightless-P*, which supports narrowband channels of 12.5 kHz, with Frequency Division and Time Division Multiple Access modes, adaptive data rate from 0.2 kbit/s to 100 kbit/s, time-synchronised aggregators, and low-cost highly energy efficient modulations; and *Weightless-W*, which is a system with star topology operating in TV white space spectrum.

On-Ramp Wireless. An emerging star in the landscape of LPWAN is On-Ramp Wireless, a company based in San Diego (USA) [11]. On-Ramp Wireless has been pioneering the 802.15.4k standard [12]. The company developed and owns the rights of the patented technology Random Phase Multiple Access (RPMA®) [13], which is deployed in different networks. Conversely to the other LPWAN solutions, this technology works in the 2.4 GHz band but, thanks to a robust physical layer design, can still operate over long-range wireless links and under the most challenging RF environments. This technology is mainly targeted to metering and SmartGrid applications.

3   The SemTech LoRa^TM Technology

This section focuses on the LoRa^TM technology, first proposed by SemTech and now being developed by the LoRa^TM Alliance [14].

3.1 LoRa^{TM} system architecture

The LoRa^{TM} system consists of three main components:

- LoRa^{TM} End-devices: sensors/actuators connected via the LoRa^{TM} radio interface to one or more LoRa^{TM} Gateways;
- LoRa^{TM} Gateways: concentrators that bridge end-devices to the LoRa^{TM} NetServer, which is the central element of the network architecture.
- LoRa^{TM} NetServer: the network server that controls the whole network (radio resource management, admission control, security, etc.).

As exemplified in Fig. 1, the network is typically laid out in a star-of-stars topology, where the end-devices are connected via single-hop LoRa^{TM} communication to one or many gateways that, in turn, are connected to a common NetServer via standard Internet technologies. The gateways relay messages between end-devices and NetServer, according to the protocol architecture represented in Fig. 2. Interestingly, *all* the gateways that successfully decode the message sent by an end-device will forward the packet to the NetServer by adding some information regarding the quality of the reception. The NetServer will hence reply to the end-device by choosing one such gateway, according to some criterion (e.g., best radio connectivity). The gateways are hence totally transparent to the end-devices, which are logically connected directly to the NetServer.

A distinguishing feature of the LoRa^{TM} network is that it envisions three classes of end-devices, named *Class A* (for *All*), *B* (for *Beacon*) and *C* (for *Continuously listening*), each associated to a different operating mode [15].

Class A defines the default functional mode of the LoRa^{TM} networks, and must be mandatorily supported by all LoRa^{TM} devices. In a Class A network, transmissions are always initiated by the end-devices, in a totally asynchronous manner. After each uplink transmission, the end-device will open (at least) two reception windows, waiting for any command or data packet returned by the NetServer. The second window is opened on a different sub-band (previously agreed upon with the NetServer) in order to increase resilience to channel fluctuations. Class A networks are mainly intended for monitoring applications, where data produced by the end-devices have to be collected by a control station.

Class B has been introduced to decouple uplink and downlink transmissions. Class B end-devices, indeed, get synchronized with the NetServer by means of beacon packets broadcast by Class B gateways, and can hence receive downlink data or command packets in specific time windows, irrespective of the uplink traffic. Class B is intended for end-devices that need to receive commands from a remote controller, e.g., switches or actuators, or need to provide data at user's request.

Finally, Class C is defined for end-devices without (strict) energy constraints (e.g., connected to the power grid), which can hence keep the receive window always open.

It is worth noting that, at the moment of writing, class A and B specifications are provided in [15], while class C specifications are still in draft form.

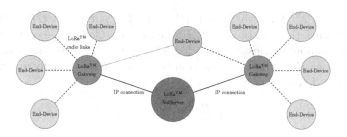

Fig. 1. LoRa^TM system architecture

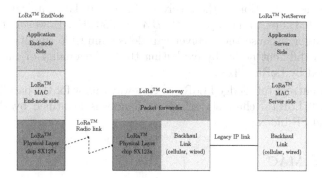

Fig. 2. LoRa^TM protocol architecture

3.2 LoRa^TM Physical Layer

The LoRa^TM radio communication is based on a proprietary modulation scheme [16], which is a derivative of *Chirp Spread Spectrum* (CSS) [17]. The innovation consists in ensuring the phase continuity between different chirp symbols in the preamble part of the physical layer packet, which enables a simpler and more accurate timing and frequency synchronisation, without requiring expensive components for generating a stable local clock in the LoRa^TM node. Furthermore, the technology supports variable data rate, thus giving the possibility to trade throughput for coverage range, or robustness, or energy consumption, while keeping a constant bandwidth.

The chip was designed to work in the bands centred at frequencies 169 MHz, 433 MHz and 915 MHz in the USA, but in Europe it works in the band centred at the 868 MHz (SRD860). The regulations in [8] require the radio emitters to adopt duty cycled transmission (1 % or 0.1 %, depending on the subband), or the so-called Listen Before Talk (LBT) Adaptive Frequency Agility (AFA), which is a sort of carrier sense mechanism that shall prevent severe interference among devices operating in the same band. According to the specifications [15], LoRa^TM only uses the duty cycled transmission option.

The LoRa^TM modulation is hence completely specified by three parameters: the bandwidth BW that, in Europe, usually is 125 kHz or 250 kHz; the so-called "spreading factor" $SF \in \{7, \ldots, 12\}$, which determines the length of the chirp symbol as $T_s = 2^{SF} T_c$, with $T_c = 1/BW$, and the parameter $CR \in \{0, \ldots, 4\}$ which determines the rate of the FEC code as $Rate\ Code = \frac{4}{4+R}$. According to [18], a chirp symbol carries SF encoded bits, coming from the interleaver, and every bit carries $Rate\ Code$ information bits. Therefore, the effective data rate of an infinitely long payload is given by [18, p. 10]

$$R_b = SF \frac{Rate\ Code}{\frac{2^{SF}}{BW}} \quad [\text{bit/s}]. \tag{1}$$

Considering that each packet is prepended with a preamble to allow for frequency and timing synchronization at the receiver, the actual data rate ranges approximately from 0.3 kbps to 11 kbps, with $BW = 250$ kHz. However, the system capacity is larger because the receiver can detect multiple simultaneous transmissions from different nodes by exploiting the orthogonality of the spreading sequences used by LoRa™ [18].

Note that current full-fledged LoRa™ Gateways allow for the parallel processing of up to 9 LoRa™ channels, where a channel is identified by the specific sub–band and SF index.

3.3 LoRa™ MAC

The MAC layer defined by the LoRa Alliance is called LoRaWAN and, according to the specifications in [15], it is basically an ALOHA protocol controlled primarily by the LoRa™ NetServer. A description of the protocol is beyond the scope of this paper and can be found in [15].

A distinguishing feature of the LoRa™ MAC is the *Adaptive Data Rate*, which allows the NetServer to adapt the transmit rate of an end-device by changing the SF index, in order to find the best tradeoff between energy efficiency and link robustness.

Another important feature is the strong security mechanisms that entail a network key and an application key, which are set up through an over-the-air activation procedure, as well as an activation by personalisation procedure (where the security parameters are set into the device at production time).

Overall the LoRa™ MAC has been designed attempting to mimic as much as possible the IEEE 802.15.4 MAC. The objective is to simplify the accommodation, on top of the LoRa™ MAC, of the major protocols now running on top of the IEEE 802.15.4 MAC, for example 6LoWPAN and CoAP. A clear analogy is the *authentication* mechanism, which is taken directly from the IEEE 802.15.4 standard using the 4–octet Message Integrity Code.

4   Discussion

Albeit still in its infancy, the landscape of the LPWAN is already crowded, with different technologies that share many commonalities but differ in some key features and design choices. A lively debate is ongoing in the scientific and technical communities to identify the characteristics that may determine the supremacy of one technology over the others. Some of the debated aspects are the following:

(a) Wideband or UNB?
(b) 2.4 GHz or sub-GHz?

For example the LoRa™ solution is wideband sub-GHz, while SIGFOX™ is UNB sub-GHz. Texas Instruments as well is supporting the UNB sub-GHz solutions [19], arguing that the wideband solutions would suffer from the interference of UNB technologies, also considering the relatively long symbol period associated with low data rates. In parallel, On-Ramp Wireless claims that the worldwide availability of the 2.4 GHz ISM band offsets the link-budget gain, estimated around 9 dB, granted by the most favourable propagation conditions of the bands centred at 868 MHz and 915 MHz. Indeed, the RPMA® developed by On-Ramp Wireless can gain about 8 dB in the link budget by exploiting antenna diversity at 2.4 GHz, thus almost completely offsetting the degradation due to the higher pathloss. However, the 2.4 GHz ISM band is now crowded with plenty of different radio emitters, and channel access contention and/or interference may be critical.

Unfortunately, to the best of the authors' knowledge, no objective comparisons (not biased by marketing) of the different solutions exist yet. Therefore, there is not yet a definite answer to these questions and, as often happens in these matters, the winning technologies will likely be determined by a number of not necessarily technical factors.

Nonetheless, we believe that the LoRa™ technology offers some advantages over the other technologies, which may make the difference in the competition to gain a leading role in the IoT market. Some of these advantages come from the technical domain, where the chirp modulation used at the PHY layer allows for long-range, robust communications, with low complexity, low power and low cost receivers, while the upper layer protocols simplify the adoption of other protocols (e.g., the security mechanisms already tested in IEEE 802.15.4 networks), and enhance the compatibility with other technologies, such as the IEEE 802.15.4 and 6LowPAN networks.

From a strategic standpoint, instead, LoRa™ takes advantage of the establishment of the LoRa™ Alliance [14], which is guiding the development and expansion of the LoRa™ technology, with subgroups dedicated not only to the technical development, but also to the marketing, strategy, and interoperability aspects. As a consequence, a strong eco-system is growing around the technology, with partners developing different parts of the systems, and integrators selling the complete solutions for both *geographical* and *residential/industrial* types of networks. Today, there are plenty of companies developing different types of end-nodes, for the most heterogeneous applications, including healthcare, streetlighting, waste management, building monitoring and control. We believe that, if this ecosystem will continue to grow and stay aligned via interoperability checks, it will be a strong driving force for the success of the LoRa™ technology.

References

1. Gubbi, J., Buyya, R., Marusic, S., Palaniswami, M.: Internet of Things (IoT): a vision, architectural elements, and future directions. Future Gener. Comput. Syst. **29**(7), 1645–1660 (2013)
2. Miorandi, D., Sicari, S., De Pellegrini, F., Chlamtac, I.: Internet of things: vision, applications and research challenges. Ad Hoc Netw. **10**(7), 1497–1516 (2012)
3. Zanella, A., Bui, N., Castellani, A., Vangelista, L., Zorzi, M.: Internet of things for smart cities. Internet of Things J. IEEE **1**(1), 22–32 (2014)
4. Anton-Haro, C., Dohler, M. (eds.): Machine-to-machine (M2M) Communications: Architecture, Performance and Applications. Elsevier, Cambridge (2014)
5. Lien, S.-Y., Chen, K.-C., Lin, Y.: Toward ubiquitous massive accesses in 3GPP machine-to-machine communications. IEEE Commun. Mag. **49**(4), 66–74 (2011)
6. 3GPP, Standarization of Machine-type Communications, 3rd Generation Partnership Project. Technical report, vol. 2.4, June 2014
7. Biral, A., Centenaro, M., Zanella, A., Vangelista, L., Zorzi, M.: The challenges of M2M massive access in wireless cellular networks. Digit. Commun. Netw. **1**(1), 1–19 (2015)
8. ETSI EN 300 220–1 V2.4.1 Electromagnetic compatibility and Radio spectrum Matters (ERM); Short Range Devices (SRD); Radio equipment to be used in the 25 MHz to 1 000 MHz frequency range with power levels ranging up to 500 mW; Part 1: Technical characteristics and test methods, ETSI 650 Route des Lucioles F-06921 Sophia Antipolis Cedex - France 2012
9. http://www.sigfox.com/. Accessed 10 August 2015
10. http://www.weightless.org/. Accessed 10 August 2015
11. http://www.onrampwireless.com/. Accessed 10 August 2015
12. IEEE Standard for Local and metropolitan area networks. Part 15.4: Low-Rate Wireless Personal Area Networks (LR-WPANs) Amendment 5: Physical Layer Specifications for Low Energy, Critical Infrastructure Monitoring Networks, IEEE Computer Society (2015)
13. Light monitoring system using a random phase multiple access system Patent No.: US 8,477,830 B2 (2013)
14. https://www.lora-alliance.org/. Accessed 10 August 2015
15. "LoRaWAN^{TM}" Specification v1.0, LoRa Alliance, Inc. 2400 Camino Ramon, Suite 375 San Ramon, CA 94583 (2015)
16. Sforza, F.: Communications system, US Patent 8,406,275
17. Berni, A.J., Gregg, W.D.: On the utility of chirp modulation for digital signaling. IEEE Trans. Commun. **21**(6), 748–751 (1973)
18. AN1200.22 LoRa^{TM} modulation basics, Revision 2, Semtech Corporation, May 2015: http://www.semtech.com/images/datasheet/an1200.22.pdf. Accessed 15 August 2015
19. http://www.ti.com/lit/wp/swry006/swry006.pdf. Accessed 10 August 2015

Analysis of Two-Tier LTE Network with Randomized Resource Allocation and Proactive Offloading

Aleksandar Ichkov[✉], Vladimir Atanasovski,
and Liljana Gavrilovska

Faculty of Electrical Engineering and Information Technologies,
Saints Cyril and Methodius University in Skopje, Skopje, Macedonia
{ichkov,vladimir,liljana}@feit.ukim.edu.mk

Abstract. The heterogeneity in cellular networks that comprise multiple base stations' types imposes new challenges in network planning and deployment. The Radio Resource Management (RRM) techniques, such as dynamic sharing of the available resources and advanced user association strategies determine the overall network capacity and efficiency. This paper evaluates the downlink performance of a two-tier heterogeneous LTE network (consisting of macro and femto tiers) in terms of rate distribution, i.e. the percentage of users that achieve certain rate in the system. The paper specifically addresses the femto tier RRM by randomization of the allocated resources (1) and the user association process by introducing novel proactive offloading scheme (2). System level simulation results show that the proposed proactive offloading scheme in the association phase improves the performance of congested networks by efficiently utilizing the available femto tier resources.

Keywords: LTE · Heterogeneous networks · Femtocells · RRM · User association · Proactive offloading

1 Introduction

The increasing need for capacity in cellular networks leads to network densification, which is one of the evolution directions for 5G networks [1]. The densification can be achieved either in space, by increasing the number of network nodes in the system, or in frequency, by utilizing different portions of spectrum in different bands.

The densification by adding new Macro Base Stations (MBSs) is an expensive solution. Additionally, the MBSs are not able to solve the problem of indoor coverage and high data rate for indoor users. Femtocells have emerged as a promising solution since the user-centric deployment of Femto Base Stations (FBSs) is inexpensive and uncoordinated. This makes them preferable for coverage and data rate improvement [2]. Network densification by adding additional femto tier of base stations that differs from the macro tier in terms of transmission power, capacity and base station spatial density, results in network heterogeneity.

© Institute for Computer Sciences, Social Informatics and Telecommunications Engineering 2015
V. Atanasovski, L.-G. Alberto (Eds.): Fabulous 2015, LNICST 159, pp. 59–65, 2015.
DOI: 10.1007/978-3-319-27072-2_8

The Radio Resource Management (RRM) of the femto tier is essential for the overall network performance. Unlike the macro tier that is a subject to frequency planning prior to actual deployment, the femto tier is usually deployed sporadically and randomly without any spatial or frequency planning [3]. Additionally, the deployment of the FBSs is usually uncoordinated with the macro tier, which further complicates the design of intelligent strategies for resource allocation and sharing [4].

Another important aspect for the overall network performance is the user-to-BS association strategy. Traditional user-to-BS association strategies are mostly BS coverage based and favor the MBSs for user association. In such cases, high portions of the femto tier resources might remain underutilized, resulting in degradations of the overall network spectrum efficiency.

Heterogeneous cellular networks aim to maximize the network capacity. The analysis of such networks requires new metrics for performance evaluation, such as the *rate distribution*, defined as the probability that a typical user in the network receives data rate beyond a predefined threshold. The rate distribution unambiguously captures the aspect of spectrum utilization efficiency in heterogeneous networks, unlike traditional network coverage based metrics.

This paper evaluates the performance of a two-tier LTE network that employs randomization of the allocated resources at femto tier, in terms of the rate distribution. Also, we introduce a novel two-step offloading scheme, which is used proactively in the user-to-BS association phase to improve the rate distribution in congested network.

2 System Topology and Radio Resource Management

The overall network system is comprised of two tiers of BSs, macro and femto, deployed over a specific area denoted with A, as shown at Fig. 1.

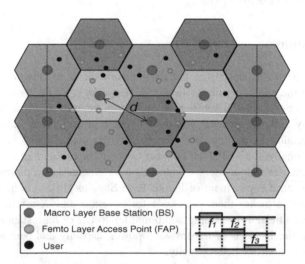

Macro Layer Base Station (BS)
Femto Layer Access Point (FAP)
User

Fig. 1. System topology and macro tier frequency allocation in the observed area

The MBSs are distributed using regular MBSs distribution, in a grid. Each MBS is at the center of hexagonal cell and the distance between two adjacent BSs is denoted as d. The set of all MBSs is denoted with M while the actual number of MBSs is denoted with N_m. The downlink transmit power of each MBS is denoted as P_m.

The FBSs are randomly distributed over the same area A, uncoordinated with the MBSs. Poisson Point Process (PPP) models the randomized and uncoordinated deployment of FBSs, as one of the most frequently used statistical distribution for modeling stochastic, two-dimensional point processes [5]. The intensity of the femto tier PPP is denoted as λ_f. The set of all FBSs is denoted as F with an average number of FBSs in the area $N_f = \lambda_f A$. The main difference between the macro and femto tier is in the transmit powers of the respective BSs, as the downlink transmit power of the FBSs is much lower than the one of the MBSs, $P_f << P_m$.

The users are assumed to be distributed according to PPP (Fig. 1), with intensity λ_u and average number $N_u = \lambda_u A$. The set of users is denoted with U.

2.1 Radio Resource Management

The radio access technology in focus is LTE's OFDMA with total system bandwidth W in MHz. The smallest resource unit that can be allocated to a single user is referred as Physical Resource Block (PRB) with $W_{PRB} = 180$ kHz of bandwidth in frequency domain and 2 slots in time domain. Thus, the total bandwidth of the system can be represented as the total number of available PRBs in the system.

The macro tier uses Hard Frequency Reuse (HFR) with Frequency Reuse Factor $K = 3$, dividing the available bandwidth on K equal continuous frequency fragments. (Figure 1). Each MBS gets one fragment containing $N_{PRB,m} = N_{PRB}/K$ PRBs and thus, a maximum of $N_{PRB,m}$ users can be associated to the MBS for downlink transmission.

The femto tier employs uncoordinated approach for resource allocation in order to mitigate the interference between different FBSs and to alleviate the cross-tier interference, as it requires minor coordination with the macro tier to determine the traffic state of the network, The femto tier divides the available system bandwidth in n_f continuous fragments of PRBs, each consisting of $N_{PRB,f} = N_{PRB}/n_f$ PRBs. Each of the FBSs randomly chooses a single fragment from the overall pool. Thus, a maximum of $N_{PRB,f}$ users can be associated to the FBS for downlink transmission.

2.2 User Resource Allocation

The user resource allocation strategy requires each BS to distribute the available physical resources fairly, using equal power allocation to each PRB, so that each user gets the maximal possible data rate with respect to the network settings and traffic load. For example, when the number of users is equal to the number of available PRBs, $N_{u,i} = N_{PRB,m}$ for $i \in M$ or $N_{u,i} = N_{PRB,f}$ for $i \in F$, each associated user is allocated a single PRB.

3 User-to-BS Association for Downlink Transmission

The user-to-BS association strategy determines which BS the user associates for downlink transmission. The common approach is that each user associates to the BS, macro or femto, that maximizes a predefined association rule.

Let $V = M \cup F$ denote the set of all BSs in the two-tier network. Each user associates with the BS k, in accordance with the following general association rule:

$$k = \arg\max_{i \in V}\{T_i Z_i^{-\gamma}\} \tag{1}$$

In (1), Z_i is the distance between the ith BS and the user, γ is the path loss exponent and T_i is referred as association weight. For example, if $T_i > > T_j$, $i \in F$, $j \in M$, then more traffic is routed through the femto tier. Thus, by adjusting T_i, the system can control the distribution of traffic among the tiers.

This paper analyzes several association strategies, depending on the value of T_i:

- *Nearest BS association* (MBS or FBS): $T_i = 1$, $\forall i \in V$
- *Cell range modification*: $T_i = P_i B_i$ and the range is extended if the bias factor $B_i > 1$ or reduced if $B_i < 1$
- *Femtocell range extension*: if the bias factor $B_i > 1$, $\forall i \in F$ and $B_i = 1$, $\forall i \in M$
- *Maximum received power association*: if the bias factor $B_i = 1$, $\forall i \in V$ then $T_i = P_i$, $\forall i \in V$

In most cases, the general rule (1) results in high number of users being associated to the MBSs. This is critical in congested networks, where there are high number of denied users by the macro tier and high portions of the femto tier resources unused. Forcing more traffic routing to the femto tier might also result in congested FBSs.

Therefore, this paper proposes a *simple two-step macro-to-femto offloading scheme* for the user association, based on the following algorithm:

Algorithm: Two-step, macro-to-femto offloading scheme
1: Number of users that send association requests to MBS i using (1) $\rightarrow N_{u,i}$
2: Step 1: *Macro layer user association*
3:      If $N_{u,i} \le N_{PRB,m} \rightarrow$ associate all users with MBS i
4:      Else If $N_{u,i} > N_{PRB,m}$
5:          Step 2: *Femto layer offloading*
6:          $\rightarrow$ Associate the best $N_{PRB,m}$ to the MBS i
7:          $\rightarrow$ Forward the rest $N = N_{u,i} - N_{PRB,m}$ users to their closest FBSs and use (1) for association

The basic idea is to allow each user, initially to send association request to the desired BS in accordance with the association rule (1). However, if the MBS does not have enough resources (PRBs) to allocate all tagged users for downlink transmission, the best $N_{PRB,m}$ are associated with the MBS (see 6:) and the remaining N users are forwarded to the femto tier to perform association with their respective, closest FBS (see 7:). The scheme can be regarded as proactive as it tries to avoid congestion in the initial association phase. Additionally, it avoids time and resource consuming re-associations of the dropped users by forwarding them to the femto tier and it is well suited for scenarios with high number of user association requests at a time.

4 Performance Evaluation

In order to evaluate the performance of such two-tier cellular network, the proposed network system is simulated in MATLAB, using realistic LTE settings.

The network is deployed over a targeted area A with a size of 25 km^2. A total number of 33 MBSs are distributed over the area, in a grid. The FBSs and the users are randomly distributed according to their respective PPPs. The system uses an overall bandwidth of 15 MHz, corresponding to 75 PRBs. At the macro tier, the total bandwidth is divided in three sub-bands, each containing 25 PRBs, regularly assigned to the MBSs with frequency reuse factor 3. Different scenarios are simulated, as the whole bandwidth at the femto tier can be divided into different number of fragments 1, 3, 5, 15 or 25, each containing 75, 25, 15, 5 or 3 continuous PRBs, respectively. Each FBS randomly choosing one fragment from the overall pool.

The paper introduces novel SINR calculation to calculate the interference from surrounding BSs with overlapping PRBs, also incorporating the number of scheduled PRBs for a particular user. For a particular user $i \in U$, the SINR is calculated as:

$$SINR_{ij} = \frac{\frac{\alpha_{ij}P_j}{N_{PRB,j}}\left\|h_{ij}\right\|^2\left\|x_{ij}\right\|^{-\alpha}}{\sum\limits_{\substack{m=1\\m\neq j\\j\in M}}^{N_m}\frac{\beta_{im}P_m}{N_{PRB,m}}\left\|h_{im}\right\|^2\left\|x_{im}\right\|^{-\alpha} + \sum\limits_{\substack{f=1\\f\neq j\\j\in M}}^{N_f}\frac{\beta_{if}P_f}{N_{PRB,f}}\left\|h_{if}\right\|^2\left\|x_{if}\right\|^{-\alpha} + N_0} \qquad (2)$$

Equation (2) represents the received SINR at the ith user that is associated to the jth BS (j is either in M or F). α_{ij} is random variable that represents the number of PRBs allocated to the user. The total transmit power from the jth base station to the ith user is $\alpha_{ij}P_j/N_{PRB,j}$, where $P_j/N_{PRB,j}$ is the transmit power on one PRB from the jth base station. h_{ij} and x_{ij} are the channel fading and the distance between the ith user and the jth BS, respectively. The first sum in the denominator denotes the interference from MBSs in the system, while the second sum denotes the interference from FBSs in the system. The random variables β_{im} and β_{if} represent the number of overlapping PRBs between the ith user and the interfering BSs, both macro and femto, respectively. The parameter N_0 is the noise power.

The rate R, for the ith user in the system, knowing the received SINR from the jth BS which the user is associated to, is calculated as:

$$R_{ij} = \alpha_{ij}W_{PRB}\log_2\left(1 + SINR_{ij}\right) \qquad (3)$$

The rate distribution Ψ, defined as the probability that certain percentage of users achieve rate higher than a predefined threshold, is calculated as:

$$\Psi = \Pr[R > \delta | R > 0] \qquad (4)$$

where R refers to the rate for the associated users only.

The goal is to maximize the average rate in the system that can be guaranteed to any associated user.

4.1   Simulation Results

The simulation scenarios analyze the rate distribution in the network for different number of femto tier spectrum fragments, n_f, and different number of FBSs. Nearest BS association strategy is used with an average number of users $N_u = 10000$. The rate distribution when the average number of FBSs is $N_f = 1000$ is shown at Fig. 2a, and the rate distribution for $N_f = 5000$ is shown at Fig. 2b. The results illustrate that there is a trade-off between attaining high data rates per user and the percentage of users that are guaranteed to achieve those rates. If the operator targets high data rate for small percentage of users, then the femto tier should use larger spectrum fragments. However, if the operator wants to guarantee a predefined, lower data rate to higher number of users, the femto tier should use smaller spectrum fragments. Using smaller spectrum fragments efficiently mitigates the inter/intra tier interference in congested network, but results in more service denied users. By rescheduling the dropped users in subsequent time slots, the network is able to guarantee higher data rates per user.

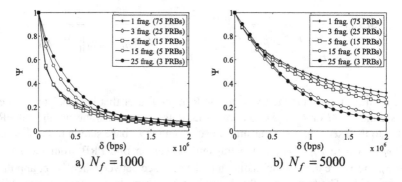

Fig. 2. Rate distribution Ψ for different number of spectrum fragments at the femto

Figure 3 shows a comparison of the performance for different user association strategies in terms of the rate distribution in congested network. The femto tier uses the smallest fragment size of 3 PRBs, as it provides best performances in congested networks (see Fig. 2a). The two-step offloading scheme significantly outperforms all other user-to-BS association strategies (see Sect. 3) around 1 Mbps for this scenario, providing better utilization of the available spectrum resources at the femto tier. However, the improvement of the two-step offloading over the other association strategies vanishes for higher data rates due to the fact that the LTE air interface is channelized system with limited resources.

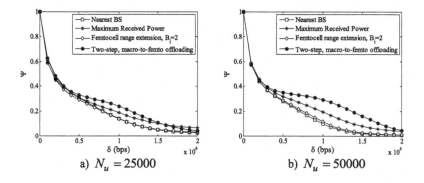

Fig. 3. Rate distribution Ψ of the system for different user association strategies

5 Conclusion

This paper analyzes the spectrum resource allocation, sharing and utilization efficiency in two-tier heterogeneous LTE networks with macro and an additional, uncoordinated, femto tier. The femto tier uses simple spectrum fragmentation and random fragment allocation to determine the operating resources. The results show that the rate distribution of the system depends on the fragment size for varying network conditions and suggests that the femto tier can dynamically adjust it. The paper also proposes novel, two-step, macro-to-femto offloading scheme at the user-to-BS association for efficient utilization of the femto tier resources. The scheme is proven to provide better rate distribution compared to existing user association strategies.

From operators' perspective, the results can be used to implement an intelligent RRM, where the fragment size at the femto tier can be dynamically adjusted according to the congestion in the network, by providing loose coordination with the macro tier.

Acknowledgments. This work was performed within the NATO SfP-984409 project "Optimization and Rational Use of Wireless Communications Bands" (ORCA). The authors would like to thank everyone involved.

References

1. Bhushan, N., et al.: Network densification: the dominant theme for wireless evolution into 5G. In: Communications Magazine. IEEE, vol. 52, no. 2, pp. 82–89 (2014)
2. Andrews, J.G., Claussen, H., Dohler, M., Rangan, S., Reed, M.C.: Femtocells: Past, present, and future. In: Selected Areas in Communications, IEEE Journal, vol. 30, no. 3, pp. 497–508 (2012)
3. Chiu, S.N., Stoyan, D., Kendall, W.S., Mecke, J.: Stochastic Geometry and Its Applications, 3rd Ediition, Aug. 2013
4. Andrews, J.G.: Seven ways that HetNets are a cellular paradigm shift. IEEE Comm. Magazine **51**(3), 136–144 (2013)
5. Singh, S., Dhillon, H.S., Andrews, J.G.: Offloading in heterogeneous networks: modeling, analysis, and design insights. IEEE Trans. Wireless Commun., **12**(5), 2484–2497 (2013)

Special Session on Emerging Technologies for Ambient Assisted Living

Cloud Based Service Bricks Architecture for Ambient Assisted Living System

Georgi Balabanov, Krasimir Tonchev, Pavlina Koleva,
Agata Manolova$^{(\boxtimes)}$, and Vladimir Poulkov

Technical University-Sofia, 8 Blvd. Kliment Ohridski, Sofia 1000, Bulgaria
{grb, k_tonchev, p_koleva, amanolova, vkp}@tu-sofia.bg

Abstract. Ambient Assisted Living (AAL) technology will play a prominent role in home care when the 65 and older age group doubles to 40 % of the US & EU population by 2050. Driven by these ongoing demographical and social changes in these countries, there is a huge interest in IT-based technologies and services that will enable independent living of people with specific needs. AAL offers a solution for caring for this section of the population both efficacious and cost-effective. In order to pave the way towards adequate AAL system architecture and overall software solution approaches, this paper will (i) briefly present architectural styles of AAL systems with some of the problems they face, (ii) describe service bricks architecture of AAL project eWALL and, (iii) discuss the software technologies used to solve some of the common problems of such systems.

Keywords: Ambient assisted living · Smart communication architecture · Intelligent systems · Personal health monitoring · Cloud services · Service bricks

1 Introduction

Ambient Assisted Living (AAL) is an emerging multi-disciplinary field aiming at providing an ecosystem of different types of sensors, computers, mobile devices, wireless networks and software applications for personal healthcare monitoring and telehealth systems [1].

Production of hardware and software infrastructures that serve as a foundation of AAL systems has been the core topic of a number of international projects in recent years – some already completed, some still running [2–4]. Even though one can find many similarities in the architectural aspects of the different smart environments and AAL platforms, there is still no widely adopted method for developing these systems. There is currently one initiative to build a reference model of open software architecture that supports different sensors and actuators [5, 6] for AAL system that is supported by many individual researchers, leaders in their fields, and related projects.

From a physical perspective the overall system topology of an AAL system will consist of different elements, ranging from portable or home sensors, over mobile or embedded systems with fairly low computational power, up to powerful computational machines and cloud services. The major challenge for the engineering of an AAL system

© Institute for Computer Sciences, Social Informatics and Telecommunications Engineering 2015
V. Atanasovski, L.-G. Alberto (Eds.): Fabulous 2015, LNICST 159, pp. 69–75, 2015.
DOI: 10.1007/978-3-319-27072-2_9

is to consider how this diversity of elements can be integrated in a seamless way to render the assistance services in a coherent way. Currently many different architectural types exist for the smart environment and AAL domains. They are described in details in [7, 8]. The main types include: service-oriented architecture (SOA), service-oriented device architecture (SODA), peer-to-peer architecture (P2P), event-driven architecture (EDA), component and connector (C2), multi-agent system (M.A.S) and blackboard. However, as reasoned about in [8], none of them can perfectly fit the requirements for AAL systems, specifically the requirement for integration to meet the different quality demands in the best possible way.

The main goal of this paper is to present an innovative new AAL cloud-based service-oriented architecture elaborated during the development of the eWALL project [9]. The main objective of eWALL project is to create a beyond-the-state-of-the-art assistive platform that will support independent living of older adults with mild cognitive and physical impairments. The primary users will be supported through in their autonomy, functional capacity and participation in society. Informal and formal caregivers are defined as secondary end-users and eWALL is planned to provide a framework for information exchange and communication between them and the primary users. eWALL provides applications in the following areas: (a) risk management and home safety, (b) eHealth and (c) lifestyle management.

The rest of the paper is organized as follows: in Sect. 2 we describe the service bricks architecture from two different views of the project. In Sect. 3 we illustrate an example from the eWALL project - Physical Activity Service Bricks and in Sect. 4 we conclude the paper.

2 Service Bricks Architecture

2.1 Component Overview

The eWALL applications offer the interface of the system to the users. As such, their significance goes beyond that of a GUI; they are the endpoints where the intelligence and the personalization of the system are exposed to the users. The eWALL service bricks provide data to all the modules of the system. They offer the low-level data coming from the end user environment, which are a product of local context understanding (what can be observed in a single room of the home of a single user at a given instant of time), to the modules that perform reasoning (either at the given instant or across time). They also offer the data from the higher-level components, which now describe the full context understanding of the system (across space, time and possibly multiple end users), to the applications. The service bricks are in between the applications and the metadata stored in the cloud Data Management Block (DMB), and act as providers of specific aggregated data, after making some reasoning on the metadata. The applications receive the aggregated data from the service bricks via JSON/REST over HTTP communication protocol. From a technical standpoint, the service bricks act as providers of specific context-related data, built by analyzing and aggregating the raw information stored in the cloud DMB, provisioned by the local sensing environments installed in the users' homes. The eWALL applications and the reasoning modules (IDSS and Lifestyle reasoners) can retrieve such aggregated data from the service bricks via JSON/REST API calls over HTTP communication protocol. This stateless approach (no data are saved during request-response cycles) combined to the HTTP protocol is an architectural choice which enables scalability of the system and flexibility in the deployment scenarios.

To overcome slow performance issues in the retrieval of data to be presented by the applications a new type of service brick, "data-management" service brick, has been introduced. This allows the architecture to better cope with the metadata coming from the sensors through the Data Management layer. Such specialized service bricks are dedicated to the preparation of data for the applications, performing proper aggregations or transformation of information in advance and in batch mode. This data is stored in a database specific to service bricks, and made available as "pre-digested" information to the higher level service bricks, named "front-end" service bricks, which serve application upon request. In addition to this, for optimizing the computational resources usage (minimizing the number of artifacts deployed on the application servers), the functionalities previously offered by separate service bricks were aggregated into a smaller number of larger service bricks, having in common the management of specific categories of metadata. We passed from a model based on many small services, each one providing a few endpoints, to a model based on a few services, each one providing many endpoints.

The low level metadata which feed the service bricks is collected and sent to the DMB by the home sensing environment, which gathers raw signal processing information and translates it into higher level metadata according to the eWALL architecture. The metadata is provided to the DMB from the home sensing environment, which collects raw signal processing information and translates it into higher level metadata.

A service brick is composed, as shown on Fig. 1, of the following software modules:

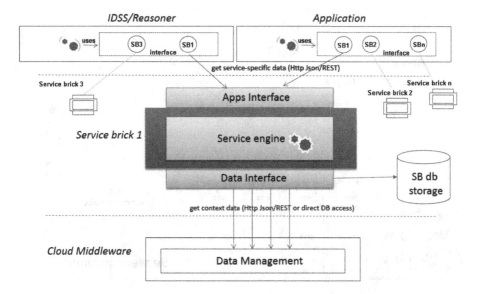

Fig. 1. Component view of a "front-end" service brick

- A northbound interface, named Apps Interface, which provides HTTP endpoints to be used by applications to collect the information provided by the service brick. The endpoints are managed by a controller module, which handles the HTTP requests with the related query parameters, checks for the correctness of the parameters and forwards the requests to the Service engine (see next point), waiting for data to be sent back to the applications.
- A *Service engine* is where the business logic of the service brick is performed. The Service engine receives the requests dispatched by the Apps Interface and applies the proper actions required to satisfy them. Typical actions consist of:
  - Getting data from the Data Management layer;
  - Applying some reasoning on such data, to compose the information required by the application;
  - Returning back such information to the Apps Interface.

  The Service engine consists of different computational modules delivering different kinds of data, either raw or already transformed data for specific time intervals.
- A *Data Interface,* which consists of an API for data access towards the Data Management layer. It queries the Data Access endpoints provided by the Data Management layer in the eWALL cloud and provides results back to the Service engine.

2.2   Deployment View

Every service brick is packaged and deployed as a *Java Web Application Archive* (war) as shown on Fig. 2. This deployment strategy allows to leverage the benefits offered by *Java servlet containers*, which are standard, consolidated, enterprise-level

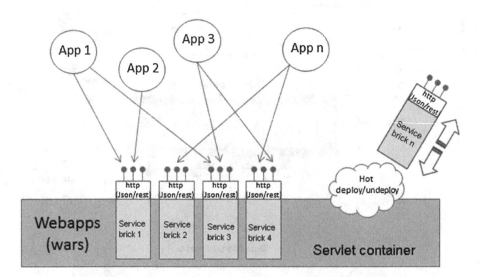

Fig. 2. Service brick deployment view

runtime environments on which Java Web Applications (in our case the service bricks) can be deployed. Servlet containers provide high reliability and management features, which allow launching stop and deploy applications independently. This permits, for *hot deployment* of applications, which basically means that it is not necessary to stop the whole application server (hence, stopping the provisioning of the services running on it) just to deploy a new service brick or an updated version of an existing one. Once a service brick is deployed, the servlet container automatically activates it and the related endpoints are made available at the specified URLs for usage by the applications. If a previous version of the service brick was already present, the servlet container automatically un-deploys it and activates the new one.

3 Physical Activity Service Bricks

The primary target users of eWALL, whether they have cognitive and/or physical impairment, have lost trust in their cognitive or physical abilities and they gradually abandon their former activities. This has an impact on their overall health and social life. The rehabilitation therapies are expensive and have certain duration; even if they are proven to be effective, patients often lack the motivation to continue the training on their own. So the physical activity application is one of the most important for the target users of this project.

Information related to physical activity of the end user is generated and made available by two dedicated service bricks:

- "Service-brick-physical-activity-dm": the data-management service brick, which runs in batch mode and analyses data coming from the accelerometer, calculates from them calories consumption, steps, kilometres walked, type of activity, inactivity and save this info in the service brick database;
- "Service-brick-activity": the front-end service brick, which provides endpoint to applications and services for retrieving the data calculated by the data-management service brick, based on query parameters.

The "service-brick-physical-activity-dm", is a component which runs on a scheduled basis. During each run, scheduled at a (configurable) rate of every 10 s, the service interprets the local context of a given end user, analysing the amount of movements he performed over a timeframe and combining it with user-specific data, with the purpose of estimating meaningful data related to physical activity. More specifically, at every iteration it performs the following operations (see Fig. 3):

- Gets the newest set of data coming from the accelerometer for each user;
- The service uses these new data to perform a set of computations and aggregations. First, it calculates the overall number of steps walked, and saves this info into the database, aggregating it by hour, day, week and month. Together with the steps, the service calculates and saves also the amount of calories consumed in every aggregation timeframe, and the related walked kilometers. Then, for each timeframe, it infers and saves the type of activity performed (one of resting, walking, running or exercising) and identifies events related to the start of activity and inactivity;

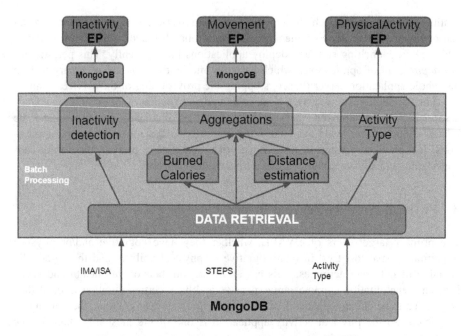

Fig. 3. Block diagram of Physical Activity service brick

- All the above information is stored in the service brick database, for every type of aggregation;
- At the end of every iteration, temporary information describing the last known status and timestamp of latest updates is stored.

The information prepared by the "service-brick-physical-activity-dm", is then made available to applications and services by the "service-brick-physical-activity". This service brick manages the date and time zone verification and formatting, and the transformation of data into JSON representation. The information delivered by the "service-brick-physical-activity", once displayed in an intuitive way on the GUI of the application, is very important to end users, as it transmits awareness about the amount of physical activity performed. The application, by comparing such data with user-specific, personalized goals (which depend on the user health profile), is able to assess the amount of activity performed and to transmit such assessment to the end user. This makes users aware that either they have done well in the last few days, or that they need to increase their physical activity.

4   Conclusion

In this paper we describe a cloud based service brick architecture developed during the work on the eWALL project as an example to demonstrate how to prepare context-aware and user adaptive services in AAL systems. The design and architectural definition of most of eWALL software components, together with their deployment model are operational and ready for end-user testing.

Acknowledgments. This work was supported in part by the Grant Agreement No: 610658, eWALL: eWall for Active Long Living" of the EU Seventh Framework Programme. The authors wish to thank the invaluable help received from all the consortium members.

References

1. Universal Open Platform and Reference Specification for Ambient Assisted Living: http://www.universaal.org/
2. Chan, M., Estève, D., Escriba, C., Campo, E.: A review of smart homes—present state and future challenges. Comput. Methods Programs Biomed. **91**, 55–81 (2008)
3. Rashidi, P., Mihailidis, A.: A survey on ambient-assisted living tools for older adults. IEEE J. Biomed. Health Inform. **17**, 579–590 (2013)
4. Fagerberg, G., et al.: Platforms for AAL applications. In: Lukowicz, P., Kunze, K., Kortuem, G. (eds.) EuroSSC 2010. LNCS, vol. 6446, pp. 177–201. Springer, Heidelberg (2010)
5. Tazari, M., Furfari, F., Fides-Valero, A., Hanke S.; Hoeftberger, O., Kehagias, D., Mosmondor, M., Wichert, R., Wolf, P., Ambient Intelligence and Smart Environments. Handbook of Ambient Assisted Living 2012
6. Augusto, J.C., Callaghan, V., Cook, D., Kameas, A., Satoh, I., Saba, T., Chorianopoulos, K., Howard, N., Cambria, E., Gupta, V.: Intelligent environments: a manifesto. Hum. Centr. Comput. Inf. Sci. **3**, 1–18 (2013)
7. Becker, M.: Assisted living systems-models, architectures engineering approaches. In: Karshmer, A.I., Nehmer, J., Raffler, H., Tröster, G. (eds.) Software Architecture Trends and Promising Technology for Ambient Assisted Living Systems. Schloss Dagstuhl-Leibniz-Zentrum fuer Informatik, Germany (2008)
8. de Morais, W.O., Lundström, J., Wickström, N.: active in-database processing to support ambient assisted living systems. Sensors **14**, 14765–14785 (2014)
9. Ewall for Active Long Living project: http://ewallproject.eu

Sensor-Based Environmental Monitoring for Ambient Assisted Living

Maria Mitoi[1], Razvan Craciunescu[1,2(✉)],
Alexandru Vulpe[1], and Octavian Fratu[1]

[1] Telecommunications Department, University Politehnica of Bucharest,
Bucharest, Romania
{maria.mitoi,razvan.craciunescu,
alex.vulpe}@radio.pub.ro, ofratu@elcom.pub.ro
[2] Center for TeleInFrastructur, Aalborg University, Aalborg, Denmark

Abstract. Home automation technologies have emerged more than four decades ago, but are undeniably a current subject of interest. Existing systems are usually highly customized, therefore expensive or very sophisticated and complicated, most of which requiring dedicated network cabling. The present paper presents a system for monitoring and control of an ordinary house in a simple and inexpensive manner. The ZigBee protocol is chosen so as to provide a reliable and secure wireless communication without additional cabling required. The data is transmitted to a computer that records and monitors any eventual threshold crossings. The control part is represented by simple means of acting upon an LED, based on data collected from the sensor network and processed accordingly.

Keywords: Arduino · Home automation · Sensor network · WEB applications · Zigbee

1 Introduction

Home automation technologies have emerged more than four decades ago, but are currently a major subject of interest. Existing systems are usually either highly customized, therefore expensive, or very sophisticated and complicated. Most of them require dedicated network cabling, often adding to the cost price. Furthermore, this solution is approachable only during the house's construction phase [1, 2].

The purpose of this paper is to develop a system for monitoring and control of an ordinary house in a simple and inexpensive manner. A centralized system will be created, in which most of the intelligence is managed via a server and network nodes' design to be kept to a minimum.

Sensor networks are ideal for any form of environmental monitoring. Due to the sensors' small size, low energy consumption and, in particular, their moderate cost, sensors can be installed in locations of interest and provide accurate reports. They will need another component to read the data and send them to a control system for processing. To achieve this, we will make use of the Arduino platform. The ZigBee protocol is chosen so as to provide a reliable and secure wireless communication without additional cable

© Institute for Computer Sciences, Social Informatics and Telecommunications Engineering 2015
V. Atanasovski, L.-G. Alberto (Eds.): Fabulous 2015, LNICST 159, pp. 76–82, 2015.
DOI: 10.1007/978-3-319-27072-2_10

required [3]. Responsibilities related to basic security functions are assigned to a server. Its role is to monitor the system's current status and provide a user interface.

This paper is directed towards such a system, using Digi XBee communication modules, database management systems and tools for creating dynamic WEB pages, in order to achieve a sensor-based environmental monitoring system for Ambient Assisted Living, through WEB applications.

The paper is organized as follows. Section 2 describes how the environmental monitoring system is implemented. Next, Sect. 3 shows the results and discusses them, while Sect. 4 concludes the paper and outlines future work.

2 Hardware and Software Implementation

Our work aims the ambient monitoring of a typical room, therefore the desired parameters to be supervised were selected among those of interest for a human observer, i.e. temperature, humidity and illuminance levels.

The data collected from the sensors is assembled into a packet to be wirelessly transmitted from one XBee radio module to the other.

The block diagram for the environmental monitoring system is depicted in Fig. 1.

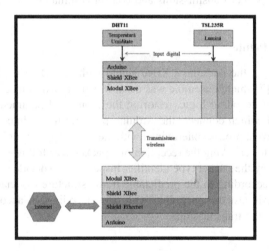

Fig. 1. Block scheme of monitoring system

2.1 Transmitting Module

The ensemble Arduino [4] - XBee shield and XBee module - sensors (Fig. 2) form the acquisition and transmission module. Clearly, their role is to monitor the room, assemble the acquired results and transmit data for further processing, while receiving control commands in reverse.

The sensors used were DHT11 [5] for temperature and humidity, respectively TSL235R [6] for illuminance. After acquiring the 3 parameters, we will proceed to assemble the package.

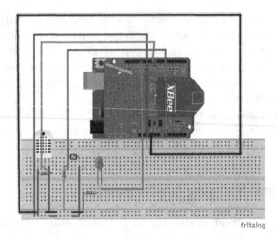

Fig. 2. XBee acquisition and transmitting module

The XBee module, accompanying the transmission module, is configured as a router, hence it fulfills the following: it expands the network, it monitors the two digital inputs, it manages packet transmissions and control commands receptions.

2.2   Receiving Module

At the reception side, the Arduino - XBee shield with the XBee module set as coordinator - Ethernet [7] shield ensemble was used. It is designed to receive and carry out the received packet decoding logic, restoring the monitored parameter values. Using the Ethernet shield, which connects the Arduino platform to the Internet, the database population is achieved, process intertwined with the WEB application's data "feeding".

The procedure for checking the reception of a packet is as follows: incoming data is checked, followed by the packet type identifier inspection (to decide on the appropriate decoding scheme, according to the predictable frame structure associated). The source address is afterwards tested, concluding with data decoding, in accordance with the known structure of the transmission.

2.3   Populating the Database

Populating the database was done in the following steps:

C.1. Create a Local Server - where databases and files allowing the WEB application to run properly will be stored; XAMPP was used for this purpose [8]. A MySQL database was likewise created.

C.2. Connect Arduino to the Internet – the Ethernet Shield [8] allows connection to an IP network; attaching this shield, Arduino can be converted into one of the two Ethernet devices, client or server. Client conversion will allow server connections and request data from the server, which is also what it is intended.

C.3. Initializing Server Connections - Effective connection to the server will be based on the server's IP address, to which to send the request, and the TCP port, in this case 80. If a successful connection is established, it performs an HTTP GET request to the server, in order to transmit the values of the three parameters, and further process them [6].

C.4. Development of PHP Scripts, in order to make changes to the database built in the previous steps (addition, deletion of data, etc.)

C.5. Building the WEB Application - PHP is capable of creating dynamic WEB pages (that can change their appearance contextually) [8]. The data was displayed in a table-fashioned manner. The table and user interface was created based on HTML, while data "fed" the application via PHP scripts, the nesting of these methods proving the claim made earlier in the paragraph.

At this point, the WEB application will display in real time (by refreshing the page) the results gathered from the acquisition node, wirelessly transmitted to the receiving node, decoded and stored in the database.

2.4   Control Interface

Monitoring the ambient parameters is fulfilled through providing qualitative and quantitative information on the environment in which the sensor network is installed. Usually, however, it is desired to act upon these parameters, therefore creating an automation system that can be easily and remotely controlled. Displaying the temperature, humidity and illuminance parameters using a WEB application allows their continuous supervision, but this can be supplemented with enabling interactive control of devices, adjustable according to a criterion of interest. The range of facilities mediated by such an approach is extremely varied: the control of a central heating system, a ventilation system, an array of switches, etc.

To emulate this concept, it was proposed to act upon an LED, having the role of an end device among those mentioned earlier, the principle being valid for any electronic device, as follows.

Acting upon a set of graphical buttons will be synonymous with the user's intention of sending a command. In this case, a file will be created that will include a value of "0", symbolizing the absence of control - because this is the prevailing state of the system, or overwrite it with an "1", indicating that a command was initialized. Arduino will query the server by opening the file, will read the value, will pack it and send it to the monitoring module installed in the room, which will decode it and act correspondingly upon the LED: will take a decision on its on- (when an "1" is decoded) or off- ("0") state.

Because, once the intended command is completed (for instance, the temperature reached the desired value, being time to stop the central heating adjustment), we proposed that, when acted upon the control button, the user is redirected to a waiting window, returning to the main application after the command's completion.

3 Results

The evolution of all 3 parameters was studied, during both daytime and nighttime, inside a laboratory environment. Figure 3 depicts data acquired from the TX module that corresponds to the particular situation of nighttime and, thus, sensors are tested in extreme conditions: the absence of light sources and proximity to a heat source.

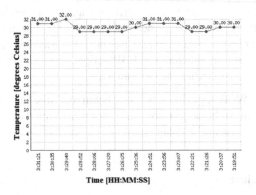

Fig. 3. Parameters'(temperature) graphical evolution over a 12 min window

At the end of the sequence described by steps C.1¬C.5, in the database stored locally, the changes in values for the 3 parameters, along with their timestamps are stored.

The developed WEB application is used to display and control the parameters. The tools provided by the WEB application are:

- Periodical statistics,
- Graphical representation of the measured values,
- Possibility to send backward commands, in order to act upon electronic devices, which could lead to the monitored parameters adjustment.

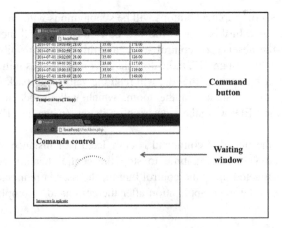

Fig. 4. Submitting a command and redirection to a waiting window

Figure 3 presents the variation of the measured values, in a 12 min window. The graphs are displayed via the developed WEB application in a WEB browser.

Intensive validation was carried out and the data from our system was compared with off-the-shelf products, such as home thermometers and lux meters. The results showed us that the system can very easily be compared in terms of accuracy and accessibility of the data.

As far as the initiating commands part is regarded, the graphical button, waiting window and results reflected upon the LED can be seen in Figs. 4 and 5. By not decoding packets of no interest for the system's proper functioning, precious time is thus saved, so the delay between the command's transmission and reception can be kept to a minimum (in our solution, the maximum delay achieved was 2 s).

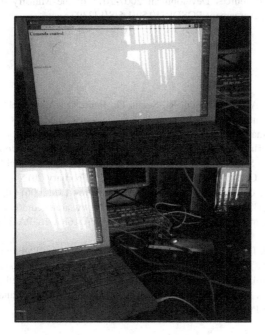

Fig. 5. Submitting a command in the web app (top) and the result of the command – led on (bottom)

4 Conclusions

The present paper presented a sensor network, designed to monitor a typical room in terms of ambient parameters, through regular reporting of the temperature, humidity and illuminance level values. The data was processed, and sent to a simple WEB application, which allowed an interactive view upon the results, and the prospective of adjusting the monitored parameters through a series of electronic devices, remotely, concept emulated by an LED. The system thus created proved to be extremely mobile and could be easily tested in various scenarios.

Future work might include the WEB application's customizing (in this project, a basic HTML code was used in order to design it), setting up 2 to more such modules to simultaneously send data to the same coordinator, replace the LED with an actual device in order to address a real-life situation.

Such a solution may find its applicability in home automation projects, for instance, Ambient Assisted Living, given the possibility to permanently monitor and adjust the indoor climate, therefore promoting a better, healthier lifestyle for people at risk.

Acknowledgments. This work has been funded by European Commission by FP7 IP project no. 610658/2013 "eWALL for Active Long Living - eWALL" and by UEFISCDI Romania under grants no. 20/2012 "Scalable Radio Transceiver for Instrumental Wireless Sensor Networks - SaRaT-IWSN", grant no. 262EU "eWALL" support project and by the Sectoral Operational Programme Human Resources Development 2007-2013 of the Ministry of European Funds through the Financial Agreement POSDRU/159/1.5/S/132397.

References

1. Mitoi, M., Vulpe, A., Craciunescu, R., Suciu, G., Fratu, O.: Approaches for environmental monitoring sensor networks. In: International Symposium on Signals, Circuits and Systems (ISSCS), Iasi, Romania, pp.1–4, 9-10 July 2015
2. Craciunescu, R., Halunga, S., Fratu, O.: Wireless ZigBee home automation system. In: Proceedings of the SPIE, Advanced Topics in Optoelectronics, Microelectronics, and Nanotechnologies VII, Constanta, Romania, vol. 9258, 21 February 2015
3. Sikora, A.: ZigBee Competitive Technology Analysis, rev 1.0 (2006) http://www.zigbee.org
4. Datasheet ATmega328P, Atmel, October 2010. http://www.atmel.com/Images/Atmel-8271-8-bit-AVR-Microcontroller-ATmega48A-48PA-88A-88PA-168A-168PA-328-328P_datasheet_Summary.pdf
5. Datasheet DHT11, D-Robotics (2010). http://www.micropik.com/PDF/dht11.pdf
6. Datasheet TSL235, Texas Instruments (1994). http://www.ti.com/lit/ds/symlink/tsl235.pdf
7. Datasheet Arduino Ethernet Shield. http://arduino.cc/en/Main/ArduinoEthernetShield
8. Allen, R., Qian, K., Tao, L., Fu, X.: Web development with JavaScript and Ajax illuminated, Jones and Bartlett Publishers (2009)

Probability of OFDM Signal Interception in eHealth Applications

Valerică Bîndar[1], Mircea Popescu[1], Valentin Grecu[1],
Răzvan Crăciunescu[2], and Simona Halunga[2(✉)]

[1] The Special Telecommunications Service, Bucharest, Romania
mpopescu@sts.ro
[2] University Politehnica of Bucharest, Bucharest, Romania
shalunga@elcom.pub.ro

Abstract. The main purpose of the research conducted in this field is to improve senior's Quality of Life using remote monitoring systems. One of the main problems of these remote systems is the sensitive personal/medical data security. As in different field of e-Health, like telemedicine, where a high data rate is requested, OFDM systems represent a suitable candidate for these areas. This paper focus is to analyze the probability of intercept (POI) for OFDM (Orthogonal Frequency Division Multiplexing) communication systems. A number of measurements are performed using a WiMAX communication signal. The measurements were conducted using two broadband spectrum analyzers and the conclusions are that the POI, for these systems, is proportional with the number of parallel receiver channels and the scanning speed of the receivers.

Keywords: Interception · Wimax · e-Health · Telemedicine · OFDM

1 Introduction. Security Issues in E-Health

The ICT domain, especially the wireless communications applications offers new possibilities for elderly people to be monitored without intruding in their day to day activities. The increase of the possible data rates that are to be transmitted over the network allows the caregivers to communicate and to address the medical/social issues in real-time. But one of the most important aspects of remote monitoring using wireless communications is the data security.

Depending on the diseases concerned and on their level, the elders may choose to store and exchange with the caregiver a lot of personal data (health information, personal preferences and habits), that may be accessible through a wireless communication network. Consequently, depending on the data transmitted through the wireless network, different levels of security need to be provided. A radio communications link can be considered to be secure if a number of technical measures have been implemented in order to minimize the probability of detection and interception probability. In the last decade, a large number of researches have been developed and their results have been published, presenting different solutions that, on the one hand, secure the radio communication link, and on the other hand, defines the threshold parameters

© Institute for Computer Sciences, Social Informatics and Telecommunications Engineering 2015
V. Atanasovski, L.-G. Alberto (Eds.): Fabulous 2015, LNICST 159, pp. 83–90, 2015.
DOI: 10.1007/978-3-319-27072-2_11

for interception receivers. In [1] the authors refers to eHealth video communications that needs to be responsive and reliable, OFDM techniques offer, at the physical layer a scalable, resilient and reliable transmission technique. In [2] the authors study the most suitable wireless technologies for eHealth applications, from WiMAX (Worldwide Interoperability for Microwave Access) to GSM/GPRS to the latest 4G networks, while in [3, 4] the authors try to evaluate the most efficient solution for implementing a reliable health service based on the 4G networks. In [5] a special emphasis is put on the security of eHealth wireless networks based on OFDM techniques. In [6] is shown that OFDMA allows a large number of users share the system by assigning each of them a subset of subcarriers or tones, while in [7] the subcarrier allocation in OFDMA is studied. In [8] a number of considerations are made regarding a CDMA-OFDMA system and its performances obtained in different propagation conditions. Researchers are continuously seeking for the best trade-off between functionality, interoperability and security of the developed systems [9].

This paper presents the interception probability for systems that uses OFDM techniques. These threats are important especially for systems that are dealing with sensitive personal or medical data. The paper is organized as follows. In Sect. 2 is evaluated the probability of interception of a WiMAX OFDM signal with a search receiver that has a number of parallel receivers that performs several scans of the received signal while in Sect. 3 are presented some practical measurements. Finally, Sect. 4 presents the eWall project as a possible implementation of such an eHealth system that uses WiMAX OFDM and a number of conclusions are highlighted.

2   Probability of Intercept for OFDM Signals

In order to intercept and detect OFDM signals the first we assume that the bandwidth of the WiMAX radio channel and the OFDMA subcarrier spacing are known. The "search" receiver has the same instantaneous bandwidth as the signal and includes a number of parallel receiver channels (denoted by M_{sc}) whose center frequency coincides with the subcarriers frequency (denoted by M_{fh}). Moreover, in order to detect an OFDMA signal its frame duration, T_s, must be larger than the receiver dwell time, T_d.

Detection of wideband signals requires a large amount of power, at least for the integration period of the receiver, T_i, (which is the sum of dwell time and the signal processing time). In addition, it and requires that the frequencies the receiver is tuned on are the subcarriers of the received signal. Assuming that at the receiver is implemented using K parallel detectors, each of them tuned on a different frequency, the probability that the wideband signal is detected in one of the K channels increases by a factor K. Thus, according to [10], the interception probability for an OFDMA signal, using a multichannel receiver in standby, is

$$P_1 = \frac{K}{M_{fh}}. \tag{1}$$

Next we assume that the receiver can perform several attempts to intercept the transmitted signal, during one frame duration T_s. Such an attempt can be considered valid only when the integration time, T_i, is less or equal then the OFDMA frame duration T_s. Therefore, the average number of valid interception attempts during T_s is given by [11]

$$\bar{n} = \frac{T_s - T_i}{T_d}. \tag{2}$$

The interception probability of wideband transmitted signals with $\bar{n}$ valid trials, during the time signal T_s, is [10]

$$P_{1n} = P_1 \cdot \bar{n} = \frac{K \cdot \bar{n}}{M_{fh}} = \frac{K}{M_{fh}} \left(\frac{T_s - T_i}{T_d} \right). \tag{3}$$

For OFDMA signals, if the total time of reception is T_t, such interception attempts can be repeated $N = T_t \cdot f_S$ times, where f_S is the frame rate. For each attempt, the interception probability is given by (3). Assuming that the receiver performs L complete scans, the probability that, in N repeated trials, we will have k correct interceptions (hits), with P success probability in each trials, is determined based on the binomial distribution and cumulative distribution function, given by [10]

$$P_N(k) \approx 1 - \sum_{l=0}^{k-1} C_N^k P^l (1-P)^{N-l} \tag{4}$$

resulting an average number of hits

$$\bar{k} = N \cdot P_N. \tag{5}$$

The relationship between the number of repeated attempts to intercept (N), the dwell time (T_d), the number of complete scans at the receiver (L), the number of reception channels (M_{sc}) the number of parallel filters (K) and frame rate (f_s) is given by [11]

$$N = \frac{M_{sc} T_d f_s L}{K} \tag{6}$$

3 Practical Estimation of OFDMA Signals Probability of Intercept

In the following we will analyze the probability of interception for WiMAX 802.16e transmissions using OFDMA signals. The following parameters are used for the transmitted signal: central frequency = 3660.5 MHz, bandwidth BW = 10 MHz, FFT size = 512, number of used carriers = 426, subcarrier spacing = 11.16 kHz, OFDMA symbol time = 100.8 μs, frame length T_s = 5 ms (for 49 symbols). A received signal containing a multiburst PUSC (partial usage of subchannels), FUSC (full usage of subchannels) zone with BPSK pilots and signals with QPSK, 16QAM, and 64QAM modulation types has been used for test purposes.

Regarding the receiver part we consider two different spectrum analyzers, with incorporated Vector Signal Analyzer, namely Agilent E3238 s system with Agilent 89600 system software and Anritsu MS2722 system. The receivers parameters are: instantaneous bandwidth = 36 MHz (for Agilent) /10 MHz (for Anritsu), dwell time = 1 ms (for Agilent) /3 ms (for Anritsu), frequency span = signal bandwidth × 1.1, center frequency = 3660.5 MHz, RBW = 1 kHz, triggering on the signal (to obtain good spectrum and time measurements on a burst signal), demodulator selected = 802.16e OFDMA -10 MHz, parallel channels $K = 32$ channels (for Agilent) /20 channels (for Anritsu), with IFBW = 10 kHz.

With (1) the detection probabilities for a single burst using a multichannel receiver are $P_1 = 6.2$ % for Agilent and $P_1 = 4$ % for Anritsu. According to (2) and (3) the detection probabilities of wideband transmitted signals, with $\bar{n} = 4$ for Agilent and $\bar{n} = 2$ for Anritsu, the probabilities of valid trials are $P_{In} = 24.8$ % for Agilent and $P_{In} = 8$ % for Anritsu. Assuming that the receiver performs a number $L = 1$ full scans and, according to (6), the number N of repeated attempts to intercept during L scans is $N = 132$. Then, the probability P_N of at k successes in N trials, where success probability in each trialis P_{In}, can beestimated using (4).

In Fig. 1a is represented the probability P_N of at least k valid interception in N repeated attempts, for an ideal case using $K = 426$ parallel channels, with a variable mean number $\bar{n} = \{2; 4\}$ of valid attempts during one hop. The blue line (1) represents this probability achieved when the Agilent spectrum analyzer is used, while the red line (2) corresponds to the same probability when the Anritsu one is used, under the same conditions. Note that the probability of at least $k = 10$ valid interceptions in $N = 132$ attempts for the Anritsu analyzer is about 50 % while for the Agilent one is 100 %. This difference is due to the fact that the Agilent analyzer has a lower dwell time than the Anritsu analyzer and, implicitly, Agilent scanning speed is higher.

Figure 1b represents, the probability of at least k valid interception in N attempts, P_N, given in (4), with success probability in each trialis P_1, supposing only one valid detection attempt per hop interval, $\bar{n} = 1$, for receivers with different number of scanning filters, K. In the following, since the Agilent spectrum analyzer performs better than the Anritsu one, the first one will be used with different number of scanning filters, K, that may be enabled at the receiver. The blue line (3) represents probability P_N of at least k valid interception in $N = 132$ attempts when the central frequencies of the parallel receiver channels K, coincides with all the subcarriers of the WiMAX radio channel. In this case, the analyzer scans 512 consecutive subcarriers and uses $K = 32$ parallel channels. The red line (2) represents the interception probability of the WiMAX signal, with at least k valid interception in $N = 132$ attempts, when the spectrum analyzer scans consecutive WiMAX subcarriers. In this situation the interception receiver is using $K = 20$ parallel channels. Finally, the green line (1) represents the probability of achieving at least k valid interception in N attempts, for WiMAX signal, when the spectrum analyzer consecutively scans only one detection channel ($K = 1$). If we compare the performances obtained in the three cases above, one can see that for $k = 10$ valid interception performed by the intercept receiver, we obtainprobability $P_N = 20.4$ % when $K = 32$ parallel channels are used (similar to Agilent

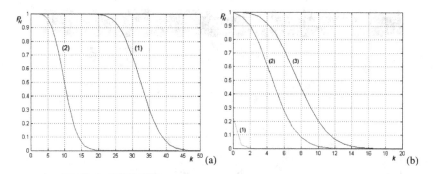

Fig. 1. (a). The probability P_N of at least k valid interception in N repeated attempts, with mean number of valid attempts by the receiver during one hop $\bar{n} = 4$ (trace 1) and $\bar{n} = 2$ (trace 2), for a ideal case using $K = 426$ parallel channels and (b) using using $K = 32$ parallel channels (trace 3), $K = 20$ parallel channels (trace 2) and single channel receiver (trace 1) (Color figure onlne)

spectrum analyzer), $P_N = 1.8$ % when $K = 20$ parallel channels are used (similar to Anritsu spectrum analyzer) and $P_N = 0$ % when only one scanning channel is used. Hence, as the receiver has more parallel channels enabled, the interception probability of the OFDMA signal is higher.

To show the accordance between analytical expression for the interception probability and the experimental results, we conducted tests to detect a real WiMAX transmission using a spectrum analyzer Agilent E3238 s including Vector Signal Analyzer Agilent 89600. The test signal was an IEEE 802.16e-compliant downlink subframe, based on a WiMAX 10 MHz profile. It contains a PUSC zone of 12 symbols followed by a FUSC zone of 10 symbols, with BPSK pilots and signals with QPSK, 16QAM, and 64QAM modulationtypes. The spectrum analyzer settings for test were: central frequency $f = 3660.5$ MHz, span 11 MHz, resolution bandwidth 3 kHz, reference level −15 dBm, 32 parallel receiver channels, detector Peak, demodulation type = IEEE 802.16e OFDMA. Sweep time and trigger delay must be set so that the complete response signal of the tag is recorded. Displaying graphs station was to stop after 10 detections.

The measurement system receives the WiMAX signal represented in Fig. 2. In the top windows are displayed: the spectrum of the signal (a), time measurements on a burst signal (b) and table with the contents of the decoded FCH (Frame Control Header) and DL-MAP (c). In this table one can see that the spectrum analyzer with settings mentioned above, was performed detection and decoding of WiMAX signal. In the bottom windows are displayed: Probability Density Function - PDF for the received signal (d), Cumulative Distribution Function - CDF (e) and Complementary Cumulative Distribution Function - CCDF (f). From the PDF trace it can be deduced that the mean value of burst signal is 27.8 mV$_{\mathrm{rms}}$, while using CDF trace, on can determine the probability corresponding to this average value of signal, resulting 47.9 %. In CCDF measurement the average power of the signal is −18.12 dBm and it can be seen that all signal's peaks with this level have probability of occurrence around 21 %. This probability of detection is very close to the theoretical value $P_N = 20.4$ %, obtained from simulations (Fig. 1b).

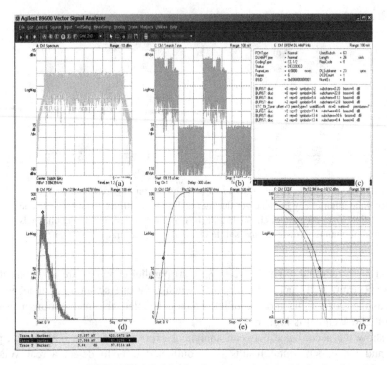

Fig. 2. Measurements of WiMAX signal in the frequency domain (a), in the time domain (b), burst analysis with DL-MAP (c) PDF (d), CDF (e) and CCDF (f) measurements of burst signal

From those results one can see that the interception probability of an OFDMA system is relatively high only if the interceptor has a relatively sophisticated dedicated measurement device. Such equipment should be multichannel receiverand with fastscan, which are characteristics that are difficult to obtain from a technical point of view. In this respect, WiMAX OFDMA proves to be a good candidate for implementing the physical layer in an eHealth system.

4   Possible Applications – the EWALL Project

The eWall for Active Long Living (eWALL) it's a project that intends to develop an architecture and appropriate methods for assisting the elderly that have health issues as Chronic Obstructive Pulmonary Disease or Mild dementia. As the quality of life has improved, the life expectancy also increased during the last years, fact that leads to an aging of the population [15]. It is well known that elderly people need special treatment and resources due to their decreasing capacity of self-caring. Thus, a high number of caregiver staff is trained for the challenge of assuring the suitable conditions, medicine, laboratory tests and - not less important – daily supervision.

Thus, in order for the Sensing environment to communicate to the eWALL cloud a secure wireless or wired solution is required. In order to find the best solution multiple tests are being performed in order to determine the system with the best intercept-free percentage. As we demonstrated in Sect. 3, OFDMA with a large number of subcarriers proved to be a suitable solution for the eWALL system, and is now under testing. Measurements have shown that the signal can be intercepted with a high probability only by using sophisticated and expensive measurement devices, while for single channel receiver the interception probability is null, showing that, from security and privacy point of view, this technique offers increased data security. Based on those remarks the OFDMA technique is used in eWALLproject to communicate between the sensing environment and the cloud.

Acknowledgment. This work has been funded by European Commission by FP7 IP project no. 610658/2013 "eWALL for Active Long Living - eWALL" and the SfP-984409 ORCA project and by the SOPHRD Sectorial Operational Programme Human Resources Development 2007–2013 of the Ministry of European Funds through the Financial Agreement POSDRU/159/1.5/S/132397.

References

1. Panayides, A.S., Antoniou, Z.C., Constantinides, A.G.: An overview of mHealth medical video communication systems. In: Adibi, S. (ed.) Mobile Health. SSBN, vol. 5, pp. 609–634. Springer, Heidelberg (2015)
2. Keikhosrokiani, P., Zakaria, N., Mustaffa, N., Wan, T.-C., Sarwar, M.I., Azimi, K.: Wireless networks in mobile healthcare. In: Adibi, S. (ed.) Mobile Health. SSBN, vol. 5, pp. 687–726. Springer, Heidelberg (2015)
3. M., S.M., A., L.A., S., G.A.: Quality of service in wireless technologies for mHealth service providing. In: Adibi, S. (ed.) Mobile Health. SSBN, vol. 5, pp. 971–990. Springer, Heidelberg (2015)
4. Park, R.C., Hoill Jung, J., Shin, D., Cho, Y.H., Lee, K.D.: Telemedicine health service using LTE-Advanced relay antenna. Pers. Ubiquit. Comput. **18**(6), 1325–1335 (2014)
5. Song, J., Ding, W., Yang, F., Yang, H., Wang, J., Wang, X., Zhang, X.: Indoor hospital communication systems: An integrated solution based on power line and visible light communication. In: Faible Tension FaibleConsommation (FTFC), 2014 IEEE, pp. 1–6. IEEE (2014)
6. Craciunescu, R., Halunga, S., Fratu, O., Vizireanu, N.: Multi User Orthogonal Frequency division Multiple Access (MU-OFDMA) performances in AWGN and fading channels. In: 11th International Conference on Telecommunication in Modern Satellite, Cable and Broadcasting Services (TELSIKS), Nis, Serbia, vol. 01, pp. 229–232, 16–19 October 2013
7. Manea, C., Craciunescu, R., Halunga, S., Voicu, C., Preda, R.: Performance evaluation of subcarrier allocation methods for OFDMA. In: Proceedings of 21st Telecommunications Forum (TELFOR), Belgrade, Serbia, pp. 260–263, 26–28 November 2013
8. Craciunescu, R., Manea, O., Halunga, S., Fratu, O., Vizireanu, D.N.: Considerations on CDMA–OFDM system performances in different channel environments for different modulation and coding scenarios. Wireless Pers. Commun. J. **78**(3), 1667–1682 (2014)
9. Raychaudhuri, K., Pradeep, R.: Privacy challenges in the use of eHealth systems for public health management. Emerg. Commun. Technol. E-Health Med. **1**, 155 (2012)

10. Papoulis, Probability, Random Variables and Stochastic Processes. McGraw-Hill, Chap. 3, 1965
11. Wout, J., Martens, L.: Performance evaluation of broadband fixed wireless system based on IEEE 802.16. In: Wireless Communications and Networking Conference, 2006. WCNC 2006. IEEE, vol. 2, pp. 978–983. IEEE (2006)
12. eWALL Project Homepage, http://ewallproject.eu/ (accessed in March 2015)

Device-Free Localization Using Sun SPOT WSNs

Konstantin Chomu[(⊠)], Vladimir Atanasovski,
and Liljana Gavrilovska

Faculty of Electrical Engineering and Information Technologies,
Saints Cyril and Methodius University in Skopje,
Rugjer Boshkovik 18, 1000 Skopje, Macedonia
{konstantin.chomu,vladimir,liljana}@feit.ukim.edu.mk

Abstract. Human presence in the vicinity of a wireless link causes variations in the link's Received Signal Strength (RSS). Device-free Localization (DfL) systems use these RSS variations in a static Wireless Sensor Network (WSN) to detect and locate people in the area of the network. The main advantage of this emerging technique is localization of people without requiring them to carry any devices. This paper investigates the feasibility of a DfL system using a Sun SPOT WSN. The system uses 16 Sun SPOT sensors and covers 4×4 m square area, which is a size of a typical living room. The sensors exchange testing messages, measure RSSs and forward the results to a host computer via a base station. The host application processes the received RSS values using the Radio Tomographic Imaging (RTI) technique and displays a real-time image with the estimated position of the person in the monitored area.

Keywords: Device-free localization · Passive RF tracking · Passive indoor positioning · Wireless sensor networks

1 Introduction

The health monitoring Wireless Sensor Networks (WSNs), which made their debut in hospitals and assisted living centers, have recently been moving into the homes of seniors in order to prolong the seniors' home stay as long as possible. This desire for independence is conceivable, but for the caregivers, it is also a reason for concern that they might fall, be physical inactive, forget to take their meds or just need assistance.

A key parameter for the estimation of people's vitality for an ambient assisted living is their activity, i.e. the detection of their everyday life motion sequences. Traditionally, computer-vision camera systems and mobile RF devices, such as body-worn transmitters and active RF tags, have been the foremost agents by which real-time human presence is tracked [1, 2]. There are also techniques that enable smartphones to track user location and motion [3]. Camera based sensors, such as Kinect, sense the light directly reflected off of users' bodies. Many of these technologies leverage well-established computer vision techniques such as epipolar geometry (two cameras view a scene from two distinct positions), but also employ other, non-traditional methods such as Time-Of-Flight

© Institute for Computer Sciences, Social Informatics and Telecommunications Engineering 2015
V. Atanasovski, L.-G. Alberto (Eds.): Fabulous 2015, LNICST 159, pp. 91–99, 2015.
DOI: 10.1007/978-3-319-27072-2_12

(TOF) measurements that have become more affordable [1]. Common challenges with these systems include field of view, low light situations and privacy concerns [4].

Recently, there are a number of techniques by which user location can be estimated without the use of any portable RF device. A passive system without any handheld devices is much more suitable and comfortable for this purpose than any other solution. In these methods, some RF signal is broadcasted, and its attenuations by the human body are measured. The values of these attenuations are used to estimate the position of the body being tracked. This technique is essentially treating the user's body as a sort of radio-wave absorbing object, thus, it is the user being tracked rather than an external RF device they are attached to. Of all technologies being developed to enable mobile Device-free Localization (DfL), the Radio Tomographic Imaging (RTI) technique has been most broadly used [5]. These systems typically require that an area of interest be outfit with a large network of sensors. In these networks, the sensor nodes create mesh topology via RF links. For each of these links a change in the Received Signal Strength (RSS) is attributed to human presence [6–8].

This paper presents the practical implementation of a DfL system with a Sun^{TM} Small Programmable Object Technology (Sun SPOT) WSN testbed platform. The paper is organized as follows. Section 2 describes the RTI technique with WSN. Section 3 describes the Sun SPOT setup. Section 4 describes the gathering of the RSS measurements. Section 5 presents the localization results and, finally, Sect. 6 gives the conclusions.

2   Radio Tomographic Imaging with WSN

RTI is technique of estimating the changes in the propagation field of a deployed WSN that covers the monitored area. Several RTI methods have been already developed [5, 9, 10]. This section describes attenuation-based RTI [5], in which the change of the propagation field to be estimated is shadowing.

In RTI DfL, the monitored area is surrounded with N sensor nodes as shown in Fig. 1(a) and divided into P pixels as shown in Fig. 1(b). The total number of links L between all sensors is $L = N(N-1)/2$.

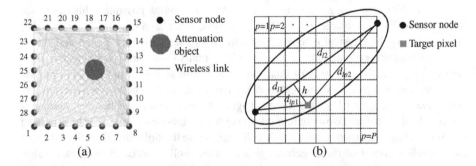

Fig. 1. Monitored area is surrounded with N sensor nodes and covered with $L = N(N-1)/2$ links (a) (in this example $N = 28$; $L = 378$), and a link between two randomly chosen nodes (b). For (b), only the pixels in the ellipse around the observed link affect its RSS measurement.

The RSS value $y_l(t)$ of each link l at time t is given as:

$$y_l(t) = T_l - S_l - O_l(t) - I_l(t) - n_l(t).\tag{1}$$

where T_l is the transmitting power, S_l is the static attenuation, $O_l(t)$ is the attenuation of the object, $I_l(t)$ is the interference, and $n_l(t)$ is the noise.

The number of pixels ($p = 1, 2,..., P$) and the number of sensors are not correlated. Figure 1(b) shows a link between two randomly chosen sensors. Only the attenuations of the pixels encompassed by the ellipse affect the link. The spatial RTI model is an ellipse having the foci located at the sensors. The RTI model defines the ellipse width.

The attenuation $O_l(t)$ caused by the objects can be considered to be the weighted sum of attenuations $x_p(t)$ from all pixels P in the monitored area:

$$O_l(t) = \sum_{p=1}^{P} A_{lp} x_p(t).\tag{2}$$

The most common type of defining the entries A_{lp} is to make them constants inversely proportional to the square root of the link length $d_l = d_{l1} + d_{l2}$ [5, 6, 8]. According to this model, the pixels that are located outside of the ellipse have their weight set to zero. This paper defines the entries A_{lp} as constants too, but takes into consideration *the pixel's distance to the link's line-of-sight h*, and the pixel's distance to the closest sensor of the link. Accordingly, the pixels that are located outside of the ellipse have their weight set to zero too. The entries A_{lp} are given as:

$$A_{lp} = \frac{1}{\sqrt{\min(d_{l1},\, d_{l2}) + \frac{d_l}{2} + h}} \begin{cases} \varphi, & \text{if } d_{lp1} + d_{lp2} \leq d_{l1} + d_{l2} + \beta \\ 0, & \text{otherwise} \end{cases}.\tag{3}$$

where φ is a constant scaling factor (often set to 1) and β is a tunable parameter controlling the ellipse width. Such extended definition of the entries A_{lp} is consequence of one assumption and one preliminary experiment, conducted before placing the final Sun SPOT setup. The assumption is that the influence of the pixel to the link decreases as h increases, and the preliminary experiment had been tried to find out how distance

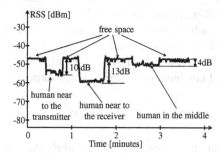

Fig. 2. Human body influence on the link's RSS measurement in different positions between the transmitter and receiver.

of the object to the sensor node (when the object lies on the line-of-sight) influences the link's RSS measurement. Figure 2 shows the influence of the human body on the link's RSS when two Sun SPOTs (transmitter and receiver) are 4 m apart and transmitting power is set to 0 dBm. The user stands in three different positions on the line-of-sight between the Sun SPOTs: near the transmitter; in the middle between the transmitter and receiver; near the receiver.

The RSSs value for free space is approximately −47 dBm. Then, when the person enters the link and stands near the transmitter, the RSS decreases for 10 dB. When the user stands near the receiver, the RSSs decrease for 13 dB relative to the free space case. When the user stands in the middle of the link, the RSSs decrease for 4 dB relative to the free space case. These measurements show that all pixels that lie along the line-of-sight of the link do not have the same influence on the link's RSS. The pixels lying closer to the sensors introduce approximately 2 to 3 times more RSS reduction compared to the pixels lying in the middle of the link. The entries A_{lp} defined with (3) take into consideration this situation and apply more weight to the pixels lying closer to the sensors.

Regarding (1), the link's RSS change Δy_l, between times t and $t + \delta$ is given as:

$$
\begin{aligned}
\Delta y_l &= y_l(t) - y_l(t + \delta) \\
&= O_l(t + \delta) - O_l(t) + I_l(t + \delta) - I_l(t) + n_l(t + \delta) - n_l(t).
\end{aligned}
\tag{4}
$$

Replacing (2) in (4) yields:

$$
\Delta y_l = \sum_{p=1}^{P} A_{lp} \Delta x_p + \varepsilon_l.
\tag{5}
$$

where $\Delta x_p = x_p(t + \delta) - x_p(t)$ is the attenuation change in the pixel p, and $\varepsilon_l = I_l(t + \delta) - I_l(t) + n_l(t + \delta) - n_l(t)$ is a random variable collating the interference and noise in link l.

A linear equation system describes attenuation in all links:

$$
y = Ax + \varepsilon.
\tag{6}
$$

where A is an $L \times P$ weighting matrix, y is $L \times 1$ vector for measured RSS changes, ε is $L \times 1$ error vector (interference and noise), and x is $P \times 1$ vector for attenuation changes.

Solution of (6) for x, gives the attenuation field in the monitored area. The attenuation object is most likely to be in the pixels with highest attenuation changes. Equation (6) describes an ill-posed problem [11, 12], i.e. a problem that need not have a solution, that may have multiple solutions, or a solution whose behavior does not change continuously with the initial conditions. Such problems can be solved by Tikhonov regularization [11, 12]. Tikhonov defines regularized solution x_λ as the minimizer of the weighted combination of the residual norm and the side constraint:

$$
\min_{x} \left\{ \|Ax - y\|^2 + \lambda^2 \|Ix\|^2 \right\}.
\tag{7}
$$

where λ is the regularization parameter which controls the weight given to minimization of the side constraint relative to minimization of the residual norm, and I is $P \times P$ identity matrix. With substitution $\Gamma = \lambda I$, an explicit solution is given by:

$$x_\lambda = \left(A^\mathrm{T}A + \Gamma^\mathrm{T}\Gamma\right)^{-1} A^\mathrm{T} y. \tag{8}$$

where x_λ is $P \times 1$ vector for estimated attenuation field caused by the attenuation object. In many cases, the matrix $(A^\mathrm{T}A + \Gamma^\mathrm{T}\Gamma)^{-1} A^\mathrm{T}$ can be precomputed, thus estimating x_λ from y becomes an inexpensive operation. This is very appealing for real time RTI systems that require frequent image updates.

3 Sun SPOT Setup

All Sun SPOTs are placed on fixed locations as shown in Fig. 3(a). The 16 nodes are around a 4×4 m square area with a node density of 1 node per m^2. Figure 3(b) shows spectrum occupancy of the room where the WSN testbed platform is placed, for the entire Sun SPOT frequency range.

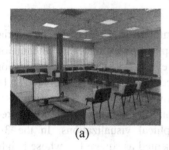
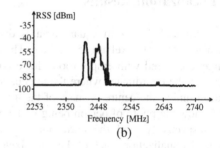

(a)   (b)

Fig. 3. Photo of 16-node Sun SPOT indoor testbed platform (a), and room spectrum occupancy (b).

The distance between each two adjacent nodes along each side is 1 m so there are 5 nodes (including one node at each corner) at each side of the square. Each of the 16 nodes is programmed to broadcasts test messages for the RSS measurement between itself and all the other nodes in the network. The base station, which is connected to the host computer, collects messages with pairwise RSS measurements from all nodes of the network. First, a calibration is performed in empty room. Then, the RTI algorithm runs on the host computer and the person enters the room and interacts with the RTI system. Since the RTI algorithm works in real time, observers can see the RTI images immediately after the person enters the network. The setup allows multiple people localization.

To avoid interference with other RF sources, the Sun SPOTs nodes measure RSSs by test messages at 2300 MHz (frequency granted to the radio amateurs). To avoid mutual interference, nodes send data messages with averaged RSSs to the base at 2480 MHz.

4   RSS Measurements

Each sensor node broadcasts a test messages to the other 15 sensor nodes at a rate of five messages per second. Each sensor node receives test messages and stores the measured RSS values from the other sensor nodes. Simultaneously with the measurement process, each sensor node sends averaged RSS measurements to the base every 1.5 s. For each link, i.e. for each pair of nodes A and B, the host application gets two RSS values. The first value gives the averaged RSS from A to B, whereas the second value gives the averaged RSS from B to A. The host application calculates the final RSS for each link (each pair of nodes A and B) by averaging the averages from A to B and from B to A. This paper defines the y vector as differences between empty room RSS links' values and the actual RSS links' values from the last calculation. The y vector is being recalculated every 1.5 s. The host application recalculates the x_λ vector at the same rate.

5   Localization Results

The monitored 4 × 4 m square area is divided into 16 × 16 pixels. The spatial dimensions of each pixel are 25 × 25 cm. The host application estimates the attenuation change, compared with empty room, for each pixel every 1.5 s. The host application calculates the coordinates where the attenuation object (the person) is estimated to be by determining the centre of mass of the 4 % pixels with the lowest RSSs. Figures 4 and 5 show the photo of person being in the corner and in the center of the monitored area, respectively, and the corresponding 3D graphical visualizations. In the 3D graphical visualization, each of the 256 pixels is presented as square bar whose height and color change (from blue to red), according to the attenuation change intense.

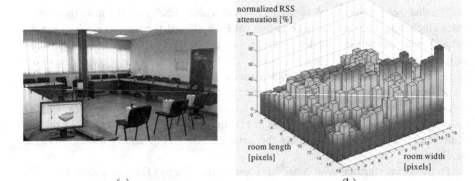

(a)   (b)

Fig. 4. Person stands in the corner of monitored area (a), with the corresponding 3D graphical visualization of the RSS attenuation (b) (Color figure online).

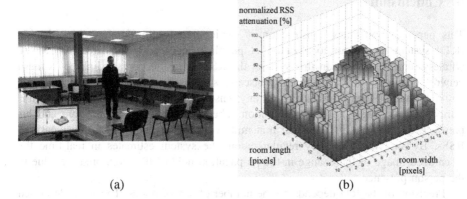

(a)   (b)

Fig. 5. Person stands in the center of monitored area (a), with the corresponding 3D graphical visualization of the RSS attenuation (b) (Color figure online).

The room coordinates are presented as room width and room length, both expressed in pixels. The resolution of the positioning procedure is one pixel. Since the human body certainly covers more than one pixel, this is adequate resolution choice.

The vertical axis on the 3D graphical visualization represents the min-max normalization of the RSS attenuation.

This paper evaluates the accuracy of the RTI system in localizing the person in different areas of the monitored area. The person stands in 9 different spots of evaluation without moving for a pre-determined amount of time, before walking to the next position. Figure 6 shows the average position estimates provided by the RTI system in each of the 9 spots of evaluation. The average localization error is 39 cm.

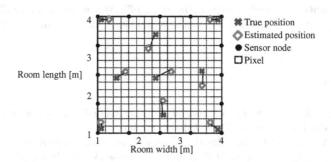

Fig. 6. The true and estimated position of the person in 9 different points of the monitored area.

When the person stands in the corners, the localization is the most accurate. The least accurate localization is when the person stands in the center of the monitored area, where the error reaches up to 60 cm. This error distribution is caused by the greater shadow fading when person stands near the transmitter or receiver than standing in the middle of the link (Fig. 2).

6 Conclusion

This paper demonstrates construction of device-free Radio Tomographic Imaging (RTI) system for indoor localization of people using readily available Sun SPOT wireless sensor network. In this system, the RSSs measured on the links of a mesh network composed of static wireless transceivers are used to accurately localize people without requiring them to wear or carry any sensor or radio device. When the system is started, the room is empty for calibration. Then, a person enters the room and his presence on the link line between transmitters and receivers changes the measured RSSs. By applying Tikhonov regularization, the system estimates in real-time the discretized image of the change in the propagation field of the monitored area due to the person presence.

Precision of the RTI depends on the number of sensor nodes. The setup described in this paper has 16 nodes, achieving an average positioning error of 39 cm in a 4 × 4 m room. The minimal error is in the corners, and the maximum error of 60 cm is in the center of the room. The biggest source of the error at the RTI is that the reflections of the RF signals are not adequately modeled. The RTI model assumes that the RF signal is mainly a line-of-sight signal. As the occurrence of reflections depends on the frequency and the properties of the possibly reflecting surfaces, the modeling of the reflection is practically unfeasible.

An advantage of the RTI is that it needs small computational effort to construct an image. All complex calculations are performed beforehand, leaving one matrix multiplication at runtime. This is essential since it makes the RTI system low-cost and easy available to the ordinary consumers, offering them precision adequate to their needs.

Future work may comprise experimentation in different setups and number of WSN nodes, introduction of spectrum agility for message broadcasting in order to alleviate potential spectrum occupancy problems etc.

Acknowledgments. This work is supported by the EC FP7 eWall project (http://ewallproject.eu/) under grant agreement No. 610658. The authors would like to thank everyone involved.

References

1. Moeslund, T.B., Granum, E.: A survey of computer vision-based human motion capture. Comput. Vis. Image Underst. **81**(3), 231–268 (2001)
2. Bulling, A., Blanke, U., Schiele, B.: A tutorial on human activity recognition using body-worn inertial sensors. ACM Computing Surveys **46**(3), Article No. 33 (2014)
3. Herrera, J., et al.: Evaluation of traffic data obtained via GPS-enabled mobile phones: The Mobile Century field experiment. Transp. Res. Part C: Emerg. Technol. **18**(4), 568–583 (2010)
4. Winkler, T., Rinner, B.: Security and privacy protection in visual sensor networks: a survey. ACM Computing Surveys **47**(1), Article No. 2 (2014)
5. Wilson, J., Patwari, N.: Radio tomographic imaging with wireless networks. IEEE Trans. Mob. Comput. **9**(5), 621–632 (2010)

6. Adler, S., Schmitt, S., Kyas, M.: Device-free indoor localisation using radio tomography imaging in 800/900 MHz band. In: International Conference on Indoor Positioning and Indoor Navigation, Busan (2014)
7. Bocca, M., Kaltiokallio, O., Patwari, N.: Radio tomographic imaging for ambient assisted living. In: Chessa, S., Knauth, S. (eds.) EvAAL 2012. CCIS, vol. 362, pp. 108–130. Springer, Heidelberg (2013)
8. Kaltiokallio, O., Bocca, M., Patwari, N.: A multi-scale spatial model for RSS-based device-free localization. IEEE Transactions on Mobile Computing, arXiv:1302.5914 [cs.NI] (2013)
9. Wilson, J., Patwari, N.: See through walls: motion tracking using variance-based radio tomography networks. IEEE Trans. Mob. Comput. 10(5), 612–621 (2011)
10. Zhao, Y., Patwari, N.: Histogram distance-based radio tomographic localization. In: 11th ACM/IEEE International Conference on Information Processing in Sensor Networks (IPSN), pp. 129–130 (2012)
11. Bal, G.: Introduction to inverse problems. In: Lecture Notes - Department of Applied Physics and Applied Mathematics, Columbia University, New York (2012)
12. Kabanikhin, S.I.: Definitions and examples of inverse and ill-posed problems. J. Inverse Ill-posed Problems 16, 317–357 (2008)

Device Gateway Design for Ambient Assisted Living

Daniel Denkovski[✉], Vladimir Atanasovski, and Liljana Gavrilovska

Faculty of Electrical Engineering and Information Technologies,
Saints Cyril and Methodius University in Skopje, Skopje, Macedonia
{danield,vladimir,liljana}@feit.ukim.edu.mk

Abstract. Cloud-based smart homes for ambient assisted living are emerging information and communication technology aiming to facilitate and improve users' lives. The design of home sensing architecture and corresponding device gateway to connect different types of perceptual and automation devices with cloud services and applications is a challenging task. This paper presents a conceptual home sensing architecture and a modular device gateway design able to combine multiple sources and clients of perceptual and actuator devices providing the required interoperability, flexibility and extensibility for such applications. Furthermore, the paper presents a home sensing environment prototype, which adopts the proposed device gateway design. The proposed design and implementation can be used in a variety of smart-home applications.

Keywords: Smart homes · Ambient assisted living · Home sensing architecture · Device gateway design · Prototype

1 Introduction

The Internet-of-Things and the cloud computing concepts are increasingly attracting academic and industrial interest lately. These technologies have a potential for support of a number of different applications and beneficiaries and are in focus of future smart-x environments. The growing need for improving various users' health, lifestyle, entertainment, convenience, comfort, energy efficiency, security etc. leads to deployment of sensing and automation devices in smart-homes and design of cloud applications to utilize the connected in-home devices.

The smart-homes for ambient assisted living incorporate different environment sensing devices such as fixed sensors for monitoring temperature, humidity, luminosity, mobility, gasses and wearable sensors for activity and vitals detection. Additionally, they may include audio visual sensing devices for monitoring presence and activities, face tracking and analytics. The smart-home environments can also integrate actuator devices to control lighting, heating, ventilation, air conditioning, and other different home appliances.

Existing of-the-shelf solutions provide device gateways [1, 2] which are usually device and/or manufacturer specific. There is lack of a generic and modular device gateway design that provides interconnection and straightforward integration of

© Institute for Computer Sciences, Social Informatics and Telecommunications Engineering 2015
V. Atanasovski, L.-G. Alberto (Eds.): Fabulous 2015, LNICST 159, pp. 100–107, 2015.
DOI: 10.1007/978-3-319-27072-2_13

different types of devices and cloud services/applications and supports multi-device (/client) operation, different communication (e.g. pull/push) and sensing capabilities.

The design and development of device gateways for home sensing environments is a complex task [3]. The device gateways must integrate different market available sensing and automation hardware from different manufacturers having diverse capabilities, physical communication interfaces and APIs. Moreover, the control of the connected devices should be interfaced with different device gateway clients, such as processing components, cloud services and applications. Finally, the home sensing environment and the device gateway in particular, should provide the required reliability for user critical applications and the required flexibility and modularity to support ease integration of new devices, services and applications.

This paper presents conceptual home sensing/automation architecture and a device gateway design that provides the abovementioned possibilities. The proposed device gateway architectural design is adopted and incorporated in a home sensing environment prototype for ambient assisted living.

2 Home Environment for Ambient Assisted Living

The home environment of cloud-controlled smart homes for ambient assisted living should comprise several hardware devices and software modules for environment perception and context extraction, data management, learning, reasoning, decision making and effectuating. The hardware performs environment sensing and system hosting, while the software components perform all remaining activities.

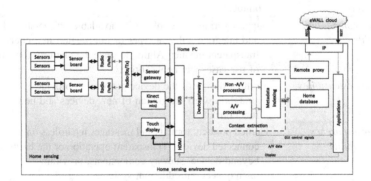

Fig. 1. Conceptual architecture of home environment for ambient assisted living

Figure 1 presents a conceptual architecture with the building blocks and components for cloud-based ambient assisted living [4], with particular focus on the home sensing environment. The chain starts with audio/visual/sensor devices for environment perception connected to a device gateway residing in a home PC, acting as a data collector and aggregator. Based on the input from the perceptual devices (e.g. temperature, accelerometer data, video/audio samples etc.), processing components perform context extraction storing processed data into a home database. A remote gateway acts as a home gateway, relaying and exposing context data to the cloud. The cloud components perform further processing in terms of learning and reasoning upon users behavior (in short/long term history), making decisions, conveying notifications, reminders and actions to improve the user's lifestyle, health, safety etc. The services and applications residing in the cloud can control actuators of different home appliances to improve the habitat and make the user's life more comfortable. This paper focuses mainly on the design of the device gateway component that acts as a unified proxy to the perceptual (cams, mics, sensor motes) and actuator devices.

2.1 Device Gateway Design for Home Sensing Environments

The device gateway should represent a single point of access to sensor measurements, audio/visual streams and metadata performing the role of a unified proxy in the home sensing architecture (Fig. 1) for cloud-based smart homes. It should integrate multiple perception devices (audio/visual and sensors) and actuator devices, relaying the raw sensing/streaming data to other relevant components. The device gateway should keep track of the connected devices and of the connected device gateway clients, handling subscription to measurement and streaming services and (re)configuration of devices. In order to provide a fully functional, easily deployable, controllable and extensible system for ambient assisted living, the device gateway should support the generic system requirements listed and explained in Table 1.

Table 1. Generic system requirements

Requirements	Comments
Flexibility, compatibility, scalability	Support various types of market available off-the-shelf devices and integrate different types of information in a client transparent manner. Ability to scale the platform for a variety of use-cases and applications.
Modularity, extensibility	Modular design of the device gateway to provide straightforward integration of new devices and new functionalities.
Unicity, transparency, interoperability	Unified protocol formats and messages regardless on the type of connected devices. Transparent operation of the hardware for beyond device gateway components, providing the ability to interconnect with different systems.
Reliability, responsiveness	Reliable communication within the platform and real-time operation. Capabilities to dynamically react and/or reconfigure devices.
Multi-device, multi-client support	Interconnection of multiple sources (sensors, audio/visual devices) and multiple destinations of perceptual information (e.g. processing components).
Maintainability, (re)configurability	Ability to easily maintain and (re)configure the system after deployment and during operation.

(Continued)

Table 1. (*Continued*)

Requirements	Comments
Remote accessibility, (re)configurability	Remote access to perceptual information and remote configuration or change of connected devices parameters.
Pull and push type of communication	Handling information subscriptions, ability to provision continuous communication and information distribution to device gateway clients. Ability to trigger specific reporting based on push/pull communication towards/from the device gateway clients.
Device registration and deregistration	Ability to register a perceptual or actuator device in the system (the registration may encompass the location, the type and the measurement capability of the device) and ability to temporarily or permanently de-register a perceptual device.

Figure 2 proposes a device gateway decomposition model satisfying the previously emphasized requirements. The suggested modular design of the device gateway embraces four main building blocks, i.e. sensor gateway controller, audio/visual device controller, actuator device controller and communication module. As highlighted in Fig. 2, the device gateway should be able to connect and control multiple controllers of the perceptual and actuator devices. The communication module is in charge of sensing, streaming data and metadata exchange with device gateway clients and facilitates the remote control of the connected devices.

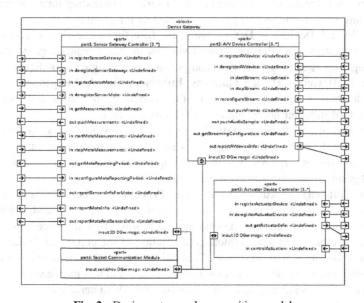

Fig. 2. Device gateway decomposition model

The *sensor gateway controller* includes multiple sensor motes handlers and the sensor gateway middleware to exchange measurements and control messages with the sensor motes. The sensor gateway controller should be able to register and deregister sensor motes, query sensor motes for instantaneous (pull) and periodic (push) measurements, keep track on the connected sensor motes and their configuration and report sensor measurements and devices metadata to device gateway clients. The sensor gateway controller can (re)configure sensor motes remotely using the communication capabilities provided by sensor gateway middleware. The particular realization of the sensor gateway middleware depends on the selected hardware and hardware drivers. The *audio/visual device controller* is decomposed into audio/visual device handler and middleware. Via the audio/visual device handler, the device gateway registers and deregisters audio/visual perception devices, keeps track on the connected devices and their configuration, (re)configures data streaming. The audio/visual device handler can start, stop and reconfigure streams and push streaming data (video frames and audio samples) to device gateway clients. The audio/visual device middleware is a device driver wrapper, which again, provides the physical communication with the device. The decomposition of the *actuator device controller* is similar to the previous two controllers. It contains an actuator device handler which registers and deregisters actuators, keeps track on the actuator information and controls the actuation utilizing the communication capabilities provided by the middleware.

Considering the conceptual home sensing architecture in Fig. 1 and the decomposition model in Fig. 2:

1. **Sensors – Device Gateway Interface**. The device gateway connects multiple sensors (motes and gateways) through this interface controlling their configuration, extracting measurements and preparing metadata for clients.
2. **Audio/Visual Devices – Device Gateway Interface**. The device gateway can connect multiple audio/visual devices via this interface requesting, stopping and reconfiguring streaming, receiving and pushing streaming data to clients.
3. **Actuator Device – Device Gateway Interface**. The device gateway connects multiple actuator devices, keeps track of the current configuration and controls the actuation of different home appliances via this interface.
4. **Device Gateway – Sensing Data Processing**. The device gateway connects multiple sensor data processing components and relays sensor measurements via this interface. This interface also handles subscriptions to sensor measurements, remote reconfiguration and measurement querying.
5. **Device Gateway – Audio/Visual Data Processing**. This interface can relay streaming data (video frames and audio samples) from multiple audio/visual perception devices to multiple processing algorithms. This interface also handles streaming subscriptions and remote configuration of the connected devices.
6. **Device Gateway – Remote Proxy**. This interface is used for remote connection of the connected home devices to cloud components. Via this interface metadata and raw sensing and streaming data can be exchanged. This interface is used for remote access/configuration of all the devices.

3   Prototype Implementation

We have selected a clean slate design of the device gateway, with the Libelium sensor networks platform [6] and the Kinect camera device [7] as underlying devices for environmental parameters perception. The current prototype [5] does not incorporate actuator devices, envisioned for future extensions and improvements.

3.1   Hardware Devices and Interoperability

The core of the Libelium's wireless sensor network portfolio is the Waspmote node [6] (i.e. a sensor mote). The sensor mote is composed of a microcontroller board (for processing purposes) and a sensor board (for attaching different sensors). Motion sensors are connected directly on the sensor nodes microcontroller. The accelerometer sensor is embedded on the sensor board microcontroller. Other sensors (air temperature, luminosity and humidity) use sensor boards. All sensor readings have very fast response time and can be queried at any desired moment. Both communication parties, i.e. the sensor motes and the sensor gateway, are equipped with XBee 868 radio modules and communicate on 868 MHz with an RF protocol. All motes have two-way communication with the sensor gateway.

Kinect is a sensor developed by Microsoft for the Xbox 360 and Xbox One game consoles. It provides control and interaction with the scene or the game, without a console controller, using specified gestures and spoken commands. The Kinect sensor incorporates several advanced technologies such as a depth infrared-based sensing, an RGB colour camera and a four-microphone array. The hardware and software provide full-body 3D motion capture, face/voice recognition capabilities. The Kinect audio/visual sensing device employs a wired USB connection to the computer. The current version of the Kinect audio/visual device implementation in the device gateway uses the libfreenect. hpp C++ wrapper to port the Kinect hardware. The implementation supports starting, stopping and reconfiguring RGB, depth and audio streaming by the device gateway and changing the tilt of the Kinect device.

3.2   Software Components

The selected platform for the device wrappers and the device gateway realization is the Linux operating system and the C++ programming environment due to the open-source availability of the device drivers. The device gateway has a modular C++ design for transparent and seamless integration of these hardware devices, adopting the decomposition model from Sect. 2. The communication module in the devices gateway (Fig. 2) is implemented with TCP/IP socket communication, with the device gateway acting as a socket server for device gateway clients. The configuration of the components and the message exchange with device gateway clients is *JSON-based (JavaScript Object Notation)* strings provided by the *JSON spirit* library.

There are currently three device gateway clients (processing algorithms) in the realized prototype. A *step counting algorithm* exploits the accelerometer data received at 20+Hz rate, to calculate the integrated modulus of body acceleration (IMA),

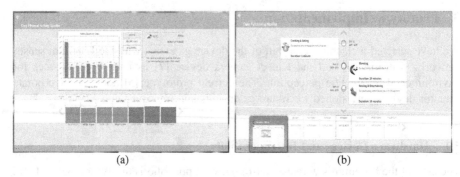

(a)   (b)

Fig. 3. Applications in the cloud (a) Daily Physical Activity Monitoring application (b) Daily Functioning Monitoring application

the integrated squared output of accelerometer (ISA) and the step counts. The results are stored in couchDB storage database in a JSON style format. An *ambient parameters storage component* receives the remaining ambient parameters, i.e. temperature, humidity, luminosity, movement, and stores the results in JSON format in the couchDB database. A *visual movement detection algorithm* uses the difference between consecutive RGB frames from the Kinect sensor to detect whether there is a movement in the surveillance area. All three device gateway clients are based on C++ realizations, acting as TCP/IP socket clients to the device gateway. They are all compiled and run in separate executables.

The remote proxy and the remaining cloud components are native java implementations using the REST API to exchange JSON based http messages. The interface between the remote-proxy and the device gateway is based on C++ → JAVA wrapping using the SWIG platform.

There are two developed applications in the cloud [5] that utilize the home environmental perception inputs, i.e. a Daily Physical Activity Monitoring application (Fig. 3(a)), operating based on the step counts and a Daily Functioning Monitoring application (Fig. 3(b)), using the ambient parameters to detect specific activities of the user (resting and entertaining in the living room, showering in the bathroom etc.).

4   Conclusions

The cloud-based smart-homes for ambient assisted living incorporate different perceptual and automation devices and cloud services and applications to ease peoples' lives, improve their lifestyle, convenience and comfort. Integrating multiple devices with different communication and sensing capabilities in a single home sensing environment is a challenging task, with respect to interoperability, flexibility, reliability aspects. This paper presented a conceptual home sensing architecture for ambient assisted living and a modular device gateway design and prototype, able to combine multiple sources and clients of perceptual and actuator devices. The proposed design and implementation can be beneficial in a variety of applications for smart-homes, especially for the elderly people, to improve their health, daily functioning and lifestyle.

Acknowledgments. This work was supported by the EC project eWall (FP7- 610658). The authors would to thank everyone involved, particularly partners from Ericsson Nikola Tesla (ENT), Athens Institute of Technology (AIT) and Technical University of Sofia (TUS), for their extensive work on the presented prototype.

References

1. Introducing the Qualcomm Smart Gateway. http://www.qca.qualcomm.com/networking/connected-home/qualcomm-smart-gateway
2. HealthCare Gateway: Simple Gateway for the Home. http://www.acutetechnology.com/products/hydra-healthcare-gateway/
3. Qualcom Comprlimentary webcast: Designing Smarter Gateways for the Internet of Everything. http://www.parksassociates.com/qualcomm-ioe-2015
4. The eWALL Consortium: D3.1.1 eWALL Networked Devices. eWALL for Active Long Living FP7 project (2014)
5. The eWALL Consortium: D6.1 Integration report. eWALL for Active Long Living FP7 project (2014)
6. Libelium Comunicaciones Distribuidas S.L. http://www.libelium.com
7. Kinect for Xbox 360. http://www.xbox.com/en-SG/Xbox360/Accessories/Kinect/kinect forxbox360

Extending Body Sensor Nodes' Lifetime
Using a Wearable Wake-up Radio

Andres Gomez[1], Michele Magno[1,2(✉)], Xin Wen[1], and Luca Benini[1,2]

[1] D-ITET, ETH Zurich, Gloriastrasse 35, 8092 Zurich, Switzerland
{andres.gomez,michele.magno,
xin.wen,luca.benini}@ee.ethz.ch
[2] DEI, University of Bologna, Viale del Resorgimento 2, 40132 Bologna, Italy

Abstract. Body Area Networks (BAN) have received significant attention in recent years and have found a wide range of applications, including wearable devices for fitness and health tracking, mobile communications, among others. Energy storage devices such as batteries continue to be a bottleneck in these small form factor devices, thus requiring advanced power management techniques to sustain devices' increasing power and lifetime demands. As radio transceivers are typically the most power hungry subsystem in wearable sensors devices, many techniques focus to reduce the communication power consumption. In this work, we focus on wake-up radios as a novel technology which can be in listening mode consuming only few nW, significantly reducing the overall power consumption of communication. We evaluate the performance of state-of-the-art wake-up receivers (WUR) in the BAN context, and the tradeoffs between its addressing capabilities, range, and sensitivity. Using in-field measurements, we quantify energy savings and estimate the resulting prolongation of the sensor node's lifetime in a wearable gait-detection application, where nodes communicate via a Bluetooth main radio.

Keywords: Body area networks · Wake-Up receiver · Energy efficiency

1 Introduction

With the rapid development of technology, increasing functionality is being integrated into wearable devices. Wearable technology is strategic in healthcare, where smart electronic devices can continuously monitor patient's vital signs and enable doctors to identify possible diseases earlier and to provide optimal treatment [1]. These new capabilities have led to increased power requirements, while wearable devices continue to trend to smaller, slimmer and lighter form factors [1]. As a result, many power and energy-aware techniques have been proposed to address these conflicting goals.

Reducing the power consumed in communication by wireless sensor nodes can be very effective, since the radio transceiver is one of the components with the highest power consumption, as shown in Fig. 1. One common way of reducing the energy consumed by the radio is duty-cycling. The node can switch the radio between active and sleep mode with predefined intervals. Low-power states are programmed to take place only when no communication is supposed to happen. However, there are some

© Institute for Computer Sciences, Social Informatics and Telecommunications Engineering 2015
V. Atanasovski, L.-G. Alberto (Eds.): Fabulous 2015, LNICST 159, pp. 108–117, 2015.
DOI: 10.1007/978-3-319-27072-2_14

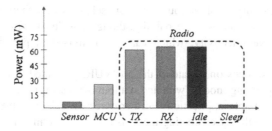

Fig. 1. Typical power consumption in wearable nodes

limitations to duty-cycling. First, devices still have to stay in idle listening during certain periods. Second, overhearing communications destined to other devices will also cost a considerable amount of energy. Third, radios have to be synchronized in order to guarantee proper communication among devices. Synchronization implies that transmitters have to wait for a sufficient amount of time before sending any meaningful data. Since receivers cannot successfully receive a message in sleep mode, they must kept ON even when no information is being sent or received. Another approach is to use asynchronous schemes, which are generally considered to be the most power efficient ones, since they practically eliminate the costly idle listening [1, 6]. Here, an ultra-low power wake-up radio receiver (WUR), usually coupled with another (main) radio, listens continuously to the transmission medium and wakes up the main radio only after a wake-up signal is detected. Naturally, there are clear trade-offs between cost (an additional receiver is needed), and the potential energy savings.

In this work, we implement a state-of-the-art WUR architecture in the context of BAN applications, perform a thorough evaluation of the WUR's range/addressing capabilities and their impact on the energy savings. To this end, a gait detection application for Parkinson's disease (PD) with one sink node and two sensor nodes is studied. Using real-world measurements of the implemented system, we calculate the prolongation of the sensor nodes' lifetimes and demonstrate the savings introduced by the WUR.

2 Related Works

To reduce communication power consumption, several techniques have been proposed for lowering or eliminating the power wasted for idle listening of the transceiver [8, 9]. Duty-cycling is a common technique to reduce the idle mode energy consumption which consists of switching from listening mode to sleep mode [8]. However, even though duty-cycling helps saving power, it can severely limit the reactivity of the devices, since radios cannot receive messages when they are off or in sleep. Asynchronous techniques have also received considerable attention because of their increased energy efficiency [3]. In [10–12], several different architectures for ultra-low-power WURs for wireless sensor network devices are presented. These works all reduce the idle listening and significantly reduce the overall network energy consumption. In [4], a novel solution consuming only 98 nW is presented. This solution uses a comparator, and a custom CMOS rectifier designed to achieve sensitivity of − 41 dBm. In [14, 19], the authors present a thorough survey of various wake-up schemes and their advantages over duty-cycling schemes. Addressing capability, though costlier in terms of power, is the only way to achieve selectivity, which can be an important parameter for certain applications.

In this work, we focus on a state-of-the-art WUR, presented in [16], and evaluate the impact of its operating modes (with and without addressing) and its performance in the context of a wearable application. Furthermore, we calculate the energy savings introduced by the WUR, by estimating the sensor node's lifetime in the gait-detection application.

3   Wake up Radio Overview

In this section, we present an overview of the communication with wake up radios in a wearable application scenario. Figure 2 shows two main wireless devices of a typical wearable system: the sink node and the sensor node (which can be also more than one), and their main components. The sensor node, which reads and processes data from a sensor, will transmit the data via the main radio (i.e Bluetooth Low Energy) only after the WUR receives a wake-up signal from the sink node. This work focuses on the battery-based sensor node, and how its lifetime can be significantly extended using a WUR.

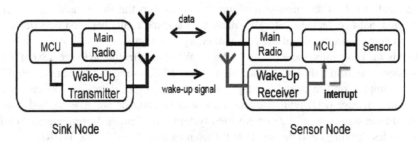

Fig. 2. Block diagram of the proposed system

Sink Node (SN). Usually body area network systems are centered on a sink node which is the node in charge to collect data from the sensor nodes and organize the network. Furthermore, it can request information from the sensor node. When no WUR is used, the communication is done via the main radio, which requires both radios (sender/receiver) to be turned on even when there is no data transmission. With WUR the main radio can be turned off when no data transmission is needed and still listen the channel with an ultra-low power radio (WUR). This is an important feature, in many wearable applications, where activation and deactivation of the main radio can be determined by the context (i.e. if the sink node detects some activity from the sensors). It should be noted that to send the wake-up signal, an additional wake-up transmitter radio is required on the sink node, meaning there is a clear trade-off between the additional cost and energy savings. Later on, in the evaluation section, we will test for two transmitter antennas with different form factors and gains, which will be important parameters for the product's design.

Sensor Node (SEN). The sensor node is usually placed on the human body to collect and process data from sensors. If no WUR is used, then the sensor node has no choice but to keep the main radio on continuously or activate it with duty cycling, dealing with the tradeoff of reactiveness and energy saving. This scenario can be seen in Fig. 3a. Using the WUR, the sensors node has the capability to be in continuously listening mode, waiting for the sink node messages and activating the main radio only when it is needed. This process can be seen in Fig. 3b. It is important to notice that as the WUR is an additional, always-on component, its power consumption has to be significant lower than the main radio (in the order or nanoWatts) to be effective. The latency is another critical feature, as the main radio has to be switched on as soon as possible. This work focuses on evaluating this wake-up process with on-the-field measurements of the maximum range and the impact that false negatives, false positives, and packet losses could have in the total energy savings of a BAN application. We will evaluate a WUR presented in [16] which consumes only around 600 nW with a latency of few microseconds. The WUR sensitivity is − 42 dBm which allows to achieve few meters with wearable antennas. The wake up radio provides two modalities with addressing and non-addressing: when using addressing mode the sink node is able to select which sensor node to wake up using an address. In the non-addressing mode, all nodes within the range of the message are woken up. The main difference lies in the length of the packet and the energy required to sample and decode the address.

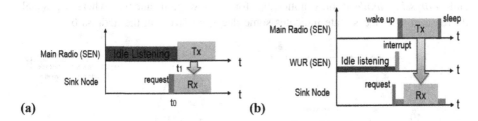

Fig. 3. Sample timeline with (a) only a main radio, and (b) with a main radio and a WUR.

4 Experimental Evaluation

In this section, we will first introduce the experimental set-up used to characterize the range and performance of the implemented WUR. The first range experiment, is done using two antenna on the sink nodes (SN). The first, shown in Fig. 4a, uses a low gain 0 dBi PCB antenna which uses only 1 cm^2 of space. A second SN with a higher gain, 7 cm long, 2 dBi antenna, shown in Fig. 4b, was also tested. In these experiments the radio was configured with On Off Key modulation for the messages and 868 MHz frequency with 1.2 Kbps and + 10 dBm power output. At the receiving part, we used a WUR with a flexible antenna by Molex [17], with a gain of 2.2 dBi as the sensor nodes have to be placed on the body. The bendable antenna, shown in Fig. 4c, measures only 1.3 cm × 10.67 cm, and can be placed directly on the node or on the body.

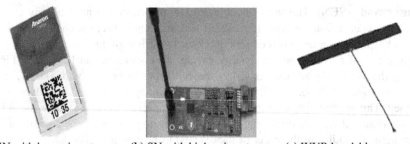

(a) SN with low gain antenna   (b) SN with high gain antenna   (c) WUR bendable antenna

Fig. 4. Antennas used for the wake-up transmitter and receiver (not to scale).

4.1   WUR Range & Performance

The first part of the experiment aims at testing the communication range of the system. The distances between the sink and sensor nodes was varied from 10 cm to 315 cm, and 1000 packets where generated 3 s apart. Afterwards, it was recorded whether the sensor node detected the wake-up signal and generated the interrupt. The results can be seen in Fig. 5. As expected, the sink node with the high gain antenna has a longer range, over 3.1 m, which is suitable for many wearable application where few meters are required. It should be noted that the difference in range between the *non-addressing* and *addressing mode* is only noticeable for the low gain antenna, where a gradual decrease in the success rate indicates some decoding errors in the address bits.

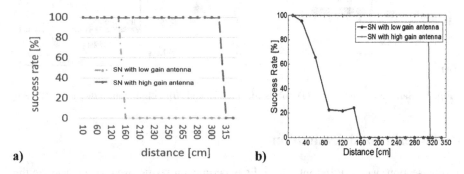

Fig. 5. WUR success rate evaluation in (a) *Non-addressing Mode*; and (b) *Addressing Mode*.

So far, it has been shown that the WUR can have a range from approx. 1.6 to 3.1 m, depending on the antenna, which is a common communication range for many BAN applications. We will now evaluate the WUR's different performance parameters using the sink node with a high gain antenna, placed at a maximum distance of 85 cm from the sensor nodes. This corresponds to the distance between the waist and feet of our test subject in standing position, as shown in Fig. 6.

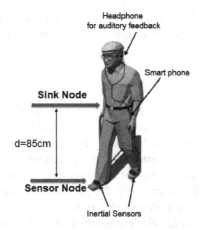

Fig. 6. Nodes worn by user in gait detection application. Modified from [7]

During the experiment, the patient will be either standing or walking, and the performance parameters were recorded. The parameters relevant to this study are:

1. False positive (FP): number of false wake-ups when not needed
2. False negative (FN): number of non-wake-ups when needed
3. Packet loss (LOSS): number of packets lost during transmission process

FPs lead to sensor nodes' unwanted wake-up of the sensors node due to an interrupt by the WUR. The wake-up process using Bluetooth is quite costly and would waste considerable energy if it tries to establish a connection when not needed. FNs occurs when the WUR is not able to detect correctly the wake up messages. FN will generate only a small latency, since the sink node use a timeout mechanism to simply re-send a second packet in order to wake up the selected sensor node. As a consequence, these two parameters are meaningful in evaluating the quality of the wake up radio systems. Figure 7a, shows the measurements when the user is standing. Here, there were no losses, false positives or negatives. This means all the messages has been received correctly. Figure 7b shows the same test except for the user who is now walking in a building. Due to the movement of the user's legs, the body occlusions, the environmental Radio Frequency noise, FN's and LOSS's now occur. It should be noted that the result is slightly worse on the right foot, because the sink node is mounted to the left

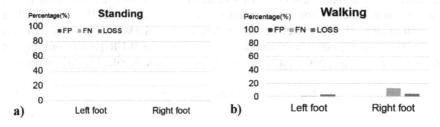

Fig. 7. On the field measurements of WUR with addressing in different conditions.

side of the user's waist and the human body occlusion is worst. More importantly, even with movement, there were no FP's, so the sensor node will incur the costly wake-up cost only when truly necessary.

4.2   Lifetime Analysis

In the last section, evaluation of energy consumption has been done in order to demonstrate quantitatively the improvement of the proposed architecture. We used a gait detection application for Parkinson's disease (PD) presented in [2, 7]. The authors of [2, 7] have presented a wearable sensor system that can assist patients by detecting gait disturbances using IMU sensors attached to their feet. When an event is detected, it triggers auditory feedback that can help the patient overcome the episode. The gait detection system is composed of three nodes, one sink node and two sensor nodes. The sink node is placed in the waist, and also contains sensors that can recognize the context: whether the patient is walking, or sitting down. The two sensor nodes are placed on the patient's feet. These nodes read the sensor data and do the feature extraction that allows the system to detect gait disturbances. However, since gait anomalies could only occur while the patient is walking, the sensor nodes could potentially enter sleep mode when the patient is sitting down. Patients with advanced Parkinson's disease tend to be seniors who spend most of their time sitting or in bed, which would allow potentially large energy savings. Since the sink node has the ability to detect when the patient is walking, only then will it send a wake-up signal to the sensor node so it can turn on the Bluetooth radio for data transmission.

Table 1. Sensor node's power consumption, with and without WUR.

Radios Used	Idle Listening Power	Transmission Power
Bluetooth	92.4 mW	135.3 mW
Bluetooth and WUR	600 nW	135.3 mW

To quantify the impact of the WUR on the lifetime of the sensor node, we will compare an initial system with only a Bluetooth 2.0 radio (BLU), and another with Bluetooth and a WUR (BLU+WUR). The former will maintain the Bluetooth radio on (in idle mode) even if the user not walking, while the latter will have it on only when the user is walking. To calculate the lifetimes of these systems, we first estimate the energy they consume with power measurements on our implemented system. These values, measured at 3.3 V, can be seen in Table 1. The Idle listening power of the node with only the Bluetooth is around 92.4 mW. This value comprises both the Bluetooth power consumption and the idle power consumption of the rest of the node. When the WUR is present the power whole node can be in deep sleep mode as the WUR can act as a wireless switch [18], then the power consumption include only the WUR power consumption (600 nW). The energy consumed in one idle to active cycle is calculated as follows:

$$E_{BT} = P_{idle,BT} * t_{idle} + P_{active} * t_{active} \tag{1}$$

$$E_{BT\_WUR} = P_{idle,BT\_WUR} * t_{idle} + P_{active} * \left(t_{active} + t_{wake\_up}\right) \qquad (2)$$

Equation (1) represents the energy consumed by the Bluetooth-only system, which is simply the sum of the idle and active energies based on their respective power consumptions, from Table 1. The idle time (t_{idle}) is the time the patient spends sitting, when the Bluetooth radio is not transmitting data and t_{active} is the time the patient spends walking, during which there is Bluetooth transmission. Equation (2) represents the energy consumed by the Bluetooth and WUR system. The main difference between these equations is the idle power, as shown in Table 1, and the inclusion of the t_{wake_up} term, which is the amount of time it takes for the Bluetooth radio to turn on and be ready for transmission. Lastly, with these energies per cycle, we can estimate the systems' lifetime when connected to a fully charged, 150 mAh Li-Ion battery, using the following equations:

$$Lifetime_{BT} = \frac{C_{batt} * V_{cc}}{E_{BT}} * \left(t_{idle} + t_{active}\right) \qquad (3)$$

$$Lifetime_{BT\_WUR} = \frac{C_{batt} * V_{cc}}{E_{BT\_WUR}} * \left(t_{idle} + t_{active} + t_{wake\_up}\right) \qquad (4)$$

Equations (3) and (4) show the lifetimes of the Bluetooth and Bluetooth+WUR systems. These can simply be thought of as the number of cycles that the battery can supply from a given initial capacity (C_{batt}). The calculation is done by assuming $t_{wake\_up} = 3\,s$, $t_{active} = 30\,min$, t_{idle} was varied from 0 to 30 min and Vcc was 3.3 V. Figure 8 shows the estimated lifetimes, in hours, as a function of the idle to active time ratio. When this ratio tends to 1, it means the device was active mode the entire time. Conversely, as the ratio tends to 0, the device spends more time in idle mode. The figure shows two lines, the blue indicates a system with only a Bluetooth ratio, and the red shows the same system with Bluetooth and WUR. Finally, the more time the patient spends sitting down, the more time the system spends in low-power mode, and the greater the energy savings.

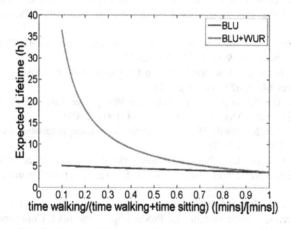

Fig. 8. Expected lifetime with and without the WUR.

5   Conclusions

This work has evaluated the feasibility of WUR for BAN nodes and its potential energy savings in a real BAN application. Thorough testing of the WUR's performance have demonstrated that its range of over 3 meters surpasses the needs of many BAN applications. Furthermore, its addressing capabilities would increase the network's selectivity and the node's lifetime, with only marginal false positives and negatives. In the studied gait detection scenario, two nodes have been attached to the body of an individual and the evaluation has been done in standing state and walking state separately. Lastly, we have calculated the energy savings introduced by the WUR and the resulting prolongation in the node's lifetime of up to 7 times, depending on the amount of time the system can be in sleep mode.

Acknowledgments. This work was supported by "Transient Computing Systems", SNF project (200021_157048), by SCOPES SNF project (IZ74Z0_160481), and ETHZ Grant funding.

References

1. Magno, M., Spagnol, C., Benini, L., Popovici, E.: A low power wireless node for contact and contactless heart monitoring. Microelectron. J. **45**(12), 1656–1664 (2014)
2. Casamassima, F., Farella, E., Benini, L.: Context aware power management for motion-sensing body area network nodes. In: Proceedings of the DATE Conference, pp. 1–6. IEEE, March 2014
3. Kerhet, A., Leonardi, F., Boni, A., Lombardo, P., Magno, M., Benini, L.: Distributed video surveillance using hardware-friendly sparse large margin classifiers. In: IEEE Conference on Advanced Video and Signal Based Surveillance, AVSS 2007, pp. 87, 92, 5–7, September 2007
4. Roberts, N.E., Wentzloff, D.D.: A 98 nW wake-up radio for wireless body area networks. In: Radio Frequency Integrated Circuits Symposium (RFIC), 2012 IEEE, pp. 373–376, 17–19, June 2012
5. Landsiedel, O., et al.: Low power, low delay: opportunistic routing meets duty cycling. In: Proceedings of the 11th International Conference on Information Processing in Sensor Networks. ACM (2012)
6. Groza, B., Murvay, S.: Efficient protocols for secure broadcast in controller area networks. IEEE Trans. Industr. Inf. **9**(4), 2034–2042 (2013)
7. Casamassima, F., et al.: A wearable system for gait training in subjects with Parkinson's disease. Sensors **14**(4), 6229–6246 (2014)
8. Jurdak, R., Baldi, P., Lopes, C.V.: Adaptive low power listening for wireless sensor networks. IEEE Trans. Mob. Comput. **6**(8), 988–1004 (2007)
9. Vodel, M., Caspar, M., Hardt, W.: Wake-up-receiver concepts-capabilities and limitations. J. Netw. **7**(1), 126–134 (2012)
10. Nilsson, E., Svensson, C.: Ultra low power wake-up radio using envelope detector and transmission line voltage transformer. IEEE J. Emerg. Sel. Top. Circuits Syst. **3**(1), 5–12 (2013)
11. Spenza, D., et al.: Beyond duty cycling: wake-up radio with selective awakenings for long-lived wireless sensing systems. In: Proceedings of the IEEE Conference on Computer Communications, pp. 522–530 (2015)

12. Alírio Soares, B., Borges Carvalho, N.: A low-power wakeup radio for application in WSN-based indoor location systems. Int. J. Wirel. Inf. Netw. **20**(1), 67–73 (2013)
13. Takahagi, K., et al.: Low-power wake-up receiver with subthreshold CMOS circuits for wireless sensor networks. Analog Integr. Circ. Sig. Process **75**(2), 199–205 (2013)
14. Jelicic, V., et al.: Analytic comparison of wake-up receivers for WSNs and benefits over the wake-on radio scheme. In: Proceedings of the PM2HW2 N. ACM (2012)
15. Gamm, G.U., et al.: Low–power sensor node with addressable wake–up on–demand capability. Int. J. Sens. Netw. **11**(1), 48–56 (2012)
16. Magno, M., Benini, L.: An ultra low power high sensitivity wake-up radio receiver with addressing capability. In: 2014 IEEE 10th International Conference on Wireless and Mobile Computing, Networking and Communications (WiMob), pp. 92, 99, 8–10 October 2014
17. Molex. Cellular 6-band Standalone Antenna 105263-002 Datasheet. 2012()
18. Magno, M., et al.: Combination of hybrid energy harvesters with MEMS piezoelectric and nano-Watt radio wake up to extend lifetime of system for wireless sensor nodes. In: Proceedings of 2013, 26th International Conference on Architecture of Computing Systems (ARCS), VDE (2013)
19. Jelicic, V., et al.: Benefits of wake-up radio in energy-efficient multimodal surveillance wireless sensor network. IEEE Sens. J. **14**(9), 3210–3220 (2014)

M2M Communications for Intraoral Sensors: A Wireless Communications Perspective

Gianpaolo Sannino[1]([⌧]), Ernestina Cianca[1], Chaffia Hamitouche[2,3], and Marina Ruggieri[1]

[1] Center for Teleinfrastructures (CTIF), University of Roma "Tor Vergata", Via Politecnico 1-00133, Rome, Italy
gianpaolosannino@gmail.com
[2] Institut Mines-Telecom, Télécom Bretagne, 29238 Brest, France
[3] Laboratoire de Traitement de l'Information Médicale, INSERM UMR 1101, 29609 Brest, France

Abstract. The use of mobile and wireless communication technologies to facilitate and improve healthcare and medical services is bringing a shift to healthcare delivery. In this context, an important application scenario is represented by dentistry applications and more generally, intraoral sensors applications. An oral sensory system that allows real-time monitoring of intraoral parameters/activities would open new opportunities for both dentistry applications and more generally wellness applications. This paper provides an overview of the possible applications of intraoral sensors wirelessly connected to external devices, outlining open challenges and research directions.

Keywords: Intraoral sensors · Wireless communications · Dentistry · mHealth

1 Introduction

The application of M2M enabling technologies to the healthcare sector is expected to be one of the major M2M market drivers [1]. The so-called mHealth, i.e. the use of mobile and wireless communication technologies to facilitate and improve healthcare and medical services is bringing a shift to healthcare delivery ensuring enhanced quality, efficiency, flexibility and cost reductions. mHealth application scenarios includes the active management of diseases such as diabetes, the support for independent aging to the elderly and the monitoring of personal fitness activities to improve health and well-being.

An emerging application scenario, which could offer great benefits both from the health and from the commercial point of view is represented by dentistry applications and more generally, intraoral sensors applications. The mouth is one of the most important organs of the human body. The stomatognathic system is made by several units (bones, nerves, vessels, muscles, ligaments, joints, teeth) that are constantly involved in functional demands (chewing, speaking, breathing). As the oral health is closely related to general health conditions, the oral cavity could be the ideal environment to place sensory systems and collect data, which could be useful in monitoring oral activities, detection of pathologies/problems and early interventions.

© Institute for Computer Sciences, Social Informatics and Telecommunications Engineering 2015
V. Atanasovski, L.-G. Alberto (Eds.): Fabulous 2015, LNICST 159, pp. 118–124, 2015.
DOI: 10.1007/978-3-319-27072-2_15

In the past two decades several devices (and related patents) have been developed allowing intraoral sensing using different mechanical and electronic sensing principles [2, 3]. However, the invasive nature of wired connections, between the oral cavity and a readout unit placed outside could be uncomfortable for the patient impairing physiological functions [2, 3]. The huge advancement in micromachining techniques has allowed the fabrication of micro-biosensors featuring wireless transmission of collected data. The reduction of the system dimensions reduces the discomfort in the oral cavity and enable easy implantation with no tissue injury while collecting real-time data. Although several intraoral sensing systems have been developed (mainly prototypes) that allow the wireless transmission of data [4–7], the potential opportunities offered by this sector have not been truly exploited yet.

In this paper, we first review the applications of wirelessly connected intraoral sensors, outlining also novel unexplored opportunities. Then, we review the use of wireless communications in this context. It is worth noting that the use of intraoral sensors from the communication point of view is analogous to other mHealth applications. Nevertheless, intraoral sensors are in the border between intra-body and wearable sensors and hence, they pose peculiar challenges, which will be outlined in the paper as well as open related research issues.

The paper is organized as follows: Sect. 2 presents several possible applications of intraoral sensors, also proposing novel application scenarios; Sect. 3 reviews the use of wireless communication for intraoral sensors applications, outlining current challenges and limits; conclusions are drawn in Sect. 4.

2 Intraoral Sensors Applications

Intraoral sensors applications can be divided: dentistry applications, i.e. applications strictly related to the "tooth" and oral health; more general sensing applications, i.e. use of sensors for sensing parameters related to human health, even if not strictly for oral or teeth health; Human-Machine-Interface (HMI), i.e. applications that use measurement of oral activity to drive/control a machine.

Dentistry Applications. A digital micro pH meter could be very useful to record the change in intra-oral pH. Since caries is caused by specific types of acid-producing bacteria when the pH at the tooth surface drops below 5.5, miniaturized sensors, which are attached to the tooth surface, allow for pH monitoring and providing real time feedback to the patients and dental experts [8]. The use of this device would be excellent for all people who show high susceptibility to the development of decay processes, especially for problems related to the altered structure of the dental enamel. This happens when some diseases which occur during the formation process of the dental enamel, i.e. the amelogenesis, may lead to hypoplastic and/or hypomineralized teeth which are less resistant to bacterial insult and to the resulting demineralization processes induced by the acid environment.

Temperature sensors, applied in a removable dental device as an occlusal splint or an orthodontic system, would be a non-invasive way to check the proper usage by the patient as prescribed by the dentist. Occlusal splint, usually employed in the treatment of bruxism (clenching and grinding) and of temporomandibular disorders is usually prescribed in adult patients to treat these diseases uncommon in young patients. The presence of a temperature sensor, would provide a way to control the frequency and duration of application of the splint, while evaluating the actual progress of the therapy and comparing different possible treatments. Orthodontic treatment performed by removable retainers are especially employed for children (from 6 to 10 years) to control the growth of the jaws and the status of the teeth in the jaw. Since young patients, the discipline of wearing the retainers over a necessary daily duration can not be presupposed and the removable retainers are mostly worn for less than the prescribed time or not at all. It is very important to consistently adhere to the prescribed regular daily application hours to achieve the planned results, thus a wireless biomonitoring would allow the dentist to take action in case of a bad compliance, avoiding additional expensive new adjustment or a new preparation of the retainer. The successful avoidance of these negative consequences of uncontrolled use results in a substantial financial and practical advantage for dentists and their patients [9].

Intraoral pressure sensors for bite-force sensing and measurement have been largely used for several applications in dentistry. They have been employed for assessing the functional state of the masticatory system, for assessing the degree and for monitoring of dental and occlusal pathologies, for the evaluation of post-surgical evolution and for comparing alternative treatments and their influence on temporomandibular disorders. In other cases, pressure sensors have been used to assess the degree of patient satisfaction with dental prostheses, both fixed and removable, in order to validate therapeutic solutions and to propose additional improvements. Furthermore these sensors, which are embedded into dental devices such as a mouth-guard, can be also used as a tool that helps to monitor and reinforce patient compliance. Measurements of intraoral bite-force become especially relevant when related to the study of bruxism, especially as a complement for polysomnographic diagnosis, which still is the most adequate procedure for monitoring the evolution of patients and comparing different possible treatments.

A different oral sensory system, which uses a small accelerometer sensor embedded inside artificial teeth, has been proposed to recognize human oral activities, since each of them produces a unique teeth motion. However it has been underestimated that each tooth has a specific function and teeth are not all involved simultaneously, so the sensor placement becomes crucial for this purpose.

This type of sensor would be very useful if applied within a fixed prosthesis, whose prerequisite for long term success, is the stillness on the support (teeth or implants) and the structural integrity.

Applications to General Human Health Conditions. The oral sensing technologies could be very useful for detecting human health general conditions too. Through the use of sensors that perform biochemical measurements, the physician may perform an early diagnosis, monitor the state of chronic diseases (diabetes, chronic kidney disease, etc.), perform specific tests, administer drugs. It would be especially helpful for elderly or physically disabled patients. However, not much work can be found in this direction.

HMI Applications. The sensors could also be used in Human-Machine-Interface applications. The tongue pressure, exerted on sensors embedded in a mouthguard, could control remote devices. This could be especially relevant when related to quadriplegic patients or with severe disabilities. In [4] the authors proposed a tongue activated wireless system to enable patients who cannot use their hands to use human-to-computer system to communicate or perform ordinary activities.

Future perspectives. A careful analysis of the literature shows how the attention of researchers has never focused on the use of prosthetic restorations, especially the implant-supported ones, as support for sensors. The benefits could be numerous. The volume of the prosthesis provides adequate space for housing the sensors, the prosthesis itself could be featured by sensors for continuous monitoring needs and early interception of mechanical and biological problems. Furthermore, the prosthesis could be used as reservoirs for drug administration in response to chemical stimuli.

These connections allow communicating with a remote station and sending data to dental experts and taking feedback. It could be useful to extrapolate these hypotheses to the clinical environment, where millions of patients worldwide are subjected annually to expensive and time consuming restorative dental treatments.

3 Wireless Communications Perspective

In all the mentioned applications, it is crucial to allow intraoral devices to communicate with the outside world in a wireless way. Wireless communication has been successfully established in several intraoral devices [4–6]. However, in [4–6] intraoral devices are used for a very specific application not related to dentistry. It is about the monitoring of the tongue pressure on the palate and in the use of it to control some devices to easy the communication of quadriplegic or patients who have had a cerebrovascular accident or other neurological disorders (e.g. Parkinson's disease). So, for instance, mobility of the patient is not considered or important in this case.

There are few works on the use of intraoral sensors for long term monitoring of oral cavity parameters [7]. However, all the mentioned works are only focused on the system operation without the in-depth study of the wireless communication. Most of them do not use a wireless standard technology but specifically designed transceivers. Wireless communication between intraoral devices and the outside world is challenging. As a matter of fact, the oral cavity is a hybrid propagation environment. It is not strictly speaking a communication "inside the body" as a sensor inside the body, depending on its anatomical location, is usually surrounded by a distinct and fairly stable tissue environment while the intraoral device is located in a constantly changing environment depending on the relative positions of the jaws and movements of the tongue, which continuously changes shape when one swallows, breathes, or speaks. On the other hand, in many cases sensors may be located close to the "outside part of the body" and, hence, a communication "over the air" might occur. Therefore, it could be possible to use all the considerable research conducted on wireless communication inside and around the human body. As intraoral devices are in contact with the gums, the tongue, or the palate, and their associated receivers may be in contact with the human body, Body Channel Communication (BCC) can be considered to be used for these devices [10]. Two BCC scenarios are capacitive and galvanic BCC working in 30–70 MHz and 0.01–1 MHz bands, respectively. Capacitive BCC uses the conductivity of the human body and works according to the principle of quasi-static near-field coupling. The current, which is formed through capacitive coupling with common ground, e.g., the earth, must have a return path. The Galvanic BCC uses an alternating current initiated from a pair of differential transmitter (Tx) electrodes, distributed in the surrounding tissue, and picked up by the receiver (Rx) electrodes. Because this method does not need ground coupling, is suitable for the implant-to-implant communication, in which both Tx and Rx electrodes are inside the body. It shows high attenuation when the signal meets skin because skin is highly resistive to alternating current and it is completely ineffective when the Rx is detached from the body. However, when applied to intraoral devices, neither of the BCC methods maintains their desired operating conditions. For capacitive BCC, coupling between the Tx and the common ground is severely attenuated because the Tx has to be located inside the mouth. For galvanic BCC, high attenuation at a skin is expected because the Tx and the Rx is located on or outside the body. Moreover, both types of BCC require special electrodes to minimize attenuation at the boundary between the device and the body. Therefore, the use of RF-based wireless communications can be considered. As a matter of fact, RF wireless communication has been successfully adopted in implantable devices such as the pacemaker and neurostimulator. However, not much work has been done for the specific case of the intraoral devices. There were a few approaches to characterize antennas working inside the mouth [11, 12]. The proper selection of the frequency band is fundamental for establishing a reliable link between intraoral devices and the outside world. The selection of the frequency is strictly related to two fundamental design elements:

1) *Size of the antenna:* the use of higher frequency allows to reduce the size of the antenna (and easy the challenging task to design an antenna fitting inside a teeth or an implant).
2) *Attenuation:* the propagation environment is pretty complex. Higher frequencies are more attenuated by the "vicinity" of the body. Gums, teeth, and the lips, which surrounds the electronics absorb and attenuate the RF signal especially at frequency around 1-10 GHz.

An important initial work on the frequency selection has been reported where authors studied three frequency bands, among the ISM bands: 433.9 MHz, 2.48 GHz, and 27 MHz. 433.9 MHz is close to the medical implant communication service (MICS) 402–405 MHz band and hence, it is expected to show similar characteristics such as low absorption from the body; 2.48 GHz has good antenna radiation efficiency in small sized antennas; 27 MHz has been considered to employ a near-field communication by inductive coupling, which can be more efficient than EM wave propagation at short distances. In addition, the human body is almost transparent to the near-field communication at 27 MHz because its wavelength is 10 m and it mainly depends on the magnetic field. Of particular interest is the frequency band 2,48 GHz, used by commercial devices based on the short range communication technology Bluetooth. Many works mention the importance to use Bluetooth for communication between intraoral sensors and a smartphone/tablet. Nevertheless, none of these works presents a prototype, mentioning that it will be the next step of the work. From the results shown in [13], 2.48-GHz band is the best choice when the device is operating in the air but its performance significantly declined when the device is located inside the mouth. The 27-MHz band showed the best performance at short distances of 39 cm with negligible interference from the dynamic intraoral environment. The 433.9-MHz band, assisted by an adaptive impedance matching that dynamically minimizes the effect of oral kinematics, showed the best overall and sufficient robustness against head orientation and relative angle between the Tx and Rx antennas.

However, an RF-based communication approach foresees the use of a battery inside the mouth, at least for those important applications that foresee a continuous monitoring. This is one of the main challenges limiting the adoption of intraoral devices for continuous monitoring. Interesting solutions for recharging the sensors are based on the use of the jaw movement that normally occurs when chewing, eating and speaking [14]. For instance, one can obtain approximately 580 J only from daily chewing, which is equivalent to an average power of approximately 7 mW [14]. However, the challenge related to the battery is not only related to the size or the way to recharge it but also to safety issues. The battery and the TX part must be "anchored" in some way to avoid that they are swallowed.

An alternative approach has been proposed in [15, 16] where a passive sensor is inserted in the mouth and read by an external device. In particular, [15] presents a sensor that detects bacteria in the body and passes a signal to a nearby receiver. They have created a removable tattoo that adheres to dental enamel by bundling the silk and gold with graphene. Moreover, they have put on the same tattoo an antenna. An external radio transmitter held nearby the device delivers a signal that causes the device to resonate and transmit back its information. The current design allows for detection at a relatively short but practical distance, roughly a centimeter. In [16], authors propose a new system for measuring human bite forces. The prototype uses a magnetic field communication scheme similar to RFID technology. The reader generates a low-frequency magnetic field that is used as the information carrier and powers the sensor. However, the need to have an external reader, in any case located very close (few centimeters) to the mouth, limits the application of this approach for continuous monitoring.

4 Conclusions

This paper has provided a review of wireless communications for intraoral sensors applications. Because the mouth is an opening into human health, an oral sensory system that would allow real-time monitoring of intraoral parameters/activities open new opportunities for both dentistry applications and more generally wellness applications (i.e., dietary tracking). While some works have been done on the use of wireless communications for intraoral sensors, to really pave the way to a systematic use of this technology, several challenges must be addressed such as need of battery, size of the antennas, propagation in a highly dynamic environment. Safety is a big concern: sensors must to be attached somewhere to avoid swallowing the device. The electronics must remain intact when wet. Moreover, while works on wireless communications for implanted sensors could be used, the intraoral environment has some specific characteristics that calls for a more in depth study of wireless communications for providing reliable links in such a highly time-varying channel.

References

1. Kartsakli, E., Lalos, A.S., Antonopoulos, A., Tennina, S., Di Renzo, M., Alonso, L., Verikoukis, C.: A Survey on M2 M Systems for mHealth: A Wireless Communications Perspective. Sensors **14**, 18009–18052 (2014)
2. Hori, K., et al.: Newly developed sensor sheet for measuring tongue pressure during swallowing. J. Prosthod. Res. **53**, 28–32 (2009)
3. Nishigawa, K., Bando, E., Nakano, M.: Quantitative study of bite force during sleep associated bruxism. J. Oral Rehab. **28**, 485–491 (2001)
4. Peng, Q., Budinger, T.F.: ZigBee-based wireless intra-oral control system for quadriplegic patients. In: IEEE EMBS, pp. 1647–1650 (2007)
5. Sardini, E., Serpelloni, M., Fiorentini, R.: Wireless intraoral sensor for the physiological monitoring of tongue pressure. In: Proceedings of the of IEEE Transducers, pp. 1282–1285 (2013)
6. Park, H., Kiani, M., Lee, H., Kim, J., Block, J., Gosselin, B., Ghovanloo, M.: A wireless magnetoresistive sensing system for an intraoral tongue-computer interface. IEEE Trans. Biomed. Circuits Syst. **6**, 571–585 (2012)
7. Kim, J.H., Jung, J.H.. Jeon, A.Y.. Yoon, S.H.. Son, J.M.. Ye, S.Y.. Jeon, G.R.: System development of indwelling wireless pH Telemetry of intraoral acidity. ITAB IEEE EMBS, pp. 302–305 (2007)
8. Kolahi, J., Fazilati, M.: Bluetooth technology for prevention of dental caries. Med. Hypotheses **73**, 1067–1068 (2009)
9. Brandl, M., et al.: A low-cost wireless sensor system and its application in dental retainers. IEEE Sens. J. **9**, 255–262 (2009)
10. Cho, N., Yoo, J., Song, S., Lee, J., Jeon, S., Yoo, H.: The human body characteristics as a signal transmission medium for intrabody communication. IEEE Trans. Microw. Theor. Tech. 1080–1086 (2007)
11. Chandra, R., Johansson, A.J.: In-mouth antenna for tongue controlled wireless devices: characteristics and link-loss. In: IEEE EMBC, pp. 5598–5601(2011)
12. Yang, C.L., Tsai, C.L., Chen, S.H.: Implantable high-gain dental antennas for minimally invasive biomedical devices. IEEE Trans on Ant. Prop. **60**, 2380–2387 (2013)
13. Park, H., Ghovanloo, M.: Wireless communication of intraoral devices and its optimal frequency selection. IEEE Trans. Microw. Theor. Techn., 3205–3215 (2014)
14. Delnavaz, A., Voix, J.: Flexible piezoelectric energy harvesting from jaw movements. Smart Mater. Struct. **23**, 1–8 (2014)
15. Mannoor, M.S., et al.: Graphene-based wireless bacteria detection on tooth enamel. Nat. Commun. **27**, 763 (2012)
16. Diaz Lantada, A., González Bris, C., Lafont Morgado, P., Sanz Maudes, J.: Novel system for bite-force sensing and monitoring based on magnetic near field communication. Sensors **12**, 11544–11558 (2012)

Special Session on Spectrum Usage: Measurements, Modeling and Optimization

Analysis and Measurements of Wi-Fi Offloading Solutions

Mădălina Oproiu$^{(\boxtimes)}$, Alexandru Vulpe, and Ion Marghescu

Telecommunications Department,
University Politehnica of Bucharest, Bucharest, Romania
elena-madalina.oproiu@sdettib.pub.ro,
alex.vulpe@radio.pub.ro, marion@comm.pub.ro

Abstract. Wi-Fi offloading allows the data traffic, coming from users of smartphones and tablets from congested areas of the 3G/HSDPA network, to be routed over a Wi-Fi network according to certain QoS and congestion parameters. In this paper a way to implement a 3G Wi-Fi offload solution in a cellular network is analyzed. Three offload algorithms that were developed by researchers from different universities are studied. Moreover, network measurements are performed on a real operator network to present current network capabilities to support 3G Wi-Fi offload. The results show that the signal of the two technologies is good enough for a controlled offload, but the network is not yet adapted to support such a transfer.

Keywords: 3G · Wi-Fi · Offload · Algorithm · Traffic · Smartphone · Mobile network

1 Introduction

Over the last years, the explosion of Wi-Fi enabled smartphones and 3G capable tablets combined with the consumer and business demand for bandwidth, real-time video and data applications have increased the data traffic on mobile networks across the world, exponentially. One of the critical challenges facing 3G and 4G Mobile Network Operators (MNOs) is how to deal with this anticipated mobile data tsunami. One solution to control this growth involves "offloading" a proportion of data traffic, typically to Wi-Fi but also perhaps to femtocells or other emerging "small cell" solutions.

3G and Wi-Fi are major communication technologies that are used by most people today. Both these technologies deliver wireless Internet access and services to users. 3G is largely used on mobile phones for purposes such as watching mobile TV, videos on demand, video calls and video conferencing [1]. Because Wi-Fi uses unlicensed shared spectrum, this has important implications for cost of service, quality of service (QoS), congestion management and industry structure.

The speed of a Wi-Fi connection varies, with download speeds as low as 1 Mbps or as high as 600 Mbps. With 3G Internet service, download speeds are approximately 1 Mbps. The average upload speed on a 3G connection is approximately 225 Kbps, depending on signal strength and network congestion and a Wi-Fi connection has upload speeds ranging from approximately 3 to more than 50 Mbps. [2]

© Institute for Computer Sciences, Social Informatics and Telecommunications Engineering 2015
V. Atanasovski, L.-G. Alberto (Eds.): Fabulous 2015, LNICST 159, pp. 127–134, 2015.
DOI: 10.1007/978-3-319-27072-2_16

An extremely important remark is that offloading it not necessarily just about managing tonnage of data, for many operators, this is actually less of a problem, but what can really hurt the network is signaling load [3]. An illustration of 3G Wi-Fi offload can be seen in Fig. 1.

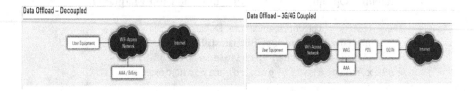

Fig. 1. Data offload decoupled and coupled architecture [4]

The paper is organized as follows: Sect. 2 reviews existing Wi-Fi offloading algorithms; while Sect. 3 presents the logical and physical Wi-Fi Mesh Topology of the Central University Library and measurements made in 3G and Wi-Fi in this zone. Results are shown and discussed in Sect. 4 and, finally, Sect. 5 draws the conclusions.

2 Wi-Fi Offloading Algorithms

A. Wiffler
Wiffler is a system designed by some researchers from the University of Massachusetts, in America. They investigated if Wi-Fi access can be used to enlarge 3G capacity in mobile environments. The system uses two key ideas: increases delay tolerance (when the offload of data is from 3G to Wi-Fi) and fast switching (when the onload of data is from Wi-Fi to 3G).

The input application data for Wiffler are:

S- the size of the transfer
D- the delay tolerance threshold among queued transfers
W: estimated Wi-Fi transfer size
c: conservative quotient–a number between 0 and ∞

Based on these input data and the characteristics of the operating environment, it decides how to distribute the data across 3G and Wi-Fi [5]:

```
if (Wi-Fi is available)

    send data on Wi-Fi and update S

if (W < S *c and 3G is available)

    send data on 3G and update S
```

B. DTP
DTP is a disruption tolerant transport layer protocol. DTP is designed by researchers from the Department of Electrical Engineering, KAIST Daejeon, South Korea. When

the mobile device is connected to a network with his physical underlying unavailable, DTP provide the illusion of continued connection. This mechanism would help the mobile application developers to focus on the application core rather than addressing the frequent network disruptions and reduce the phone network costs. DTP is very useful because supports reliable data delivery on a packet level and it doesn't require any support from the network infrastructure. DTP prototype can be implemented like a user-level UDP library. In terms of functionality DTP is compatible with TCP. [6]

C. HotZones

"HotZones" was designed by a group of researchers from Switzerland and is an algorithm for energy efficient offloading of 3G networks. This is assisted by predictions made by the operator and exploits delay tolerance trying to download contents when users are close to Wi-Fi APs [7].

In the process of HotZones selection, an operator first extracts typical mobility profiles of its subscribers: User Mobility Profiles (UMPs). A UMP is an array of 24 elements, which contains the most visited cell by a user for each hour of the day. With the UMPs created, an operator sorts cells based on the average number of daily visits. Then, a set of HotZones H is chosen, so that a cell with the highest number of daily visits is added first to the set, the second most visited cell is added second, etc. The cardinality of the set H is a tradeoff between the cost of the Wi-Fi deployment and targeted benefits. Because the target is delay-tolerant offloading it makes sense to focus on cells with a high number of daily visits. Once the set of HotZones H is created, an operator sends it to each user, with her UMP.

Parameters used in the HotZones algorithm:

$s_r^u(t)$ - the collection of pending requests of a user u (the user's requests that are still not served at time t).

c - the current cell of the user u.

D - the maximum delay users permit

τ_r - a timer with timeout equal to D, is set by the application

Using these parameters, the application on user's smartphone performs algorithm described below every TP minutes [7]:

```
if ( Sᵘᵣ(t)≠∅) then
    if (c∈ H) then
        Turn on Wi-Fi interface;
        Try to serve all r∈ Sᵘᵣ(t) via Wi-Fi
        // a success with probability p
    else
        Get τᵘₕ=time before u enters a cell ∈ H;
        for all r∈ Sᵘᵣ(t) do
            if (τᵣ expires in ≤ τᵘₕ) then
                Serve r via 3G;
            else
                Do nothing
            end if
        end if
    end if
end if
```

We can observe that the application is based on the user's UMP for the prediction of possible Wi-Fi transfer opportunities within the allowed delay D. If such an opportunity is doesn't appear, the pending requests in the set $s_t^u(t)$ are served immediately through 3G, in order to minimize delivery delays.

D. Comparison Between the Three Algorithms

One of the main characteristics of the three algorithms is that they can reduce 3G usage by offloading a big quantity of data from 3G to Wi-Fi (their goals are to reduce costs and to reduce load in 3G congested cells).

There are situations when is also necessary to onload data from Wi-Fi to 3G because Wi-Fi characteristics are unable to support some applications, with strict QoS requirement, as: VoIP or video conferencing or because there isn't Wi-Fi coverage in that area or Wi-Fi signal is very poor. For these situations Wiffler algorithm with its idea about fast switching is very useful.

The Wiffler and HotZones algorithms are assisted by predictions about Wi-Fi connectivity and they both utilize delay tolerance, but in the case of HotZones the delay has bigger values. A common disadvantage of these algorithms is that the prediction is done with no pre-programmed knowledge about the environment.

By the measurements analyzed above result that DTP and HotZones algorithms reduce battery consumption coming from 3G transfers. This is a welcome improvement because today, one of the biggest problems of smartphones is their high energy consumption. Another advantage of HotZones algorithm is that it offers best offloading performance during the hours when a 3G network is most heavily loaded. Also, HotZones needs a small investment in Wi-Fi APs because it requires 34 times less Wi-Fi cells than the real-time offloading. DTP is very useful because it supports reliable data delivery on a packet level and it does not require any special support from the network infrastructure. All the three algorithms analyzed reduce the per-byte cost of data transfers.

3   Analysis and Measurement Setup

From the analysis of algorithms presented in Sect. 2, we concluded that to seek ways to implement offload in our network, we must first do a study about the performances of the two technologies: 3G and Wi-Fi. For this reason we chose to make the measurements of the latency and speed of the two technologies in the area of the Central University Library (BCU) in Bucharest, Romania. The mobile network is operated by Orange Romania (ORO).

The physical topology of the Wi-Fi environment is presented in Fig. 2, containing the path from end-user terminal client to required Internet services. The Internet connection and MPLS are represented as a cloud and detailed topology is presented until first ORO Customer Edge (CE) /Provider Edge (PE). Wi-Fi management devices involved in this topology such as Wireless LAN Controller (WLC) or Wireless Control System (WCS), are represented, in the topology, as being isolated.

The IP address scheme for client SSID, management and interconnects as well as involved VLANs is used, as provided by mobile operator: Router "ar1-bi0739" to

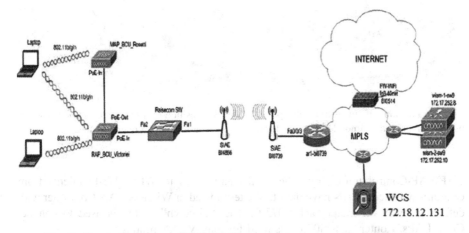

Fig. 2. Physical topology of BCU Wi-Fi network [source: mobile operator docs]

Switch "Raisecom" interconnect uses VLAN 15 and subnet 172.31.106.216/30; WLAN "Orange_WiFi" uses VLAN 210 and subnet 192.168.4.0/22;LAP (Lightweight Access Point) uses VLAN 16 and subnet 10.199.19.128/29.

The logical Topology of BCU is illustrated in Fig. 3. The green line indicates the control-plane traffic (LWAPP/CAPWAP tunnel from each LAP to the WLC) and the red line represents the client traffic from SSID Orange_Wi-Fi. Cisco LAPs use function in bridge mode with SSID "Orange_WiFi" being centrally switched.

The 802.11b/g/n client traffic is encapsulated in CAPWAP-Data traffic from the MAPs and it is sent to WLC. Also the 802.11a/n management traffic is encapsulated in

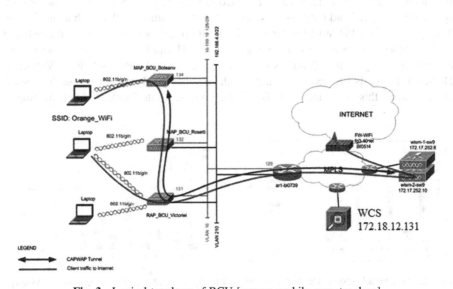

Fig. 3. Logical topology of BCU [source: mobile operator docs]

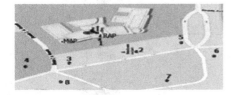
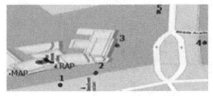

Fig. 4. Position of measurements points used in first scenario [mobile operator docs]

Fig. 5. Position of measurements points used in first scenario [mobile operator docs]

CAPWAP-Control traffic from the MAPs and sends to WLC. Wi-Fi clients from centrally switched VLAN have their traffic terminated in Wireless LAN Controller with default gateway on router "ar1-bi0739". The "raisecom" switch is used to connect Cisco LAPs. Router "ar1-bi0739" is used for inter-VLAN routing.

Measurements were made in 3 different setups with the help of Speed-Test application (this application tests the internet connection and has as results: the latency in ms, download and upload speed of the connection, in Mbps). They were taken at points marked on the map in Fig. 4.

These points were chosen considering the 3G network topology and Wi-Fi in this location (described above). The same measurements were done on the same points, with the same devices, but in different days for testing the accuracy of the Speed Test application and the reasoning for choosing the position of measurement points.

4   Results

Results from the measurements are presented in Figs. 6, 7 and 8 in terms of download speed, upload speed and ping response time. It is seen from these that both technologies have good values, but Wi-Fi is far superior to 3G in terms of the considered metrics.

Very good results in Wi-Fi are obtained in Point1 and Point5. We can observe, on the map from Fig. 4, that Point1 is very close to the central AP: RAP_BCU_Victoriei. However, Point5 is situated far from the both APs, has good results because the line of sight between this point and RAP_BCU_Victoriei isn't interfered. In this technology,

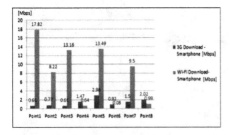
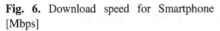

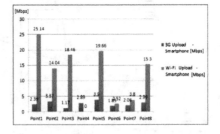

Fig. 6. Download speed for Smartphone [Mbps]

Fig. 7. Upload speed for smartphone [Mbps]

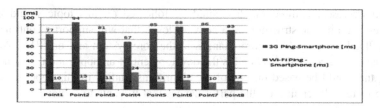

Fig. 8. Latency (ping) for smartphone [ms] -different technologies

the worst results were obtained in point 6 as line of sight between it and the two APs is interfered by the statue of Carol I.

The value of pings is also very good in this technology, in average 13 ms. From the graphics we can observe that in terms of latency, download and upload speed Wi-Fi is better than 3G. 3G technology results are also good, average values of 1.36 Mbps download, 2.57 Mbps upload and 82.65 ms ping is good even to very good.

In this area, if we have congestion in 3G network, we could successfully do a 3G Wi-Fi offload as Wi-Fi network signal is good enough to handle. Otherwise, if we have too many users in Wi-Fi or the users have applications that require QoS, Wi-Fi 3G onload would be the best solution. So the signal level of the two technologies is good enough for a controlled offload.

We also consider another scenario with the points of measurement presented in Fig. 5. First we are sitting in Point 1 near Rap_BCU_Victoriei and the smartphone is set in Wi-Fi (very close to the AP) and then we move in Point 2, Point 3 and when we moved in Point 4 we observed that Wi-Fi signal is very poor and the ping response time increases radically. In point 5 (near 3G antenna) the Wi-Fi signal is lost and the device switches automatically to 3G.

The 3G coverage is higher, so it is more difficult to lose the signal. The Wi-Fi signal has good value but has the disadvantage of more often losing the signal when the device is out of range of the APs. These measurements was made to show that there is a primitive offload (transition in Point5 of Wi-Fi to 3G) in network but this isn't a controlled offload and doesn't take into account all aspects required to realize a pure offload. For example it is possible to be in Wi-Fi coverage and the signal is weak (but not missing) and the device detects 3G coverage nearby and switches to 3G. It is possible that the 3G network can have too many users and the signal received by the device is very weak, and upload and download values to be smaller than initial values of Wi-Fi. Doing this uncontrolled transition we deplete the device's battery faster (consumption in 3G is higher).

5   Conclusions

From these measurements, we obtained that, in the measured areas, of interest to the mobile network operator, latency and UL/DL speed are superior in Wi-Fi than 3G. So, in this area, a Wi-Fi 3G offload can be done, but unfortunately it isn't currently controlled (doesn't take account aspects of QoS and network management).

A future research direction that could be followed on this topic would be the implementation of one structure, on a network level, that will support a controlled 3G Wi-Fi offload (this would require changes in the core system and on SIM). Another way to achieve a controlled offload is the development of an application for Android / iPhone, that could be based on one of the algorithms studied in this paper or a combination thereof depending on the performances that it wants to achieve.

Acknowledgment. We thank Ana Rosu from Orange Romania for help with the measurement set up, and for help with collecting data in Bucharest. This work was supported by the department Development and Innovation from Orange Romania and it has been funded by the Sectorial Operational Programme Human Resources Development of the Ministry of European Funds through the Financial Agreement POSDRU/187/1.5/S/155420.

References

1. http://www.buzzle.com/articles/3g-vs-wifi.html
2. Mobile Data Offloading through Wi-Fi, Commissioned by Proxim Wireless (2010)
3. Disruptive Analysis, "Carrier Wi-Fi Opportunities", Commissioned by iPass Inc, August 2011
4. Wi-Fi Data Offload –Turning Challenge into Opportunity, Commissioned by Motorola
5. Augmenting Mobile 3G Using Wi-Fi, http://research.microsoft.com/pubs/135671/mobisys2010-wiffler.pdf
6. A Disruption-tolerant Transmission Protocol for Practical Mobile Data Offloading, Department of Electrical Engineering, KAIST, Daejeon, South Korea
7. Energy Efficient Offloading of 3G Networks, Nikodin Ristanovic, Jean-Yves Le Boudec, Augustin Chaintreau and Vijay Erramilli

Case Study Analysis of DTV Signal Reception Near Large Water Surface

Pero Latkoski[1(✉)], Liljana Gavrilovska[1], Lidija Paunovska[2],
and Pavlos Lazaridis[3]

[1] Faculty of Electrical Engineering and Information Technologies,
Saints Cyril and Methodius University in Skopje, Skopje, Macedonia
{pero,liljana}@feit.ukim.edu.mk
[2] The Agency for Electronic Communications, Skopje, Macedonia
lidija.paunovska@aec.mk
[3] Alexander Technological Educational Institute of Thessaloniki,
Thessaloniki, Greece
pavloslazaridis@hotmail.com

Abstract. Today many different propagation models predict the coverage area of digital television (DTV) services providing various level of precision on case-by-case manner. These models tend to be very inaccurate in situations that are not nominal to the appropriate propagation model definition. The general aim of this paper is to investigate the possible problems related to the near-large-water-surface DTV reception and its prediction. The work involves a case study radio spectrum measurements and signals calculation utilizing existing propagation models. In particular, the paper provides a numerical comparison of calculated and measured TV signal levels for several points near the Dojran Lake on both sides of the Macedonian-Greek border. The values reveal significant dependence between the receiving signal strength and the antenna height, as well as its micro-location, which prove that such locations represent a big challenge for coverage area prediction and control.

Keywords: DTV · Reflection · Water surface · Propagation model · Measurements

1 Introduction and Related Work

The implementation of digital television systems requires precise radio wave prediction and planning. Calculating the propagation of radio signals can answer some crucial questions related to the DTV system operation, such as: Could the system operate correctly, i.e. will the required signal intensity/quality of service over required distance/area, given the geographic/climatic region and time period be on a satisfactory level? Furthermore, the planning of the DTV system is necessary for avoiding possible coexistence problems with other systems, which can result in degradation of service quality and/or service range/area due to potential radio interference. Generally, DTV system planners need a reliable propagation model that will suit for different terrains and variety of conditions [1].

© Institute for Computer Sciences, Social Informatics and Telecommunications Engineering 2015
V. Atanasovski, L.-G. Alberto (Eds.): Fabulous 2015, LNICST 159, pp. 135–141, 2015.
DOI: 10.1007/978-3-319-27072-2_17

Modeling and signal coverage predictions are also essential for efficient utilization of the radio spectrum, as well as for performance optimization of the existing systems. For example, a reliable model of predicting path loss helps in reducing load on base stations and helps in designing digital broadcasting networks including TV services [2]. For these reasons, the authors of [2] have considered Mauritius Island as a case study analysis. From the observations and results obtained, it is concluded that the existing empirical models are not accurate and therefore cannot be used in this case since the target area is small and is characterized as tropical and mountainous. The authors found that a general limitation of existing models is that they are developed for limited categories of land (open area, sub-urban and urban areas). Therefore the path loss analysis is conducted and tested using several models. But, before developing novel models, the paper proposes defining of small and homogenous regions and areas, each with specific propagation model.

Similarly, the territory of Republic of Macedonia characterizes with wide range of geographical varieties, including high hills and mountains, wide plateaus, deep canyons and valleys, as well as shoreline features around several natural and artificial lakes. This implies propagation models tuning in order to precisely fit for different regions and areas, including possible reception problems anticipation. So far, we have analyzed a highly urban area of the capitol Skopje [3], but it is obvious that the near water surface areas tend to be the most challenging region type, and this paper provides the initial findings for this kind of region analysis.

The reminder of the paper is organized as follows. Section 2 contains the theoretical background related to the near water surface propagation of radio signals. The case study description is included in Sect. 3, which also provides the results of the conducted measurements and calculations. Finally, Sect. 4 provides the conclusions and future work.

2 Theoretical Background

When radio waves impinge a flat surface, the surface reflects them in the same manner as light waves. In general, the strength of the reflected wave depends upon the angle of incidence (the angle between the incident ray and the horizon), frequency, polarization and surface's reflecting properties [4]. Radio waves of all frequencies are reflected by wide flat surfaces. In such situations, a phase change of the wave occurs. The amount of the change varies with the polarization of the wave and with the conductivity of the Earth, reaching a maximum of 180° for a horizontally polarized wave reflected from wide water surface (considering to have infinite conductivity), which is exactly the case of DTV signals received near a lake.

When direct waves (those traveling from transmitter to receiver in a straight line) and reflected waves arrive at the receiver antenna, the total signal is the vector sum of the two. If the signals are in phase, they reinforce each other, producing a stronger signal. If there is a phase difference, the signals tend to cancel each other, the cancellation being complete if the phase difference is 180° and the two signals have the same amplitude. This interaction of waves is called wave interference. A phase difference may occur because of the change of phase of the reflected wave, or because of the longer path it follows. The second effect decreases with greater distance between transmitter and receiver.

The 2-ray ground reflection model is a useful propagation model that is based on geometric optics, and considers both direct path and a ground reflected propagation path between transmitter and receiver (Fig. 1) [5]. This model has been found to be reasonably accurate for predicting the large-scale signal strength over distances of several kilometers for communication systems that use tall towers (heights which exceeds 50 m), as well as for line-of-sight microcell channels in urban environments.

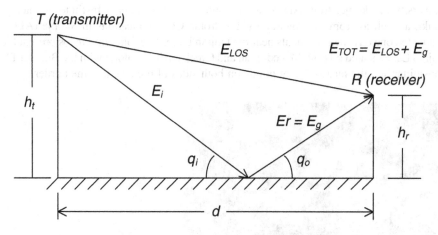

Fig. 1. Two-ray ground reflection model [5]

In most communication systems the maximum T-R separation distance is at most only a few tens of kilometers, and the earth may be assumed to be flat. The total received E-field, E_{TOT}, is then a result of the direct line-of-sight component, E_{LOS}, and the ground reflected component E_g.

Referring to the Fig. 1, h_t is the height of the transmitter and h_r is the height of the receiver. When the T-R separation distance d is very large compared to $h_r + h_t$, the received E-field can be calculated as

$$E_{TOT}\left(d, t = \frac{d''}{c}\right) \approx \frac{E_0 d_0}{d}[\cos\theta_\Delta - 1] \tag{1}$$

where d is the distance over a flat earth between the bases of the transmitter and receiver antennas, E_0 is the free space E-field (in units V/m) at a reference distance d_0 from the transmitter, and $-\Delta$ is the phase difference between the two E-field components at the receiver, calculated as

$$\theta_\Delta = \frac{2\pi\Delta}{\lambda} \tag{2}$$

and

$$\Delta = d'' - d' \approx \frac{2h_t h_r}{d}. \tag{3}$$

3 Case Study and Results

In order to investigate the problems related to DTV signal propagation and reflections from wide water surface, a team involving members from the Ss Cyril and Methodius University in Skopje, from Alexander Technological Educational Institute of Thessaloniki, as well as from the Agency for Electronic Communications in Skopje (AEC), conducted one day measurements near the Dojran Lake. The following maps present the Dojran Lake located on both Macedonian and Greek territory, along with the Boskija TV transmitter and the measurement points on both sides of the lake and the border.

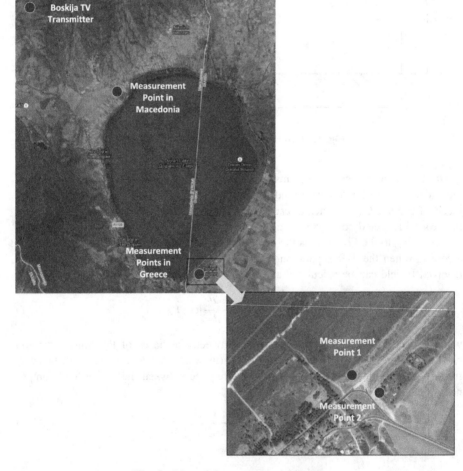

Fig. 2. Map of the measurement locations

The measurement locations on the Macedonian side and on the Greek side differ significantly in terms of their relative position to the TV transmitter and the lake location. The measurement location in Macedonia has an unobstructed line-of-sight communication with the TV transmitter and there are no significant sources of reflections. Figure 3 displays the transmitter location (on the left), as seen from the measurement point in Macedonia and the measurement location itself (on the right).

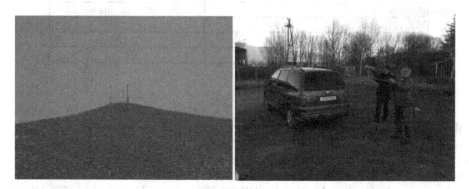

Fig. 3. Boskija transmitter (on the left) seen from the measurement point in Macedonia (on the right)

The measurement location in Greece has also line-of-sight with the transmitter location, but the Dojran Lake lies in between these two locations. This suggests that there is a high possibility for signal reflection from the lake surface, which implies using of several micro locations for measurement on this particular site (see the map in Fig. 2). Figure 4 depicts the Dojran Lake shore (on the left) and one of the measurement micro-locations on the Greek side of the lake (on the right).

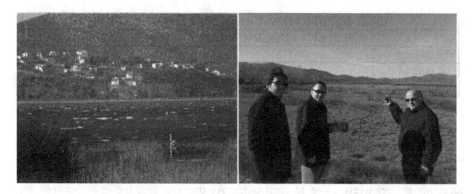

Fig. 4. Dorjan Lake shore (on the left) and measurement point in Greece (on the right)

Table 1 provides the flat terrain distances between the Boskija transmitter and the three measurement points (one in Macedonia: *MK point* and two in Greece: *GR point 1* and *GR point 2*), as well as the terrain height above the see level for each of these locations.

Table 1. Characteristics of the measurement locations

	Distance from TX [km]	Terrain Height [m]
Boskija TX	/	706 + 40 (Antenna tower)
MK point	4.946	158
GR point 1	12.66	149
GR point 2	12.7	151

As one can see from Table 1, *GR point 1* and *GR point 2* are separated for about thirty meters, but also there is a height difference of the terrain between these to points of about 2 meters.

The Boskija TV transmitter broadcasts several digital multiplexes, among which for this case study two are of particular interest: on TV channel 21 (474 MHz) signals belonging to the DigiPlus Multimedia (DIGIPLUS) and on TV channel 34 (578 MHz) signals belonging to the Macedonian Public Broadcasting Company (JPMRD). Both of these transmissions were analyzed at the target points by means of calculations and measurement. AEC provided the calculation tool, which in this case was *LStelcom* calculator, while the measurements were conducted using the latest Rohde and Schwarz FSH 8 spectrum analyzer.

Table 2 presents the obtained results as a difference between the measured and calculated values of the field strength for each of the locations. For the purpose of calculation, the tool used the Longley-Rice propagation model.

Table 2. Case Study results

ERROR [dB] = MEASUREMENT - CALCULATION		
	CH 21 (474 MHz) DIGIPLUS	CH 34 (578 MHz) JPMRD
MK point	-1.791	-1.421
GR point 1	-2.071	-1.681
GR point 2	-5.441	-8.941

The results reveal that in general the Longley-Rice propagation model overestimates the receiving signal strength for all target points. Furthermore, the difference in the values for the two points located in Greece is significantly high, although those two locations are relatively close to each other. As one can see, the error between the measurements and calculations for *GR point 1* and *GR point 2* varies from 1.6 up to 9 dB. The main reason for these variations is the different impact of the signals reflection from the lake surface, which causes different values of the total received signal at the two measurement points on the Greek side of the lake. It is obvious that the micro-location of the receiving TV antenna can significantly influence the receiving signal level, which in some cases can cause reception degradation.

4 Conclusions and Future Work

Near lake areas prove to be very challenging in providing satisfactory reception level of television signals. Although, DTV system is in a way "immune" to signal reflections, this is not completely true, as for many towns located close to large water surfaces, e.g. lakes or the sea, reflections are strong and there are rather large reflecting angles, given the relatively short distances from the transmitters. The measurements in this case study reveal that small variations in receiving antenna height or antenna location relative to the water surface boundaries, cause significant signal level variations up to 10 dB. This implies the necessity for custom-made propagation models that will be used in the TV coverage prediction for near water areas. There are few methods to overcome the problem with near lake TV signal reception, but in the end the most effective one tends to be a simple shielding of the reception antenna from the reflected beam, by lowering it and using the roof of buildings to prevent the reception of the reflected signal.

In order to provide more precise numerical values related to the near lakes TV signal reception and the related phenomena, the future work will include more measurement campaigns, as well as propagation model tuning in order to provide close matching of the calculated and measured values.

Acknowledgment. This work was supported by the Public Diplomacy Division of NATO in the framework of Science for Peace through the SfP-984409 Optimization and Rational Use of Wireless Communication Bands (ORCA) project [6]. The authors would like to thank everyone involved.

References

1. Ebdelli, M.H.: Radio wave propagation and planning. In: CoE/ARB Workshop On Transition from Analog to Digital (Digital Terrestrial Television: Trends, Implementation & Opportunities), Tunisia – Tunis, 12 – 15 March 2012
2. Armoogum, V., Soyjaudah, K.M.S., Mohamudally, N., Fogarty, T.: Propagation models and their applications in digital television broadcast network design and implementation. In: Bouras, C.J. (ed.) Trends in Telecommunications Technologies, 1 March 2010. ISBN 978-953-307-072-8
3. Denkovska, M., Latkoski, P., Gavrilovska, L.: Optimization of spectrum usage and coexistence analysis of DVB-T and LTE-800 systems. Wireless Pers. Commun., 1–18. Springer (2015). ISSN: 0929-6212
4. Sadiku, M., Sagliocca, J., Soriyan, O.: Elements of Electromagnetics, 3rd edn. Oxford University Press Inc., New York (2001)
5. Rappaport, T.S.: Wireless Communications: Principles and Practice, 2nd edn. Prentice Hall, Upper Saddle River (2002). ISBN 10: 0130422320, 13: 9780130422323
6. http://orca.feit.ukim.edu.mk

Performance Analysis of MUSIC and Capon DOA Estimation Algorithms in Cognitive Radio Networks

Cosmina-Valentina Năstase[⊠], Octavian Fratu, Alexandru Martian, and Ion Marghescu

Telecommunications Department, University Politehnica of Bucharest,
Iuliu Maniu 1-3, 061071 Bucharest, Romania
cosmina@radio.pub.ro, ofratu@elcom.pub.ro

Abstract. Many spectrum sensing algorithms have as a purpose determining if the primary users (PUs) are present or absent, by using statistical signal characteristics. However, for a better management of a cognitive network, additional information about PUs, such as their position, is required. Motivated by these requirements, this paper investigate the performance of MUSIC and Capon algorithms in Cognitive Radio networks context and show that the MUSIC algorithm is highly accurate and stable while also providing a high angular resolution compared to the Capon algorithm.

Keywords: DOA · Cognitive network · MUSIC · Capon

1 Introduction

In cognitive radio (CR) systems, when the licensed users let temporarily free some parts of the spectrum, secondary users (SU) are allowed to opportunistically reuse them. In accordance with this purpose, SUs must be able to perform spectrum sensing in order to identify primary user (PU) presence or absence [1].

There are many recent papers in literature where the performance of DoA methods is analyzed [2–4], but few of them includes these studies in the cognitive radio network context [5–7]. Motivated by these considerations, in this paper we concentrate on PU localization methods based on direction-of-arrival (DoA) estimates.

2 DOA Estimation Algorithms

Knowledge about the positions of the primary users is necessary for the secondary network, as it can be used to implement power control mechanisms, to design routing protocols for location-aware and to handle mobility of the SUs. For this reason spectrum-sensing devices should be able not only to detect primary signals, but also to localize their sources [8]. The DoA of primary signals can be estimated in different ways, for example by directional antennas or antenna arrays. In the second case, the sensors are equipped with multiple antennas, or they consist of multiple users cooperating with each other ("virtual arrays") [8].

© Institute for Computer Sciences, Social Informatics and Telecommunications Engineering 2015
V. Atanasovski, L.-G. Alberto (Eds.): Fabulous 2015, LNICST 159, pp. 142–148, 2015.
DOI: 10.1007/978-3-319-27072-2_18

2.1   System Model

We consider an uniform linear array (ULA) of N sensors, as shown in Fig. 1, and n primary users signals $\{s_i(t); i = 1,\ldots,n\}$ impinging from distinct unknown directions $\{\theta_i\}$[2]. The array observation vector $y(t)$ can be expressed as:

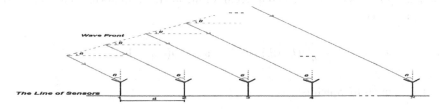

Fig. 1. The uniform linear array scenario

$$\mathbf{y}(t) = \mathbf{A}\mathbf{s}(t) + \mathbf{w}(t) = [y_1(t),\ldots,y_N(t)]^T \tag{1}$$

where

$$\mathbf{A} = [\mathbf{a}(\theta_1),\ldots,\mathbf{a}(\theta_n)] \tag{2}$$

$$s(t) = [s_1(t),\ldots,s_n(t)]^T \tag{3}$$

$$\mathbf{w}(t) = [w_1(t),\ldots,w_n(t)]^T \tag{4}$$

In the above equations, $\mathbf{A}$ is the matrix of the steering vectors, $\mathbf{s}(t)$ is the PU signals vector, $\mathbf{w}(t)$ is the additive white noise vector and $\mathbf{a}(\theta_i)$ is the steering vector written as:

$$\mathbf{a}(\theta_i) = \left[1, e^{-jw_c\tau_{1,i}},\ldots,e^{-jw_c\tau_{N,i}}\right]^T \tag{5}$$

with $w_c = \frac{2\pi c}{\lambda}$ and λ the wavelength of the PU signals.

Let denote the distance between two consecutive sensors, then:

$$\tau_{k,j} = (k-1)\frac{d\sin\theta_i}{c}, \quad \theta_i \in \left[-\frac{\pi}{2},\frac{\pi}{2}\right] \tag{6}$$

where c is the velocity of the impinging waveform, the superscript T denotes the transpose and λ is the signal wavelength. The covariance matrix for $y(t)$ is:

$$\mathbf{R} = E\left[\mathbf{y}(t)\mathbf{y}^H(t)\right] = \mathbf{A}E\left[\mathbf{s}(t)\mathbf{s}^H(t)\right]\mathbf{A}^H + E\left[\mathbf{w}(t)\mathbf{w}^H(t)\right] = \mathbf{A}\mathbf{S}\mathbf{A}^H + \sigma^2\mathbf{I}_N \tag{7}$$

where σ^2 is the noise variance, $\mathbf{I}_N$ is the $\mathbf{N} \times \mathbf{N}$ identity matrix, H is the Hermitian operator and $\mathbf{S}$ is the $\mathbf{n} \times \mathbf{n}$ primary users signals covariance matrix [2].

Having the array model derived above, the problem of DOA estimation can be reduced to that of the $\{\theta_k\}$ parameters estimation.

2.2   Capon Algorithm and Beamforming Technique

The Capon algorithm is based on a filter bank and beamforming technique. The principle of the beamforming method is to steer the array in one direction at a time and measure the output power. The key of the Capon's method is to minimize the power contributed by noise and any signals coming from other direction than desired [5]. Considering h as being the weighting vector of the filter, the following condition must be accomplished:

$$\min_{h} \left(h^H \mathbf{R} h\right) \textbf{ subject to } \left|h^H \mathbf{a}(\theta)\right| = 1,$$

the solution of which is:

$$h = \frac{\mathbf{R}^{-1}\mathbf{a}(\theta)}{\mathbf{a}^H(\theta)\mathbf{R}^{-1}\mathbf{a}(\theta)} \tag{8}$$

The Capon DOA estimates are obtained as the locations of the n maximum peaks of the function:

$$\mathbf{P}_c(\theta) = \frac{1}{\mathbf{a}^H(\theta)\mathbf{R}^{-1}\mathbf{a}(\theta)} \tag{9}$$

2.3   MUSIC Algorithm

The MUSIC (Multiple Signal Classification) algorithm is one of the most used in various treatments such as array processing [9]. MUSIC deals with the decomposition of the covariance matrix into two orthogonal matrices, i.e., signal-subspace and noise-subspace [4]. The following equation shows this decomposition:

$$\mathbf{R} = \mathbf{V}\mathbf{\Lambda}\mathbf{V}^H \tag{10}$$

where Λ is the eigen values diagonal matrix and V is the matrix of the eigenvector. Let $\mathbf{V}_n$ be the matrix constructed of the corresponding n signal eigenvectors and $\mathbf{V}_w$ be the matrix containing the remaining $N - n$ noise eigenvectors.

Thus, the MUSIC Pseudospectrum is given as:

$$\mathbf{P_M}(\theta) = \frac{1}{\mathbf{a}^H(\theta)\mathbf{V}_w\mathbf{V}_w^H\mathbf{a}(\theta)} \tag{11}$$

and the DOA estimates are obtained as the locations of the n largest peaks of the function.

3 Simulation Results

3.1 Accuracy Analysis

For the accuracy analysis of the algorithms mentioned above, we simulated in Matlab, for each method, a scenario with three radiant sources and a ULA system (Fig. 2).

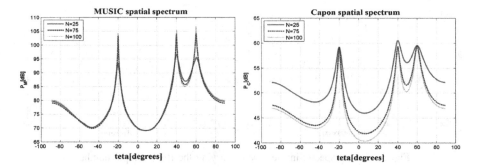

Fig. 2. Spatial spectra in sensors number variation case

We chose for the covariance matrix of PU signals the following value: $S = [1 \quad 0.6 \quad 0.8 \, ; 0.6 \quad 1 \quad 0.5; 0.8 \quad 0.5 \quad 1]$, an observing samples number of $U = 400$, the angles that had to be estimated were $\theta = [-20°, 40°, 60°]$ and 2000 trials were run.

The sensors number variation The simulation parameters in this case were $N = [25, 75, 100]$, $d = \lambda/2$, the samples number of Inverse Fast Fourier Transform $M = 1000$ and a $SNR = 20dB$

For obtaining the exact values of estimated values, we also developed the Root versions of the Capon and MUSIC algorithms. From the Table 1, it can be observed that the most accurate estimates are provided by MUSIC method, which presents the lowest deviations from the expected values.

Table 1. The mean values and the deviations from the required angles in the case of varying the sensor's number.

θ		$-20°$	$40°$	$60°$	Δ_{θ_1}	Δ_{θ_2}	Δ_{θ_3}
N = 25	Capon	-19.9006	39.8000	60.2806	0.0994	0.2000	0.2806
	MUSIC	-20.0256	40.0668	60.0164	0.0256	0.0668	0.0164
N = 75	Capon	-19.9745	39.9538	60.0439	0.0255	0.0462	0.0439
	MUSIC	-20.0089	40.0194	59.9683	0.0089	0.0194	0.0317
N = 100	Capon	-19.9802	39.9656	60.0356	0.0198	0.0344	0.0356
	MUSIC	-20.0063	40.0157	59.9740	0.0063	0.0157	0.0260

Sample number variation of the Inverse Fast Fourier Transform. The simulation parameters were $M = [100, 500, 1000]$, $d = \lambda/2$, $N = 75$ and $SNR = 20dB$. The spatial spectrum values in dB increase with increasing the samples number of Inverse Fast Fourier Transform. The best estimations are given by MUSIC algorithm (Fig. 3).

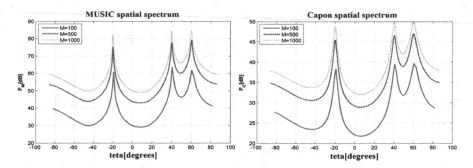

Fig. 3. Spatial spectra in the case of varying the IFFT sample number

Table 2. The mean values and the deviations from the required angles in the case of varying the IFFT sample number

θ_i		$-20°$	$40°$	$60°$	Δ_{θ_1}	Δ_{θ_2}	Δ_{θ_3}
M = 100	Capon	-19.9746	39.9541	60.0450	0.0254	0.0459	0.0450
	MUSIC	-20.0091	40.0198	59.9696	0.0091	0.0198	0.0304
M = 500	Capon	-19.9752	39.9555	60.0419	0.0248	0.0445	0.0419
	MUSIC	-20.0102	40.0219	59.9650	0.0102	0.0219	0.0350
M = 1000	Capon	-19.9749	39.9541	60.0439	0.0251	0.0459	0.0439
	MUSIC	-20.0097	40.0198	59.9681	0.0097	0.0198	0.0319

3.2   Resolution Analysis

For this simulation, there were used: $d = \lambda/2$, $N = 75$, $M = 1000$ and the angles that must be estimated equal with $\theta = \left[-20°, 25°\right]$ and $SNR = [10, 20, 30]dB$.

3.3   Cramer Rao Lower Bound

The simulations where run considering $\theta = \left[-20°, 40°, 60°\right]$ and three values for $SNR = [-10, 0, 10]dB$ and $f_s = d/\lambda * \sin\theta$, with formula $\text{var}\left(\hat{\theta}\right) \geq \left(\frac{\partial g(f_s)}{\partial f_s}\right)^2 \Big/ - E\left[\frac{\partial^2 \ln p(x; f_s)}{\partial f_s^2}\right]$

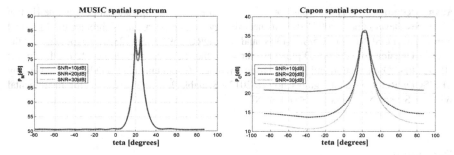

Fig. 4. Spatial spectra in SNR variation

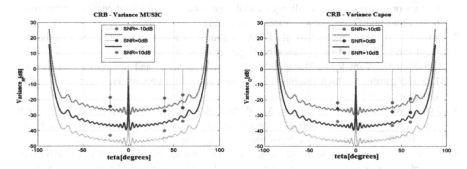

Fig. 5. The estimated angles variances and CRB in SNR variation

4 Conclusion

In this paper, the Direction of Arrival of the primary user signal has been studied and the performace of the MUSIC and Capon angle estimation algorithms was analyzed (Fig. 4).

The simulation results clearly indicate that the performance of the two DOA algorithms improves with more elements in the array, with higher samples number of IFFT and greater SNR. The MUSIC algorithm provides the best mean values of the estimated angles and the lowest deviations from the real values of the estimated angles, in condition of correlated PU signals. The Capon method is also very sensitive to *SNR* variation in terms of resolution, while the MUSIC method provides very good precision in estimations of the required PU directions. By contrast, the MUSIC algorithm requires a precise calibration, being sensitive to the sensor's position (Fig. 5).

Results highlight a new posibility of multiplexing primary and secondary users into the same geographical area with the aim of increasing channel capacity and improving frequency reuse capability. Knowing the primary users DoA, the SUs can transmit in other directions than the PUs. The results can be widely used in the design of smart antenna system and recommend the MUSIC method as the first option in advanced implementations (Table 2).

Acknowledgment. This work has been funded by the Sectorial Operational Programme Human Resources Development 2007-2013 of the Ministry of European Funds through the Financial Agreement POSDRU/159/1.5/S/134398 and POSDRU/159/1.5/S/132395, supported by the NATO Division of Public Diplomacy through the Science for Peace Research Project SfP-984409 "Optimization and Rational use of Wireless Communication Bands"(ORCA) and by UEFISCDI Romania under grants no. 20/2012 "Scalable Radio Transceiver for Instrumental Wireless Sensor Networks - SaRaT-IWSN".

References

1. Penna, F., Wang, J., Cabric, D.: Cooperative localization of primary users by directional antennas or antenna arrays: challenges and design issues. In: IEEE International Symposium on Antennas and Propagation - Proceedings (2011)
2. Devendra, M., Manjunathachari, K.: DOA estimation of a system using MUSIC method. In: Signal Processing And Communication Engineering Systems (2015)
3. Bakhar, V.M., Vani R.M., Hunagund, P.V.: Implementation and optimization of modified MUSIC algorithm for high resolution DOA estimation. In: International Microwaves and RF Conference (2014)
4. Abdalla, M., Abuitbel, M., Hassan, M.: Performance evaluation of direction of arrival estimation using MUSIC and ESPRIT algorithms for mobile communication systems. In: 6th Joint IFIP Wireless and Mobile Networking Conference (2013)
5. Dhope, T., Simunic, D.: On the performance of DoA estimation algorithms in cognitive radio networks: -a new aproach in spectrum sensing. In: 36th International Convention on Information & Communication Technology Electronics & Microelectronics (2013)
6. Dhope, T., Simunic, D., Dhokariya, N., Pawar, V., Gupta, B.: Performance analysis of angle of arrival estimation algorithms for dynamic spectrum access in cognitive radio networks. In: Advanced in Computing Communications and Informatics (2013)
7. Zhaoo, Y., Anagnostou, D., Huang, J., Sohraby, K.: AoA based sensing and performance analysis in cognitive radio networks. In: National Wireless Research Collaboration Symposium (2014)
8. Penna, F., Cabric, D.: Bounds and tradeoffs for cooperative DoA-only localization of primary users. In: IEEE Global Telecommunications Conference (2011)
9. Oumar, O.A., Siyau, M.F., Sattar, T.P.: Comparison between MUSIC and ESPRIT direction of arrival estimation algorithms for wireless communication systems. In: International Conference on Future Generation Communication Technology (2012)

Power Allocation Algorithm for LTE-800 Coverage Optimization and DVB-T Coexistence

Marija Denkovska, Daniel Denkovski$^{(\boxtimes)}$, Vladimir Atanasovski, and Liljana Gavrilovska

Faculty of Electrical Engineering and Information Technologies,
Saints Cyril and Methodius University in Skopje, Skopje, Macedonia
denkovska_marija@yahoo.com,
{danield,vladimir,liljana}@feit.ukim.edu.mk

Abstract. Power control in LTE wireless networks is essential for efficient co-channel interference management. Due to the non-convexity of the problem, the the global maximization of the weighted sum rate through power allocation is difficult to achieve. Moreover, the digital switchover and the reallocation of the upper UHF band (790–860 MHz) for LTE-800 cellular networks contribute for the necessity to control the aggregate interference caused to the DVB-T service. This paper develops an algorithm for optimal power allocation for the LTE system, which targets minimization of the adjacent channel interference onto the DVB-T system and capacity/coverage optimization of the LTE-800 macro cells. The algorithm adopts the local d.c. (difference of convex functions) programming approach and constraints the power based on the relevant DVB-T adjacent channel protection ratios (PRs). The simulation results emphasize the significance of the proposed algorithm, revealing substantial performance gains compared with the case of no power control, in terms of capacity per pixel, coverage probability and probability for pixel DVB-T service degradation.

Keywords: LTE-800 · BS · PR · Macro-cell power allocation · Coverage/capacity optimization · DVB-T coexistence

1 Introduction

Inter-cell co-channel interference (ICI) still remains a crucial issue in the LTE macro-cell deployment and is the dominant LTE aggregate capacity/coverage limiting factor, especially for the cell-edge users [1, 2]. The power allocation is one of the most important resource allocation and interference management approaches capable of reducing or completely eliminating the ICI for cell-edge users and, subsequently, increasing the overall LTE system coverage and capacity. Achieving sum rate/through put maximization through power control is an open problem in interference-limited wireless networks due to the non-convex coupling of the mutual interferences into the optimization problem formulation. There are several research efforts in the area of sum rate maximization. Most of them try to convexify the power allocation problem using approximations [3] in different SNR regimes. The remaining employ more advanced

© Institute for Computer Sciences, Social Informatics and Telecommunications Engineering 2015
V. Atanasovski, L.-G. Alberto (Eds.): Fabulous 2015, LNICST 159, pp. 149–155, 2015.
DOI: 10.1007/978-3-319-27072-2_19

methods of: multiplicative fractional linear [4], geometric [5] or local D.C. [6] (difference of two convex functions/sets) programming to make the problem convex and solve it.

The digital switchover and the reallocation of the upper UHF band (790–860 MHz) for LTE-800 cellular networks lead to interference concerns [7–9], especially for the DVB-T receivers. They operate in near spectral proximity to the LTE systems and are subject to extensive out-band interference from the LTE downlink transmissions (791–821 MHz). This stems from the fact that most current off-the-shelf DVB-T receivers are still designed to receive signals in the full UHF band. The DVB-T coexistence problems are becoming substantial as the number of LTE-800 macro-cell deployments increases (thus, increasing the aggregate interference). These problems can be efficiently solved by constraining the transmitted power of the LTE-800 macro cell transmissions and, hence, controlling the aggregate interference caused to the DVB-T service.

This paper presents a novel power optimization algorithm for capacity/coverage optimization of LTE-800 macro-cells that efficiently solves the DVB-T aggregate interference issues. The proposed power allocation algorithm adopts the local D.C. programming approach [6] aiming to maximize the capacity of macro-cell-edge users, whilst limiting the aggregate out-band interference caused to DVB-T receivers in interference-critical geographical areas.

2   System Model and Algorithm Description

The paper assumes a system model with an LTE-800 network deployment comprising M macro base stations exploiting the fully allocated DL band (as part of the digital dividend 1) for high spectral efficiency. Let $p: = (p_1, p_2,..., p_M)$ be the downlink transmit power vector, where p_i is the transmitted power of BS i. The power-based coverage optimization algorithm of the LTE-800 network operates in an iterative

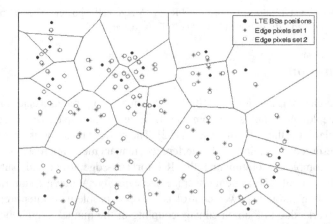

Fig. 1. LTE edge pixels selection criterion for two different algorithm iterations (The blue colored circles denote the LTE BSs while the green and red colored marks represent the two consecutive edge pixels sets) (Color figure online)

manner, starting from the maximum possible downlink transmit power for each LTE macro-cell: $p_0 := (p_{1max}, p_{2max}, \ldots, p_{Mmax})$.

2.1   Coverage Optimization Problem

The algorithm selects a set of critical edge pixels (users) between each pair of Voronoi neighboring base stations in a single iteration (Fig. 1). These pixels satisfy a selected target $SINR_t$, based on the previous LTE BS power allocations. In every current iteration, the proposed algorithm performs the weighted sum rate optimization for all of the N edge-users using local D.C. programming [6], inherently increasing the aggregate area covered with $SINR > SINR_t$ (the aggregate LTE coverage area), as well as the overall system capacity.

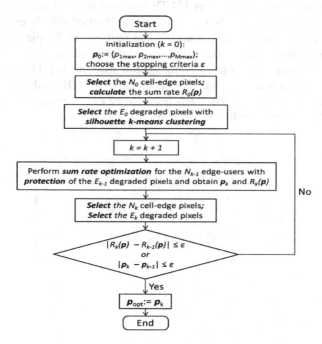

Fig. 2. Flowchart algorithm description

2.2   DVB-T Protection Constraint

The protection of the critical DVB-T pixels is performed as a subject to the weighted sum rate optimization. The DVB-T aggregate interference constraints are derived based on the relevant DVB-T Protection Ratios - PRs (extensively evaluated by the European regulatory bodies [7, 8]). This paper uses the derived protection ratios in [7] to assess the DVB-T service degradation in the pixels. In each iteration, the algorithm, first, clusters the degraded pixels based on silhouette k-means clustering [10] and, afterwards, selects the lead pixel in each cluster (with the most dominant aggregate interference) based on the previous power allocations per LTE BSs. In the concurrent operation, the algorithm tends to satisfy the PRs for all lead pixels (Fig. 2).

3 Simulation Results

Targeted performances for evaluation are *capacity per pixel, coverage probability* and *probability for pixel DVB-T service degradation*. The proposed algorithm is compared with case of no power control assuming LTE operation with max transmit power.

The DVB-T system modeling is based on the Longley-Rice propagation model along with terrain effects in order to predict the received DVB-T signal strength. It exploits relevant operating parameters obtained from the Agency for Electronic Communications (AEC) of the Republic of Macedonia [11].

The simulation scenario considers M LTE base stations, randomly distributed with Poisson Point Process (PPP) in the target area, and collocated with the existing DVB-T transmitters. The evaluation area considers the territory of Skopje (the capital of Macedonia) with dimensions 15 km × 19.5 km and a pixel size of 30 m × 30 m (Fig. 3). The LTE channel gains incorporate the propagation losses predicted by Okumura-Hata propagation model, whereas the occupied bandwidth is 10 MHz at the lowest possible LTE frequency, with nearest DVB-T proximity (worst case scenario) and the Effective Isotropic Radiated Power (EIRP) is 59 dBm [12].

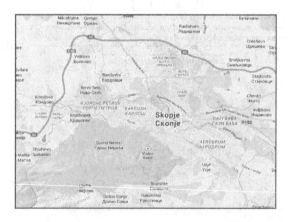

Fig. 3. Skopje city map (in the considered area of the simulations, Fig. 4)

The simulation analysis applies the algorithm for optimal power allocation with $SINR_t$ = 10 dB (selected arbitrarily, to provide a satisfying LTE service quality), and obtains the transmit power set p while taking the DVB-T PRs (in presence of fully loaded LTE base stations operations, representing the worst case scenario) as constraints in the optimization problem. The quantitative assessment relies on a Monte Carlo observation with 100 trials.

Figure 4 illustrates the spatial distribution of the capacity per pixel for the cases with and without algorithm for optimal power allocation. Both the figures Figs. 4a and b reveal the significant gain in capacity with the introduction of algorithm for proper and optimal power allocation for the LTE-800 base stations. Figure 5 presents the coverage probability as a function of the SINR, i.e. the cumulative distribution of the output SINR throughout the evaluation area. It proves that the power allocation algorithm further enhances the base stations coverage in interference-limited networks, regardless of the significant limitation due to the DVB-T service protection.

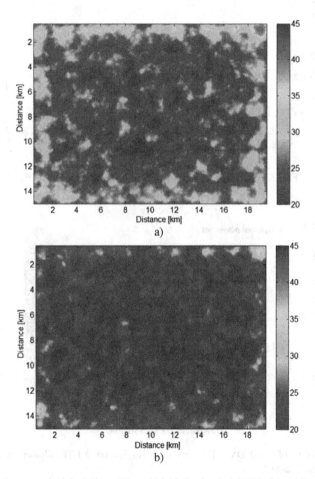

Fig. 4. Capacity per pixel in Mbps ($M = 100$, fully loaded LTE) (a) with optimal power allocation algorithm (b) without power allocation (with max transmit power)

Figure 6 depicts the probability of pixel DVB-T service degradation targeting the degradation on 9 consecutive DVB-T channels (52–60 channels). In this calculation, a pixel is declared as degraded if the channel specific DVB-T PR on any of the inspected channels is violated. The figure reveals the significant reduction of the degradation probability when utilizing the optimal power set, since the optimization problem includes the DVB-T service protection as a constraint.

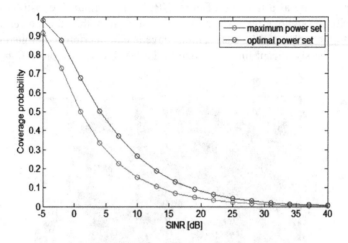

Fig. 5. Coverage probability (M = 100, fully loaded LTE)

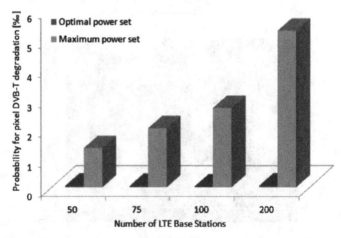

Fig. 6. Probability of pixel DVB-T degradation [in ‰] on 9 LTE adjacent and consecutive DVB-T channels (52–60)

4   Conclusions

This paper presents a developed algorithm for optimal power allocation aiming to maximize the capacity of macro-cell-edge users and minimize the DVB-T service degradation due to aggregate interference. The simulation results reveal the significant benefits of the introduction of optimal power allocation, whilst enabling the required protection of the coexisting DVB-T network in the UHF band. They provide performance gains in terms of capacity per pixel and coverage and pave the way for possible trade-offs in order to optimize the performances in general.

Acknowledgments. This work was performed within the NATO SfP-984409 project "Optimization and Rational Use of Wireless Communications Bands" (ORCA). The authors would like to thank everyone involved.

References

1. Elayoubi, S.E., Ben Haddada, O., Fourestie, B.: Performance evaluation of frequency planning schemes in OFDMA-based networks. IEEE Trans. Wirel. Commun. **7**, 1623–1633 (2008)
2. Ning, G., Yang, Q., Kwak, K.S., Hanzo, L.: Macro- and femtocell interference mitigation in OFDMA wireless systems. In: IEEE Global Communications Conference (GLOBECOM) 2012 (2012)
3. Tan, C.W., Chiang, M., Srikant, R.: Fast algorithms and performance bounds for sum rate maximization in wireless networks. IEEE/ACM Trans. Netw. **21**(3), 706–719 (2013)
4. Qian, L., Zhang, Y.J., Huang, J.W.: MAPEL: achieving global optimality for a non-convex wireless power control problem. IEEE Trans. Wirel. Commun. **8**(3), 1553–1563 (2009)
5. Chiang, M., Tan, C.W., Palomar, D.P., O'Neill, D., Julian, D.: Power control by geometric programming. IEEE Trans. Wirel. Commun. **6**(6), 2640–2651 (2007)
6. Kha, H.H., Tuan, H.D., Nguyen, H.H.: Fast global optimal power allocation in wireless networks by local D.C. programming. IEEE Trans. Wirel. Commun. **11**(2), 510–515 (2012)
7. ERA Technology Report: Assessment of LTE 800 MHz Base Station Interference into DTT Receivers, July 2011
8. OFCOM Technical Report: Technical analysis of interference from mobile network base stations in the 800 MHz band to digital terrestrial television, June 2011
9. ECC Report 159. Technical and Operational Requirements for the Possible Operation of Cognitive Radio Systems in the 'White Spaces' of the Frequency band 470–790 MHz, January 2011
10. Kaufman, L., Rousseeuw, P.J.: Finding Groups in Data: An Introduction to Cluster Analysis. Wiley, Hoboken (1990)
11. Agency for Electronic Communications (AEC) of the Republic of Macedonia. www.aec.mk
12. Holma, H., Toskala, A.: WCDMA for UMTS: HSPA Evolution and LTE. Wiley, New York (2010)

Special Session on Indoor Positioning: Enabler for Ubiquitous, Smart Architectures

Cooperative Multipath-Assisted Navigation and Tracking: A Low-Complexity Approach

Josef Kulmer$^{(\boxtimes)}$, Erik Leitinger, Paul Meissner, and Klaus Witrisal

Graz University of Technology, Inffeldgasse 16c, 8010 Graz, Austria
{kulmer,erik.leitinger,paul.meissner,witrisal}@tugraz.at

Abstract. Wireless localization has become a key technology for cooperative agent networks. However, for many applications, it is still illusive to reach the desired level of *accuracy* and *robustness*, especially in indoor environments which are characterized by harsh multipath propagation. In this work we introduce a cooperative low-complexity algorithm that utilizes multipath components for localization instead of suffering from them. The algorithm uses two types of measurements: (i) *bistatic* measurements between agents and (ii) *monostatic* (bat-like) measurements by the individual agents. Simulations that use data generated from a realistic channel model, show the applicability of the methodology and the high level of accuracy that can be reached.

Keywords: Cooperative localization · Multipath propagation · Indoor localization and tracking

1 Introduction

Location awareness is a key component of many future wireless applications. However, achieving the needed level of accuracy is still elusive in many cases, especially in indoor environments which are characterized by harsh multipath conditions. Promising candidate systems thus either use sensing technologies that provide remedies against multipath or they fuse information from multiple information sources [1,2].

In *Multipath-assisted indoor navigation and tracking (MINT)* [3,4] multipath components (MPCs) can be associated to the local geometry using a known floor plan. In this way, MPCs can be seen as signals from additional (virtual) anchors (VAs). Ultra-wideband (UWB) signals are used because of their superior time resolution facilitating the separation of MPCs. Hence, additional position-related information is exploited that is contained in the radio signals. All other—not geometrically modelled—propagation effects included in the signals constitute interference to the useful position-related information and are called diffuse multipath (DM) [5]. Insight on the position-related information that is conveyed in the signals can be gained by an analysis of performance bounds, such as the Cramér-Rao lower bound (CRLB) [4]. In [4], the CRLB for cooperative MINT was derived using *bistatic* measurements between agents and *monostatic* measurements from an agent itself. The same measurement model will be used in this

© Institute for Computer Sciences, Social Informatics and Telecommunications Engineering 2015
V. Atanasovski, L.-G. Alberto (Eds.): Fabulous 2015, LNICST 159, pp. 159–165, 2015.
DOI: 10.1007/978-3-319-27072-2_20

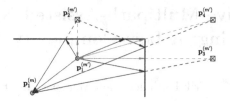

Fig. 1. Illustration of multipath geometry using VAs for (i) bistatic transmissions (blue) between an agents and for (ii) a monostatic measurement (gray) by an agent (Color figure online).

work. Cooperation between agents is another method to increase the amount of available information [6] and thus to reduce the localization outage. In this work, we present a low-complexity variant of [7] that is based on data-association (DA) and extended Kalman filtering (EKF) [8]. The method relies on the same factor graph as presented in [7], but in contrast it just uses the extracted MPC delays and complex path amplitudes[1] instead of the complete received signals. The key contributions of this paper are (i) incorporate VAs into a joint state space with the agents, and (ii) formulate the cooperative algorithm that uses DA of MPC delays with according VAs and an EKF for tracking the joint state of the agents and the according VAs.

2   Problem Formulation

We assume M agents at positions $\mathbf{p}_1^{(m)}$ with $m \in \mathcal{N}_m = \{1, 2, \ldots, M\}$, which cooperate with one another. As outlined in the introduction, every agent conducts a monostatic measurement, meaning it emits a pulse and receives the multipath signal reflected by the environment, and conventional bistatic measurements with all other agents and the fixed anchors. All bistatic and monostatic measurements are distributed such that every agent is able to exploit information from any of its received and/or transmitted signals.

Figure 1 illustrates the geometric model for multipath-assisted positioning. A signal exchanged between the agents m' and m at positions $\mathbf{p}_1^{(m')}$ and $\mathbf{p}_1^{(m)}$, respectively, contains specular reflections at the room walls, indicated by the black lines. These reflections can be modeled geometrically using VAs $\mathbf{p}_k^{(m')}$, mirror images of the anchor w.r.t. walls that can be computed from the floor plan [3]. We call this the bistatic setup. If the agents are equipped accordingly, they can use monostatic measurements, indicated by the gray lines. Here, the node at $\mathbf{p}_k^{(m')}$ acts as anchor for itself with its own set of VAs.

---

[1] These are used to compute online, the reliability measure of the MPCs in form a signal-to-interference-plus-noise-ratio (SINR) that is used to compute the according MPC's delay uncertainty.

2.1 Signal Model

In this Section, we simplify the setup—for the ease of readability—to a single (fixed) anchor located at position $\mathbf{p}_1 \in \mathbb{R}^2$ and one agent at position $\mathbf{p} \in \mathbb{R}^2$. Note that two-dimensional position coordinates are used throughout the paper, for the sake of simplicity. A *baseband* UWB signal $s(t)$ is exchanged between the anchor and the agent. The corresponding received signal is modeled as [4]

$$r(t) = \sum_{k=1}^{K} \alpha_k s(t - \tau_k) + (s * \nu)(t) + w(t) \tag{1}$$

where $\{\alpha_k\}$ and $\{\tau_k\}$ are the complex amplitudes and delays of the deterministic MPCs, respectively. We model these delays by VAs at positions $\mathbf{p}_k \in \mathbb{R}^2$, yielding $\tau_k = \frac{1}{c}\|\mathbf{p} - \mathbf{p}_k\| = \frac{1}{c}d(\mathbf{p}_k, \mathbf{p})$, with $k = 1 \ldots K$, where c is the speed of light and $d(\cdot)$ is the Euclidean distance. K is equivalent to the number of visible VAs at the agent position $\mathbf{p}$. We assume the energy of $s(t)$ is normalized to one.

The DM $(s * \nu)(t)$ is modeled as a zero-mean Gaussian random process which is non-stationary in the delay domain and colored due to the spectrum of $s(t)$. For DM we assume uncorrelated scattering along the delay axis τ, hence the auto-correlation function (ACF) of $\nu(t)$ is given by $K_\nu(\tau, u) = \mathbb{E}_\nu\{\nu(\tau)[\nu(u)]^*\} = S_\nu(\tau)\delta(\tau - u)$, where $S_\nu(\tau)$ is the PDP of DM at the agent position $\mathbf{p}$. The DM process is assumed to be quasi-stationary in the spatial domain, which means that $S_\nu(\tau)$ does not change in the vicinity of position $\mathbf{p}$ [4]. Finally, $w(t)$ denotes an additive white Gaussian noise (AWGN) process with double-sided power spectral density (PSD) of $N_0/2$.

2.2 Channel Estimation

The arrival time estimation $\hat{\tau}_{k,n}^{(m,m')}$ at time step n between two agents at positions $\mathbf{p}_{1,n}^{(m)}$ and $\mathbf{p}_{1,n}^{(m')}$, where $m, m' \in \mathcal{N}_m$, is realized as an iterative least-squares approximation of the received signal [8]. The according path amplitudes $\hat{a}_{k,n}^{(m,m')}$ are estimated using a projection of the received signal $r_n^{(m,m')}(t)$ onto a unit-energy pulse $s(t - \hat{\tau}_{k,n}^{(m,m')})$. The number of estimated MPCs $\hat{K}_n^{(m,m')}$ should be chosen according to the number of expected specular paths in an environment. The finite set of measured delays is written as $\mathcal{Z}_n^{(m)} = \bigcup_{m'} \mathcal{Z}_n^{(m,m')} = \bigcup_{m'}\{\hat{d}_{k,n}^{(m,m')}\}_{k=1}^{\hat{K}_n^{(m,m')}}$, where $\hat{d}_{k,n}^{(m,m')} = c\hat{\tau}_{k,n}^{(m,m')}$.

2.3 Data Association (DA)

The set of expected MPC delays $\mathcal{D}_n^{(m,m')} = \{d(\mathbf{p}_{n,k}^{(m')}, \mathbf{p}_{1,n}^{(m)}) : \mathbf{p}_{n,k}^{(m,m')} \in \mathcal{A}_n^{(m,m')}\}$ is computed from the distances of each VA in $\mathcal{A}_n^{(m,m')}$ to the predicted position $\mathbf{p}_{1,n}^{(m)}$ of agent m at time step n. As $\mathcal{D}_n^{(m,m')}$ and the set of measured delays $\mathcal{Z}_n^{(m,m')}$ are sets of usually different cardinalities, i.e. $|\mathcal{Z}_n^{(m,m')}| = \hat{K}_n^{(m,m')} \neq$

$|\mathcal{D}_n^{(m,m')}| = K_n^{(m,m')}$, no conventional distance measure is defined and therefore there is no straightforward way of an association. We employ a well-known multi- target miss-distance, the *optimal sub-pattern assignment* (OSPA) metric [9]. As described in [8,10], after the DA was applied for all agents, the following union sets are defined: (i) the set of associated discovered (and optionally a-priori known) VAs $\mathcal{A}_{n,\text{ass}}^{(m)} = \bigcup_{m'} \mathcal{A}_{n,\text{ass}}^{(m,m')}$, (ii) the corresponding set of associated measurements $\mathcal{Z}_{timestepsym,\text{ass}}^{(m)} = \bigcup_{m'} \mathcal{Z}_{n,\text{ass}}^{(m,m')}$.

3   State Space and Measurement Model

The state dynamics are characterized by a linear, constant-velocity motion model. Each agent $\mathbf{x}_n^{(m)}$ is described by its position $\mathbf{p}_{1,n}^{(m)}$ and velocity $\mathbf{v}_{1,n}^{(m)}$ according to $\mathbf{x}_n^{(m)} = [(\mathbf{p}_{1,n}{}^{(m)})^\mathrm{T}, (\mathbf{v}_{1,n}{}^{(m)})^\mathrm{T}]^\mathrm{T}$. The position of the agent is mirrored at a each wall segment in order to obtain the positions of the corresponding VAs $\mathbf{p}_{k,n}^{(m)}$. The orientation of the wall segments determine the relation between the movement gradients of the agent and the corresponding VAs. We describe this relation by introducing a VA transition matrix $\mathbf{P}_k^{(m)}$ (cf. [4]). The state space model for agent m is thus characterized by

$$\tilde{\mathbf{x}}_n^{(m)} = \underbrace{\begin{bmatrix} \mathbf{F} & \mathbf{0}_{4 \times 2K_n} \\ \mathbf{0}_{2K_n \times 2}\,\mathbf{P}^{(m)} & \mathbf{I}_{2K_n \times 2K_n} \end{bmatrix}}_{\tilde{\mathbf{F}}^{(m)}} \tilde{\mathbf{x}}_{n-1}^{(m)} + \underbrace{\begin{bmatrix} \mathbf{G} \\ \mathbf{0}_{2K_n \times 2} \end{bmatrix}}_{\tilde{\mathbf{G}}^{(m)}} \mathbf{n}_{a,n}, \tag{2}$$

with

$$\mathbf{F} = \begin{bmatrix} 1 & 0 & \varDelta T & 0 \\ 0 & 1 & 0 & \varDelta T \\ 0 & 0 & 1 & 0 \\ 0 & 0 & 0 & 1 \end{bmatrix}, \quad \mathbf{G} = \begin{bmatrix} \frac{\varDelta T^2}{2} & 0 \\ 0 & \frac{\varDelta T^2}{2} \\ \varDelta T & 0 \\ 0 & \varDelta T \end{bmatrix},$$

$\tilde{\mathbf{x}}_n^{(m)} = [\mathbf{x}^{\mathrm{T}}{}_n^{(m)}, \mathbf{p}^{\mathrm{T}}{}_{2,n}^{(m)}, \dots \mathbf{p}^{\mathrm{T}}{}_{K,n}^{(m)}]^\mathrm{T}$ and $\mathbf{P}^{(m)} = [\mathbf{P}_2^{\mathrm{T}\,(m)}, \dots, \mathbf{P}_{K_n}^{\mathrm{T}\,(m)}]^\mathrm{T}$ with dimensions $(2K_n \times 2)$. Under the assumption of independent movement of the agents, the motion model finally results in

$$\underbrace{\begin{bmatrix} \tilde{\mathbf{x}}_n^{(1)} \\ \vdots \\ \tilde{\mathbf{x}}_n^{(M)} \end{bmatrix}}_{\hat{\mathbf{x}}_n} = \begin{bmatrix} \tilde{\mathbf{F}}^{(1)} & & \mathbf{0} \\ & \ddots & \\ \mathbf{0} & & \tilde{\mathbf{F}}^{(M)} \end{bmatrix} \underbrace{\begin{bmatrix} \tilde{\mathbf{x}}_{n-1}^{(1)} \\ \vdots \\ \tilde{\mathbf{x}}_{n-1}^{(M)} \end{bmatrix}}_{\tilde{\mathbf{x}}_{n-1}} + \begin{bmatrix} \tilde{\mathbf{G}}_n^{(1)} \\ \vdots \\ \tilde{\mathbf{G}}_n^{(M)} \end{bmatrix} \mathbf{n}_{a,n}. \tag{3}$$

The according linearized measurement model is defined as

$$\begin{bmatrix} \tilde{\mathbf{z}}_n^{(1)} \\ \vdots \\ \tilde{\mathbf{z}}_n^{(M)} \end{bmatrix} = \begin{bmatrix} \tilde{\mathbf{H}}_n^{(1)} & & \mathbf{0} \\ & \ddots & \\ \mathbf{0} & & \tilde{\mathbf{H}}_n^{(M)} \end{bmatrix} \begin{bmatrix} \tilde{\mathbf{x}}_n^{(1)} \\ \vdots \\ \tilde{\mathbf{x}}_n^{(M)} \end{bmatrix} + \tilde{\mathbf{n}}_{z,n}. \tag{4}$$

where $\tilde{z}_n^{(m)}$ stacks the monostatic measurements from the m-th agent and the bistatic measurements to all other agents. The stack vector $\tilde{n}_{z,n}$ contains the according measurement noise with covariance matrix $\mathbf{R}_n$ described in [8]. The linearized column-wise stacked measurement matrices $\tilde{\mathbf{H}}_n^{(m)} = [(\tilde{\mathbf{H}}_n^{(\eta=1,m)})^\mathrm{T}, \ldots,$ $(\tilde{\mathbf{H}}_n^{(\eta=M,m)})^\mathrm{T}]^\mathrm{T}$ are described in (5), with $m, \eta \in \mathcal{N}_m$ and $m \neq \eta$. The matrices $\mathbf{H}_{\xi,\mu,n}^{(\eta,\eta,m)} = [\frac{\partial d(\mathbf{P}_{\mu,n}^{(\eta)}, \mathbf{P}_{1,n}^{(m)})}{\partial x_{\xi,n}^{(\eta)}}, \frac{\partial d(\mathbf{P}_{\mu,n}^{(\eta)}, \mathbf{P}_{1,n}^{(m)})}{\partial y_{\xi,n}^{(\eta)}}]$ define the derivatives of the distance measurements w.r.t. the x-and y-position coordinates. The upper-left sub-block of (5) holds the derivatives of the monostatic measurements w.r.t. the m-th agent position. The upper diagonal sub-block holds the according derivatives w.r.t. to the monostatic VA positions of the m-th agent. The lower-left sub-block holds derivatives of the bistatic measurement equations to all other agent positions and according VA positions ($\eta = 1 \ldots M$ and $m \neq \eta$) w.r.t. the m-th agent position. The lower-right diagonal sub-block holds the equivalent derivatives w.r.t. to the according bistatic VA positions.

$$
\tilde{\mathbf{H}}_n^{(\eta,m)} = \begin{bmatrix}
\mathbf{H}_{1,2,n}^{(m,m,m)} \, 0 \, 0 \, \mathbf{H}_{2,2,n}^{(m,m,m)} \cdots & 0 & \cdots & 0 & \cdots & 0 \\
\vdots & \vdots & \vdots & \vdots & \vdots & \vdots & \vdots & \vdots & \vdots \\
\mathbf{H}_{1,K_n,n}^{(m,m,m)} \, 0 \, 0 & 0 & \cdots \mathbf{H}_{K_n,K_n,n}^{(m,m,m)} \cdots & 0 & \cdots & 0 \\
\mathbf{H}_{1,1,n}^{(\eta,m,m)} \, 0 \, 0 & 0 & \cdots & 0 & \cdots \mathbf{H}_{1,1,n}^{(\eta,\eta,m)} \cdots & 0 \\
\vdots & \vdots & \vdots & \vdots & \vdots & \vdots & \vdots & \vdots & \vdots \\
\mathbf{H}_{1,K_n,n}^{(\eta,m,m)} \, 0 \, 0 & 0 & \cdots & 0 & \cdots & 0 & \cdots \mathbf{H}_{K_n,K_n,n}^{(\eta,\eta,m)}
\end{bmatrix}
\tag{5}
$$

4   Results

We evaluate the performance of the proposed algorithm in terms of localization error and computational time using synthetic data in a two-dimensional space. The transmit signal consists of a raised-cosine pulse with a roll-off factor of $R = 0.6$, a pulse duration of $T_\mathrm{p} = 0.5$ ns and unit energy. The received signals of the monostatic and bistatic measurements are modeled according to (1). Each reflection attenuates the pulse by $3\,\mathrm{dB}$. The free-space loss is modeled according to Friis' transmission equation. The parameters of the DM are set according to [4] and the power of the additive white noise is set to $N_0 = 2 \cdot 10^{-16}\,\mathrm{W/Hz}$. In order to achieve a fair comparison to the proposed method in [7] we choose the same parameter setup and simulation scenario as shown in Fig. 2. Three agents m move independently along trajectories under partly non-line-of-sight conditions where we assume a given start position. Figure 2 shows an example of the estimated agent positions $\hat{\mathbf{p}}_{1,n}$, $\hat{\mathbf{p}}_{2,n}$ and $\hat{\mathbf{p}}_{3,n}$ using the proposed EKF-based algorithm are indicated for every 5-th position. At each time step n the agents run monostatic and bistatic measurements to the neighboring agents. The utilized likelihood function of [7, Eq. (8)] simplifies the proposed system model (Sec. III in [7]). We accounted this by changing the likelihood function to

Eq. (7) of [7]. Further, [7] undermines the uncertainty of the neighboring beliefs by reducing the size of the neighboring particles to the mean value (see Sect. 5 of [7]). We omit this simplification.

The maximum number of extracted MPCs is limited to $K_n^{(\cdot,\cdot)} = 12, \forall n$ (see Sect. 2.2). The initial position of each VA $\mathbf{p}_{k,n}^{(m)}$ as well as the corresponding VA transition matrix $\mathbf{P}_k^{(m)}$ are calculated in advance. Figure 3 illustrates the cumulative distribution function (CDF) of the localization error of the proposed algorithm (CoMINT EKF) compared to [7] of ten trajectory realizations—each evaluated with 50 monte carlo runs. The comparison reveals the strong influence on performance of localization error and computational demand [7] regarding its implementation scheme of message passing (i.e. particle or parametric message representation and scheduling). Choosing a sample-based message representation the localization error reduces with increasing number of particles on the cost of computational complexity. Denoting N as the number of particles representing the message passing scheme [7], faces a complexity of $\mathcal{O}(MN^2)$ [11]. The proposed method has a complexity of $\mathcal{O}(M^2 K_n^3)$ determined by the data association stage [9]. Since the number of particles N is much higher compared to the number of extracted MPC $K_n^{(\cdot,\cdot)}$ the proposed method outperforms [7] in terms of computational complexity. We proof this claim by comparison of the average computational time for localization scaled to the proposed method. Depending on the number of particles the average computational time of the proposed method speeds up by a factor of approximately 217, 756 and 2355 for 100, 250 and 500 particles, respectively.

The gain in terms of computational time is established by the assumption of Gaussian distance errors. Figure 3 indicates the influence of this assumption by comparison to [7] with different number of particles of 100, 250 and 500. The proposed method reaches a performance comparable to [7] with a number of particles from 100–250 where 90 % of the errors are located within 2 cm.

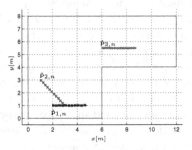

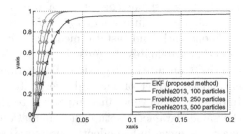

Fig. 2. Simulation scenario as in [7] with three agents moving along different trajectories.

Fig. 3. CDF of the localization error of the proposed algorithm (CoMINT EKF) (blue) compared to [7] with a different size of 500 (gray), 250 (red) and 100 (black) particles of each agent (Color figure online).

5 Conclusions

We have presented a new low-complexity algorithm for cooperative localization of agents using multipath information. The simulation results show that bistatic as well as monostatic measurements contribute a significant amount of information for localizing the agents with a high level of accuracy. The simulation results pinpoint also the robustness, i.e. low level of localization outages, of the cooperative algorithm when multipath information is used from both types of measurements. The most important attained fact it that the proposed low-complexity algorithm reaches almost the same performance than the particle-based method using several orders of magnitude less computational resources.

References

1. Shen, Y., Mazuelas, S., Win, M.: Network navigation: theory and interpretation. IEEE J. Sel. Areas Commun. **30**, 1823–1834 (2012)
2. Conti, A., Dardari, D., Guerra, M., Mucchi, L., Win, M.: Experimental characterization of diversity navigation. IEEE Syst. J. **8**, 115–124 (2014)
3. Meissner, P.: Multipath-Assisted Indoor Positioning. Ph.D. thesis, Graz University of Technology (2014)
4. Leitinger, E., Meissner, P., Ruedisser, C., Dumphart, G., Witrisal, K.: Evaluation of position-related information in multipath components for indoor positioning. IEEE J. Sel. Areas Commun. (2015)
5. Michelusi, N., Mitra, U., Molisch, A., Zorzi, M.: UWB sparse/diffuse channels, Part I channel models and bayesian estimators. IEEE Trans. Sig. Process. **60**, 5307–5319 (2012)
6. Wymeersch, H., Lien, J., Win, M.Z.: Cooperative localization in wireless networks. Proc. IEEE **97**, 427–450 (2009)
7. Froehle, M., Leitinger, E., Meissner, P., Witrisal, K.: Cooperative multipath-assisted indoor navigation and tracking (Co-MINT) using UWB signals. In: IEEE ICC Workshop on Advances in Network Localization and Navigation (2013)
8. Meissner, P., Leitinger, E., Witrisal, K.: UWB for robust indoor tracking: weighting of multipath components for efficient estimation. IEEE Wirel. Commun. Lett. **3**, 501–504 (2014)
9. Schuhmacher, D., Vo, B.T., Vo, B.N.: A consistent metric for performance evaluation of multi-object filters. IEEE Trans. Sig. Process. **56**, 3447–3457 (2008)
10. Leitinger, E., Meissner, P., Lafer, M., Witrisal, K.: Simultaneous localization and mapping using multipath channel information. In: 2015 IEEE International Conference on Communications Workshops (ICC) (2015)
11. Lien, J., Ferner, U.J., Srichavengsup, W., Wymeersch, H., Win, M.Z.: A comparison of parametric and sample-based message representation in cooperative localization. Int. J. Navig. Obs. **2012** (2012)

On the Applicability of Multi-wall Multi-floor Propagation Models to WiFi Fingerprinting Indoor Positioning

Giuseppe Caso and Luca De Nardis[(✉)]

DIET Department, Sapienza University of Rome, Rome, Italy
{caso,lucadn}@newyork.ing.uniroma1.it

Abstract. *Virtual* fingerprints have been proposed in the context of WiFi Fingerprinting Indoor Positioning systems in order to reduce the effort dedicated to offline measurements. In this work, the use of Multi-Wall Multi-Floor indoor propagation models to generate such virtual fingerprints is investigated. Experimental results show that different trade-offs can be obtained between model accuracy and measurement efforts and that good accuracy can be guaranteed while significantly reducing the complexity of the offline measurement phase.

Keywords: Indoor positioning · Fingerprinting · Propagation modeling · Multi-Wall Multi-Floor

1 Introduction

Among many proposed and investigated approaches for the implementation of indoor positioning systems, the fingerprinting technique is one of the most popular ones [1,2]. Fingerprinting operates in an offline phase, during which Received Signal Strength (RSS) values (fingerprints) from WiFi Access Points (APs) detected in the area of interest are collected at previously selected positions, referred to as Reference Points (RPs), and an online phase, during which the location of a target device is estimated as a function of the positions of the RPs that best match the RSS values measured by the device.

Accuracy and complexity of fingerprinting algorithms mainly depend on two issues: (1) careful planning of the offline phase, particularly in terms of RPs locations and number of requested measurements, and (2) selection of estimation algorithms used in the online phase.

Regarding the offline phase, the goal is to achieve satisfactory trade-off between accuracy and efforts and time dedicated to this phase. From this point of view, several previous works propose the generation of *virtual* fingerprints through the use of indoor propagation models [3–6]. Assuming to know the exact locations of the APs and the environment planimetry, empirical propagation models provide a good compromise between model accuracy and complexity. Such models rely on a set of measurements in order to estimate site-specific model propagation

© Institute for Computer Sciences, Social Informatics and Telecommunications Engineering 2015
V. Atanasovski, L.-G. Alberto (Eds.): Fabulous 2015, LNICST 159, pp. 166–172, 2015.
DOI: 10.1007/978-3-319-27072-2_21

parameters, that are then used to create the virtual RPs fingerprints. Among empirical propagation models, Multi-Wall Multi-Floor (MWMF) models are widely considered as a pragmatic and concrete solution, given their analytical simplicity [4,7,8].

Moving from the above observations, the goal of this work is to explore the trade-off between complexity and efforts in the collection of real measurements and the accuracy of the MWMF model in generating virtual RPs. The analysis is carried out based on experimental results obtained in the testbed deployed at the Department of Information Engineering, Electronics and Telecommunications (DIET) of Sapienza University of Rome.

The rest of the paper is organized as follows: Sect. 2 briefly reviews the analytical foundations of MWMF indoor propagation models. Section 3 introduces the strategies proposed for the MWMF propagation parameters evaluation; Sect. 4 firstly presents the testbed used for the experimental analysis (Sect. 4.1) and then the results obtained by applying the strategies for the virtual RPs fingerprints creation (Sect. 4.2). Finally, Sect. 5 concludes the paper and presents future research lines.

2 Multi-wall Multi-floor Propagation Models

It is widely recognized that indoor propagation characteristics greatly differ from the outdoor ones, mostly because of the indoor environmental peculiarities, such as shorter Tx-Rx distances, different power ranges, presence of walls, furniture, and so on. In the context of modeling the indoor propagation, empirical narrowband models are widely used; they are characterized by simple analytical formulas embedded with site-specific propagation parameters, the latter obtained through a procedure of model fitting based on a set of real measurements.

Multi-Wall Multi-Floor is a family of empirical narrow-band models [7,8]; they differ from each other in the number and the variety of objects taken into account in modeling the signal propagation. MWMF models take the following generic form in the evaluation of the path loss in a Tx-Rx link:

$$PL_{MWMF} = PL_{OS} + A_{MWMF} \quad [dB]. \tag{1}$$

The PL_{OS} term relates the signal attenuation to the Tx-Rx distance d and the so-called path loss exponent γ, as follows:

$$PL_{OS}(d, \gamma) = l_0 + 10\gamma \log(d) \quad [dB], \tag{2}$$

where the constant l_0 is a reference path loss for $d = 1$ m and γ is the path loss exponent (for free space conditions, $\gamma = 2$ and $l_0 \approx 40.22$ dB @ 2.45 GHz). The A_{MWMF} term models the attenuation due to obstacles in the Tx-Rx direct path and its definition characterizes the MWMF model. Focusing on a 2D propagation (Tx and Rx on the same floor), A_{MWMF} can be formulated as follows:

$$A_{MWMF} = l_c + \sum_{n=1}^{N_{obj}} \sum_{i=1}^{I_n} N_{n,i} l_{n,i} \quad [dB], \tag{3}$$

Table 1. A_{MWMF} parameters description.

Parameter	Description
l_c	Constant loss
N_{obj}	Number of different families of objects
I_n	Number of types of objects considered for family n
$N_{n,i}$	Number of objects of family n and type i
$l_{n,i}$	Loss due to objects of family n and type i

with parameters, related to both signal propagation and environment topology, described in Table 1.

Given the model, a set of M real measurements, and, for each m-th measurement (with $m = 1, 2, \ldots, M$), the set of topological parameters $\mathcal{T}_m$, a least square fitting procedure allows to obtain the set of propagation parameters $\mathcal{S}$ that minimize the difference between the measurements and the estimations. The propagation parameters included in $\mathcal{S}$ may differ from one MWMF model to the other and can in general include parameters belonging to both the $\mathsf{PL_{OS}}$ and A_{MWMF} terms [7,8]. The set adopted in this work will be explicitly defined in Sect. 4.1. In general, the optimization problem can be defined as follows:

$$\{\mathcal{S}\}_{\mathsf{opt}} = \underset{\{\mathcal{S}\}}{\operatorname{argmin}} \quad \left\{ \sum_{m=1}^{M} |P_m - (\mathsf{EIRP} - \mathsf{PL_{MWMF}}(d_m, \mathcal{T}_m, \mathcal{S}))|^2 \right\}, \qquad (4)$$

where, for the m-th available measurement, P_m is the power measured at the Rx, given a Tx at distance d_m isotropically radiating a power equal to EIRP, and $\mathsf{PL_{MWMF}}(d_m, \mathcal{T}_m, \mathcal{S})$ is the MWMF estimated path loss as described in (1), (2) and (3).

3   MWMF Models for Virtual RPs Fingerprinting

As previously introduced, the MWMF model can be used for the creation of virtual RPs fingerprints for indoor positioning purposes: given the area of interest $\mathcal{A}$, the number N of RPs to be created and the number L of APs at known positions within and around $\mathcal{A}$, the goal is to create, for each RP_n, a $L \times 1$ fingerprint $\hat{s}_n$ in which the component $\hat{s}_{l,n}$ is the estimated RSS for the transmission link from the l-th AP to the n-th RP. In order to do so, the MWMF model must be calibrated on a set of real measurements, as indicated in (4). The accuracy of the model will however depend on the strategy in the selection of the measurements and on the number of such measurements. In this paper, four different selection strategies are investigated in order to explore the trade-off between the model accuracy and complexity in the generation of the fingerprints.

Strategy I: No Fitting. This strategy relies on the use of generic parameters taken from literature for an indoor environment, without any site-specific fitting. Although this strategy is expected to provide limited accuracy, it is by far the simplest to implement and will be considered as the baseline for the perfomance evaluation of the other strategies.

Strategy II: Mockup Fitting. In this strategy, the propagation parameters obtained in a mockup environment $\mathcal{A}'$ (given a set of N'_{real} measurements taken in it, from a set of L' APs at known positions within and around $\mathcal{A}'$) are used to generate the fingerprints in the objective environment $\mathcal{A}$. This strategy has the advantage of allowing the generation of virtual RPs in multiple environments provided that a mockup environment with similar propagation characteristics can be found.

Strategy III: Environment Fitting. In this strategy, a set of N_{real} measurements from the L APs is collected in the environment $\mathcal{A}$. Such measurements are used to perform a global optimization procedure aiming at determining a set of model propagation parameters to be used for all APs.

Strategy IV: Specific AP Fitting. In this strategy, again, a set of N_{real} measurements from the L APs is collected in the environment $\mathcal{A}$. In this case, however, an optimization procedure is carried out for each AP, by considering only the measurements for the specific AP. This strategy is expected to provide the best possible accuracy at the additional price of collecting measurements in the objective environment (compared to Strategy II) and performing different and dedicated optimization procedures (compared to Strategies II and III).

4   Results and Discussions

4.1   Testbed Implementation

Experimental analysis have been carried out at the first two floors of the DIET Department, covering an area of 10×55 m^2 each. $L_1 = 6$ and $L_2 = 7$ WiFi APs working @ 2.4 GHz were placed inside the 1-st and the 2-nd floor countertops, respectively. $N_1 = 65$ and $N_2 = 69$ RPs were identified, uniformly distributed on the two floors, and the fingerprints for each RP were measured. In order to average out fluctuations, $q = 5$ measurements were taken for each RP.

In the analysis presented in this Section, the first floor was adopted as the objective environment $\mathcal{A}$ and the strategies defined in Sect. 3 were applied for modeling the N_1 RPs defined on this floor, for the $L_1 + L_2$ APs. Moreover, the environmental characteristics and the set $\mathcal{S}$ of propagation parameters used in the 2D propagation optimization procedure are reported in Table 2.

As defined in Sect. 3, Strategy I requires to extract propagation parameters from literature: in the following, propagation parameters presented in [8] were

Table 2. Model parameters setting.

N_{obj}	2 (walls, doors)
I_{walls}	1
I_{doors}	1
S	$\{\gamma, l_c, l_{wall}, l_{door}\}$

used. As for Strategy II, the II floor of the DIET Department was used as mockup environment with measurements in the N_2 RPs in this floor including RSSs from the L_2 APs deployed in the same floor. For Strategy III and IV, a total of $N_1 \times L_1$ measurements are available in the testbed. Out of this, a fraction ρ was used for the fitting procedure, selected so to preserve the uniform distribution of the considered measurements in the area. Note that for Strategy II and Strategy III this corresponded to $N'_{real} = \lceil \rho \times N_2 \times L_2 \rceil$ and $N_{real} = \lceil \rho \times N_1 \times L_1 \rceil$ measurements being used for the global fitting procedures, respectively. In Strategy IV, on the other hand, L_1 fitting procedures were carried out, each one using $N_{real} = \lceil \rho \times N_1 \rceil$ measurements. ρ was used as a tunable parameter determining how many measurements were used in the optimization procedure for each strategy, and results of the analysis as a function of ρ are presented in Sect. 4.2.

4.2   Results

The performance analysis was carried out by evaluating the cumulative distribution function (CDF) of the estimation error $\epsilon = |\hat{s}_{l,n} - s_{l,n}|$, where $\hat{s}_{l,n}$ indicates the estimated RSS for the (l, n) AP-RP pair, as already defined in Sect. 3, while $s_{l,n}$ is the measured RSS for the same pair. Due to space limitations, results are presented for a single AP in a 2D propagation (from one of the L_1 APs to the N_1 RPs), but similar results have been obtained for the other APs at the 1-st floor and for the 3D propagation case (from the L_2 APs to the N_1 RPs).

Figure 1 presents the CDFs of ϵ for Strategy II (1a), III (1b) and IV (1c) and different values of ρ ranging from 0.01 to 1. Results show that, in all strategies, after a sharp improvement as ρ is increased from 0.01 to 0.1 (in particular for Strategy IV, since it works with a single measurement with $\rho = 0.01$), the performance increase is less and less relevant as ρ increases from 0.1 to 1; this clearly suggests that few uniformly distributed measurements are in most cases sufficient for obtaining a reliable estimation of the propagation parameters. In particular, Strategy II (1a) shows a higher variability and unpredictability than Strategies III and IV (1b, 1c), due to the fact that the use of different sets of mockup measurements lead to different approximations of the objective environment propagation parameters, and it cannot be assumed that the use of the entire set of mockup measurements leads to the best approximation of the objective environment propagation parameters.

Finally, Fig. (1d) compares the errors obtained with the four strategies (including the baseline Strategy I), with ρ set to 0.5. The results show that all

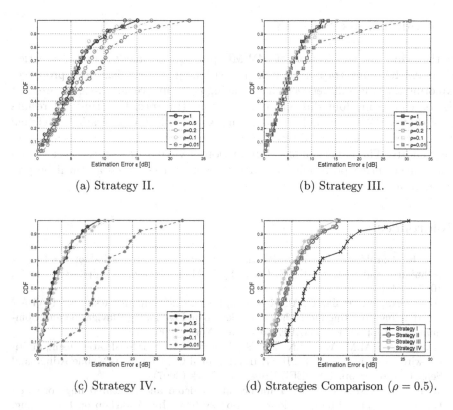

(a) Strategy II.

(b) Strategy III.

(c) Strategy IV.

(d) Strategies Comparison ($\rho = 0.5$).

Fig. 1. CDFs of ϵ for a given AP.

strategies show a significant performance improvement compared to the baseline (Strategy I). Results also show that Strategy IV leads to the best performance while Strategy II and III achieve comparable and still satisfactory accuracies.

Results highlight that if a good amount of measurements were taken in the objective environment, Strategy III is less appropriate than Strategy IV, given that the latter reaches higher accuracy by using the same set of measurements and dividing them in different optimization procedures. On the other hand, with the aim of minimizing the offline phase efforts, Strategy II performance, closely comparable with Strategy III, demonstrates that a good RSS estimation and, in turn, a reliable creation of virtual fingerprints, can be obtained by using a set of measurements and parameters taken from a mockup area. Strategy II might prove particularly useful and cost-effective in multiple floors buildings, where, taken a specific floor as mockup for the others, a single measurements campaign and fitting procedure are carried out, and then used to create a specific set of virtual fingerprints for each of the other floors, with a significant reduction in measurement efforts.

5 Conclusions

In this work the application of MWMF propagation models to the creation of virtual RPs fingerprints for indoor positioning systems has been proposed, exploring the trade-off between the modeling performance and the measurement efforts, comparing four different optimization strategies. Experimental results show that a MWMF model is a promising solution in the generation of virtual RPs as it guarantees a good trade-off between modeling accuracy and measurement efforts. The impact of the introduction of virtual RPs on the accuracy of WiFi fingeprinting positioning is currently being investigated and will be presented in future work.

References

1. Liu, H., Darabi, H., Banerjee, P., Jing, L.: Survey of wireless indoor positioning techniques and systems. IEEE Trans. Syst. Man. Cybern. C Appl. Rev. **37**(6), 1067–1080 (2007)
2. Honkavirta, V., Perälä, T., Ali-Löytty, S., Piché, R.: Comparative survey of WLAN location fingerprinting methods. In: Workshop on Positioning, Navigation and Communication, pp. 243–251. IEEE Press, New York (2009)
3. Hossain, A.K.M.M., Van, H.N., Jin, Y., Soh, W.-S.: Indoor localization using multiple wireless technologies. In: IEEE International Conference on Mobile Adhoc and Sensor Systems, pp. 1–8. IEEE Press, New York (2007)
4. Widyawan, K.M., Pesch, D.: Influence of predicted and measured fingerprint on the accuracy of rssi-based indoor location systems. In: Workshop on Positioning. Navigation, and Communication, pp. 145–151. IEEE Press, New York (2007)
5. Chintalapudi, K., Iyer, A.P., Padmanabhan, V.N.: Indoor localization without the pain. In: International Conference on Mobile Computing and Networking, pp. 173–184. ACM Press, New York (2010)
6. Eleryan, A., Elsabagh, M., Youssef, M.: Synthetic generation of radio maps for device-free passive localization. In: IEEE Global Communications Conference, pp. 1–5. IEEE Press, New York (2011)
7. COST Action 231: Digital mobile radio towards future generation systems. Technical report, European Commission (1999)
8. Borrelli, A., Monti, C., Vari, M., Mazzenga, F.: Channel models for IEEE 802.11b indoor system design. In: IEEE International Conference on Communications, pp. 3701–3705. IEEE Press, New York (2004)

Time Reversal in UWB Ad-Hoc Networks with No Power Control and Inter-symbol Interference

Flavio Maschietti[1]($\boxtimes$), Jocelyn Fiorina[2], and Maria-Gabriella Di Benedetto[1]

[1] DIET Department, La Sapienza, University of Rome,
Via Eudossiana 18, 00184 Rome, Italy
flavio.maschietti@gmail.com, gaby@acts.ing.uniroma1.it
[2] Département de Télécommunications, Centrale-Supélec,
3, rue Joliot-Curie, 91192 Gif-sur-Yvette, France
jocelyn.fiorina@centralesupelec.fr

Abstract. Time Reversal is well-known in Impulse Radio Ultra Wideband communications (IR-UWB) for its ability to improve performance and complexity both in noise limited scenarios and multiuser interference (MUI) limited ones. In an ad-hoc uncoordinated network, where no power control is possible, no users' channels are known, or no elaborate multiple access techniques can be deployed, Time Reversal is imperfect. In this paper, a comparative analysis between conventional Rake schemes and Time Reversal ones is made in order to evaluate robustness towards the absence of the mentioned operations.

Keywords: UWB · Impulse radio · Time Hopping · Time Reversal · Ad-Hoc paired networks · Multiuser interference · Inter-symbol interference

1 Introduction

Time Reversal (TR), a prefiltering technique based on reversed channel impulse responses, can be used in UWB communications to lighten the burden on the receiver. This precoding technique has several attractive properties.

In fact, Time Reversal can alter the statistical properties of multiuser interference. In [2], the influence of Time Reversal on multiuser interference in centralized networks was shown: the focusing properties of TR make multiuser interference more impulsive, with a narrower distribution and a higher kurtosis, which lead to a performance increase.

Moreover, in [3], the advantages guaranteed by Time Reversal in the context of positioning based on DOA estimation were highlighted.

In literature, numerous performance studies of UWB communications with Time Reversal precoding exist. Nonetheless, these studies are evaluated under strong assumptions: particular network topologies, centralized and synchronous communications. A comprehensive example is found in [4], where Time Reversal power controlled, synchronous transmissions are compared to conventional ones.

© Institute for Computer Sciences, Social Informatics and Telecommunications Engineering 2015
V. Atanasovski, L.-G. Alberto (Eds.): Fabulous 2015, LNICST 159, pp. 173–180, 2015.
DOI: 10.1007/978-3-319-27072-2_22

Often, other assumptions on the frame length are aimed to make inter-symbol interference (ISI) and multipath dispersion negligible.

All these assumptions are made to facilitate the evaluation of theoretical expressions, but further investigation need to be made for more complex scenarios.

Other studies such as [5–7], evaluated multiuser interference and its associated measures in UWB realistic scenarios, but without entering into Time Reversal details and comparisons.

In particular, in [5] the effect of power control on multiuser interference is shown, whereas in [6] it is highlighted that multiuser interference in a UWB non-power controlled network strongly depends on spatial densities of the users, besides their number and bitrates.

In [7], ISI/IFI is considered in a single user Time Hopping UWB context: a closed-form expression is given for its variance, highlighting its non-gaussianity.

Moreover, in [8], a discrete time model was presented to investigate and compare robustness towards channel estimation errors both in precoded and non-precoded transmissions in a centralized symbol-synchronous network, where all transmission are directed to a base station, *i.e.* a common sink.

These and other studies provide a valid working basis for this work, whose principal aim is to evaluate the performance of ad-hoc UWB networks where both precoded (TR) and non-precoded transmissions are exploited and where pairs of nodes communicate independently. It could represent a special kind of sensors network, suitable for UWB applications.

This restriction implies absence of power control, synchronization, estimation of users channels and efficient multiple access technique.

In this scenario, Time Reversal is imperfect, leading to correlation losses and interference gain. This work aim to compare conventional non-precoded schemes and Time Reversal ones in order to evaluate robustness towards these limitations.

2   System Model

An ad-hoc network where K pairs communicate in an uncoordinated manner, *independently* from each other, is considered.

A generic transmitter emits data, which is encoded into a sequence of information bearing symbols b_n. Considering just one frame - *i.e.* a fixed n - the transmitted signal when no prefiltering is used is:

$$x(t) = b_n \sqrt{E_x} p(t - nT_s - mT_c) \tag{1}$$

where T_s is the frame period, T_c is the chip time and $p(t)$ is the waveform associated with the m-th symbol of the generic user, as common in IR-UWB communications. E_x is the transmitted energy, which will be consider equal to 1 in the following expressions.

In general, $p(t)$ is the UWB pulse and has band $[-\frac{W}{2}, \frac{W}{2}]$, *i.e.* its spectrum is zero for $|f| > \frac{W}{2}$.

The transmitted spread-spectrum signal $x_k(t)$ of each user propagates over a multipath channel with impulse response $h_k(t)$, which distorts the signal.

The demodulator for user k estimates its symbols by considering users $j \neq k$ as unknown interference over user k.

In the adopted model, the receiver is a single user detector, which does not take in account a joint multiuser detection.

2.1   Single User Channel

If the transmission does not foresee prefiltering and a single b - *i.e.* one frame - is emitted, the received signal is:

$$y(t) = x(t) + n(t) = b \sum_{k=0}^{N-1} s[k]p(t - kT_c) * h(t) + n(t) \qquad (2)$$

where the *spreading* sequence $s = (s[0], \ldots, s[N-1])^T$ is made explicit.

Assuming $T_c = \frac{1}{W}$, and finite *delay spread* channels, Eq. (2) is rewritten as:

$$y(t) = b \sum_{k=0}^{N-1} s[k] \sum_{l=0}^{L} h[l]p(t - (l + k)/W) + n(t) \qquad (3)$$

that follows also from $p(t)$ - and therefore $p(t) * h(t)$ - being bandlimited to $\frac{W}{2}$.

The spreading sequence is a Time Hopping code, for which all $s[k]$ are zero, except one. Hence, $\|s\|^2 = 1$.

The Discrete Model. An equivalent discrete model is obtained when Eq. (3) is projected onto $\{p(t - \frac{k}{W}) : k = 0, \ldots, (N + L - 1)\}$:

$$y = Cxb + n \qquad (4)$$

where C is a convolution matrix with dimensions $(N + L) \times N$, having assumed a causal and finite UWB channel with $L = \frac{T_d}{T_c}$.

In general, when prefiltering is adopted - with prefiltering impulse response $h_p(t)$ - the Eq. (4) generalizes to:

$$y = CPxb + n \qquad (5)$$

where P is a convolution matrix with dimensions $(N + 2L) \times (N + L)$ and where n includes both thermal noise and inter-symbol/frame interference, with the latter arising from multipath replicas due to previous frames.

Receiver Structure. In the case of Eq. (4), the conventional optimal receiver is a matched filter, *i.e.* an All-Rake receiver when a multipath channel is considered. Knowing the spreading sequence x and the channel matrix C, a valid statistic for b is obtained as:

$$z^{AR} = \frac{Cx^T}{\|Cx\|}y = \frac{Cx^T}{\|Cx\|}(Cxb + n) \qquad (6)$$

When prefiltering is adopted, the receiver is a 1-Rake receiver matched on the overall impulse response, *i.e.* an autocorrelation of the channel:

$$z^{TR} = e_{L+j_x}^T y = e_{L+j_x}^T CPxb + e_{L+j_x}^T n \tag{7}$$

where $e_{L+j_x}^T$ denotes the canonical vector with a one in the $L + j_x$ coordinate, *i.e* the peak in the time reversed impulse response.

As well-known, in a single user scenario, there is no performance difference between an All-Rake receiver and a TR 1-Rake one.

2.2 Multiuser Channel

The direct extension of Eq. (5) to K transmitters is as follows:

$$y = \sum_{k=1}^{K} C_k P_k x_k b_k + n \tag{8}$$

where C_k and P_k are the channel and the precoding convolution matrices for the user k, with same dimensions as in Eq. (5).

Receiver Structure. In the multiuser case, the receivers are equivalent to those seen for the single user case. Without prefiltering, an All-Rake receiver gives the following decision variable:

$$z_k^{AR} = \frac{(C_k x_k)^T}{\|C_k x_k\|} y = \sum_{j=1}^{K} \frac{(C_k x_k)^T}{\|C_k x_k\|} C_j x_j b_j + \frac{(C_k x_k)^T}{\|C_k x_k\|} n$$

$$= \|C_k x_k\| b_k + S_k + I_k + \nu_k \tag{9}$$

where the k-th pair is the reference one. S_k and I_k represents the *interframe interference* and the *multiuser interference*, and $\nu_k \sim \mathcal{N}(0, \frac{N_0}{2})$ is filtered thermal noise.

In the multiuser case, the equivalence between the two schemes does not hold.

3   Simulation Results

This chapter presents the results obtained after the simulations. A *reference* pair in the network is chosen to evaluate the performance. In the proposed model, two performance measures are considered.

In the *uncoded* regime, the BER - *i.e.* bit error ratio - is taken into account. In the *coded* regime, *mutual information* with Gaussian inputs, which maximize differential entropy of the receiver output random variable, along with *spectral efficiency*, is considered.

There are various parameters which are common to each simulation: users channels are derived from a discretized version of the IEEE 802.15.3a model,

LOS (0–8 m), which is suitable for the presumed applications of an ad-hoc UWB network. In particular, the *delay spread* of each channel is fixed at 50 ns, which includes the most essential replicas. Each channel is considered to be *stationary* in the observation time. All simulations are done assuming perfect channel knowledge, *i.e.* perfect CSI, except where otherwise specified.

In each iteration, at least 5000 frames are considered, divided in N chips whose length is 1 ns. The transmitted waveform is adapted to the chip length. Channels and users positions, thus network arrangement, are modified throughout the Monte Carlo experiments.

In order to consider *asynchronism* between users, each interfering signal is shifted in time. Perfect timing is instead assumed between each receiver and its intended transmitter.

3.1 Single User

The single user case is useful to focus on ISI/IFI interference, which is reduced as the frame length is increased: a smaller number of multipath replicas overlap successive frames, *i.e.* successive symbols.

In fact, each frame can include a time guard at its end to make ISI/IFI negligible: that works, although with a high price in terms of bitrate, since a UWB channel has a delay spread of 50–100 ns on average.

Considering ISI/IFI and concerning Time Reversal, it is important to notice the better robustness to interframe interference in 1-Rake receivers, which outperform all the others. Indeed, interframe interference cause a significant degradation in TR-UWB communications above all, where a larger transmitted waveform - close to doubling the length of the received signal - is adopted. Moreover, Time Reversal increases signal power, making IFI/ISI more strong (Fig. 1).

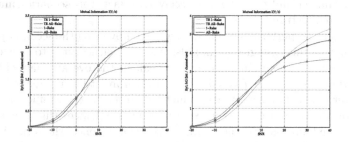

Fig. 1. Mutual information vs SNR with $N = 5, 10$. Single user case.

3.2 Multiuser

In the multiuser case, simulations showed that multiuser interference is in general not Gaussian, irrespective of precoding and receiving stages, confirming other studies. This is due to the impulsive nature of TH-UWB signals.

Dependence on Spatial Density. Due to absence of power control, multiuser interference PDFs strongly depends on the network area. In particular, more impulsive PDFs were reached as the network area increased. Along with Time Reversal schemes, a higher kurtosis - which is a measure of Gaussian-likeness - compared to conventional schemes was reached only for areas bigger than 4 m². So, Time Reversal resulted less robust to the *near-far* problem.

Two Fictitious Scenarios. In fact, when a fictitious power control (PC) was implemented, a drastic improvement in terms of mutual information was obtained in TR communications which were able to outperform conventional ones, as it can be seen in the example case with $K = 10$, $N = 20$, depicted in Fig. 2.

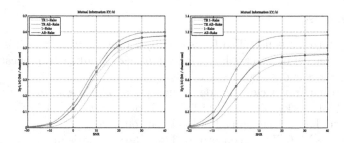

Fig. 2. Mutual information vs SNR with $K = 10$, $N = 20$ with and without PC.

Another fictitious scenario was then considered. TR is in general based on the channel through the intended receiver: in this case, the interfering signals which arrive to the reference receiver are not subjected to a peaked overall impulse response. Instead, this happens when TR is based on the channel between the generic transmitter and the reference receiver. In fact, this scenario simulates a centralized architecture.

Surprisingly, no performance increase was seen by using the second option. In fact, although in this case greater impulsiveness is reached, it is to consider that interfering signals are emphasised by the peak in the overall channel impulse response, which is *anyway* selected with a high prob. at the reference receiver.

Moreover, ISI/IFI of other pairs - which cannot be cancelled since no channel is known by the reference receiver expect its one - enhances this phenomenon: more peaks are found in reference frames. As a consequence, the result is just to increase the interfering power, through the presence of the autocorrelation peak.

Robustness to Channel Estimation Errors. Lastly, simulations showed that TR schemes are the most degraded ones under channel estimation errors. In this case, ISI/IFI cannot be completely cancelled, even in the reference pair: as seen in the single user case, TR is the least robust scheme to this type of interference. Moreover, along with TR All-Rake, the performance is degraded by the double estimation required both in transmission and reception (Fig. 3).

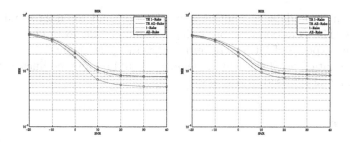

Fig. 3. BER vs SNR with $K = 10$, $N = 20$ and load $= 0.5.\tau = 0, 0.01$.

4 Conclusions and Future Investigations

This work highlighted differences between Time Reversal transmissions and non-precoded ones, along with Rake receivers, in an ad-hoc *uncoordinated* network.

In order to evaluate these techniques, a discrete time model was adopted: results were divided in single and multiuser cases.

In the single user case, the importance of ISI/IFI was underlined. Time Reversal increases both length and power of signals, leading thus to small robustness towards this kind of interference.

In the multiuser case, due to power-unbalance, multiuser interference PDFs were found to be dependent on the *spatial density* of interfering users. Increasing the network area, a greater impulsiveness was reached.

Indeed, simulations reported that kurtosis was higher in non-precoded transmissions as the network area was smaller. Precoded transmissions showed smaller robustness to the *near-far* problem. This result suggested to use *power control* in order to improve TR communications.

Another fictitious scenario was then considered: Time Reversal was based on the channel between the generic transmitter and the reference receiver. In this case, there is maximum correlation and a *peak* in the overall impulse response to which the signals of each user are subjected to.

A decrease in performance was seen under this TR scheme. An interfering Time Reversal signal is in fact more disturbing here, since precoding increases its power. The presence of ISI/IFI enhances this phenomenon.

As a final step, robustness towards channel estimation errors was evaluated. Channel estimation errors bring ISI/IFI back in the reference user frames, while decrease signal/mask correlation at each receiver. Time Reversal communications experienced the greatest performance losses - due to worse robustness to ISI/IFI.

So, effective channel estimation techniques, along with an appropriate control of ISI/IFI, are crucial to Time Reversal application in ad-hoc UWB networks.

Further investigations which could be made to enrich this work are: the development of more powerful ISI/IFI removal techniques. In particular, TR could be improved to combat ISI/IFI in the transmitter side, with the adoption of superior precoding matrices. The evaluation of more complex receivers, capable to exploit and to adapt to multiuser interference, and to endorse multi-frame processing. The consideration of coding techniques, for example a repetition code, at the expense of bitrate, to improve overall performance.

The evaluation of all these improvements should require modifications to the discrete time model used in this work.

References

1. Di Benedetto, M.-G., Giancola, G.: Understanding Ultra Wide Band Radio Fundamentals. Prentice Hall, Upper Saddle River (2004)
2. Fiorina, J., Capodanno, G., Di Benedetto, M.-G.: Impact of time reversal on Multi-User interference in IR-UWB. In: IEEE International Conference on Ultra-Wideband (2011)
3. De Nardis, L., Fiorina, J., Panaitopol, D., Di Benedetto, M.-G.: Combining UWB with Time Reversal for improved communication and positioning. Springer Telecommun. Syst. **52**, 1145–1158 (2013)
4. Popovski, K., Wisocki, B.J., Wisocki, T.A.: Modelling and comparative performance analysis of a time-reversed UWB System. EURASIP J. Wireless Commun. Networking. **2007**, 62–62 (2007)
5. Panaitopol, D.: Ultra wide band Ad-Hoc sensor networks: a Multi-Layer analysis. Supélec and National University of Singapore (2011)
6. Giancola, G., De Nardis, L., Di Benedetto, M.-G.: Multiuser interference in power-unbalanced ultra wide band systems: analysis and verification. In: IEEE Conference on Ultra Wideband Systems and Technologies (2003)
7. Deleuze, A.-L., Ciblat, P., Le Martret, C.J.: Inter-symbol/inter-frame interference in time-hopping ultra wideband impulse radio system. In: IEEE International Conference on Ultra-Wideband (2005)
8. Ferrante, G.C.: Shaping Interference Towards Optimality of Modern Wireless Communication Transceivers. La Sapienza, University of Rome (2015)

UWB and Time-Reversal Techniques Positioning System for Railway Application

Bouna Fall[1,2], Fouzia Elbahhar[1,2(✉)], Adil Elabboubi[1,2],
Marc Heddebaut[1,2], and Atika Rivenq[1,3]

[1] University of Lille Nord de France, 59000, Lille, France
Fouzia.boukour@ifsttar.fr
[2] LEOST, IFSTTAR, 59666 Villeneuve d'Ascq, France
[3] UVHC, IEMN-DOAE, 59313 Valenciennes, France

Abstract. This paper studies a new techniques for localization system in railway transport using UWB radio and Time Reversal technique (TR) techniques. Communication and localization in rail applications represents a permanent and evolutionary need, motivated by the improvement of the quality and safety of transports. Ultra wide band appears as a very suitable technology for this kind of application, due to its large bandwidth, also to its good resistance to the interference and to multipath. Time Reversal channel pre-filtering facilitates signal detection and helps increasing the received energy in a targeted area. In this paper, we evaluate the characteristics of spatio-temporal focusing of time reversal on the one hand, and secondly we compare systems without time reversal UWB location and tracking systems with time reversal UWB in terms of error localization. These studies are conducted in simulation and experimentation.

Keywords: UWB · Time reversal · Focusing · TDOA · Localization

1 Introduction

Usually, ground to train radiocommunication exploits access points installed along the track, exchanging data with mobile equipment installed on the trains [1]. Either proprietary radio modems derived from existing standards are used. Currently, all these radio modems operate sinusoidal sources of signals occupying radio channels over a limited bandwidth.

For the train localization process, drifts of the train odometer, usually composed of a wheel turn counter and a Doppler radar that continuously calculate the position and velocity data, are periodically compensated by ground balises installed between the rails. Balises are working as kilometer-markers and transmit their absolute localization to passing trains. The requested localization accuracy is important and should allow, for example in automated urban subways, vehicles to repeatedly stop in front of station doors, thus, necessitating a few centimeters localization accuracy.

This paper proposes a new approach for railway track-to-train short range communication simultaneously providing accurate localization information. Breaking with the recalled conventional approaches, an association between Ultra Wide Band (UWB)

V. Atanasovski, L.-G. Alberto (Eds.): Fabulous 2015, LNICST 159, pp. 181–187, 2015.
DOI: 10.1007/978-3-319-27072-2_23

radio and Time Reversal (TR) techniques constitutes the heart of the work outlined in this paper.

The paper will described the results obtained in the context of this railway perspective. It is organized as follows. Section 2 describes the proposed railway balise. Using different configurations, Sect. 3 develops a simulation study of the TR characteristics and UWB-TR coupled system. Section 4 presents the used experimental TR-UWB setup and the associated experimental results. Finally, conclusions are provided in Sect. 5.

2 System Description

2.1 New Balise Proposal

Conventional balises are located between the rails. They have the form of a rectangular parallelepiped, as shown in Fig. 1. The train, passing over the balise, can briefly exchange information with the ground, reads its absolute localization from this track kilometer marker and, therefore, compensates for the drift of its proprioceptive localization sensors [4, 5].

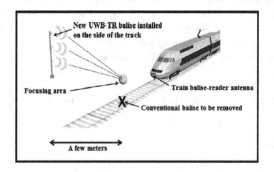

Fig. 1. TR-UWB proposed new railway balise

In many railway systems, these balises constitute the only equipment remaining on the track, between the rails, and it could prove worthwhile to remove this last equipment in order to facilitate track maintenance, for example rail replacements.

As presented in Fig. 1, in our proposal, the conventional balise situated between the rails is removed and replaced by the new balise, installed on a pole, on the side of the track, and a few meters away. This new balise focuses the radiofrequency energy coming from the pole transmitters to an area situated over the rails, right over the removed conventional balise location. Therefore, this new balise does not interfere anymore with track maintenance operations, but still develop a maximum of radio frequency signal at this particular location over the rails. Several transmitters are coupled on the pole; three can be seen in Fig. 1 to get a multiple source transmitter. This insures transmitter redundancy as well as, when correctly configured, space focusing. One single receiver or train-balise reader is used, located in front of the train. This configuration is usually denoted as a Multiple Input, three transmitters, Single Output, one receiver, MISO 3×1 system.

2.2   Time Reversal

In such situations, a TR system should be able not only to compensate for the multipath effect, but also to improve radio communication parameters by taking advantage of the energy distributed in the reflected signals [6]. Usually, the following TR process is used. Firstly, the channel impulse response (CIR) is measured between the transmitter (Tx) and the receiver (Rx) and the corresponding Channel State Information (CSI) is then loaded into Tx. Secondly, the selected signal and the impulse response are reversed in time and transmitted by Tx in the propagation channel, up to Rx. This process, can be mathematically described by noting s(t) the transmitted pulse, h(t) the complex impulse response of the channel and h*(−t) the complex conjugate of the time reversed version of h(t); y(t) the received signal without TR and $y_{RT}(t)$, the received signal with TR at the receiver; one has:

$$y(t) = s(t) \otimes h(t) \tag{1}$$

$$y_{RT}(t) = s(t) \otimes h * (-t) \otimes h(t) \tag{2}$$

Where $\otimes$ represents the convolution operation and n(t) is the Gaussian noise. From Eq. (2), we deduce the equivalent impulse response heq(t) which corresponds to the autocorrelation function of the channel:

$$heq(t) = h * (-t) \otimes h(t) \tag{3}$$

2.3   Temporal and Spatial Focusing

Temporal focusing (TF) and Spatial Focusing (SF) are characteristics associated to TR. To study TF, one can evaluate the Focusing Gain (FG), which is defined as the ratio of the spectrum power of strongest amplitude peak in TR received, to the strongest peak received by a conventional UWB system. The focusing gain can be written as:

$$FG_{[dB]} = 20 \log_{10} \left(\frac{\max(|y_{RT}(t)|)}{\max(|y(t)|)} \right) \tag{4}$$

Since the signal level is increased in the receiving area, higher FG could potentially translate into higher communication range and higher precision of localization. As an example, the study of SF considering a simple transmitter to receiver configuration is performed the following way. The channel impulse response (CIR) of the intended receiver located in position p_0 is noted $h(p_0,t)$. The CIR of the unintended receiver located in position p_i ($i \neq 0$) is noted $h(p_i, i \neq 0)$. The equivalent CIR of the intended receiver is then given by:

$$heq(p_0, t) = h * (p_0, -t) \otimes h(p_0, t) \tag{5}$$

While the equivalent impulse response of the unintended receiver is given by:

$$heq(p_1, t) = h * (p_0, -t) \otimes h(p_1, t) \tag{6}$$

SF is then evaluated as the ratio of the strongest peak power received by the intended receiver to the strongest peak received by the unintended receiver. The SF parameter can be written as:

$$SF_{[dB]} = 20 \log_{10} \left(\frac{\max(|heq(p_0, t)|)}{\max(|heq(p_1, t)|)} \right) \tag{7}$$

3   Evaluation of the TR Characterizatics in a Multi-antenna Configuration

In this section, we evaluate the contribution of TR in this configuration in terms of FG and SF. Firstly, their expressions are determined in the general case of a MISO nx1 configuration then, the simulation results are presented for cases MISO 3 × 1.

The study of FG is performed for channel models exploiting the ray channel approach channel model. The ray channel model is presented in [5]. It is set by considering a transmitter (Tx) to receiver (Rx) distance d0. The propagation domain is bounded by a first horizontal surface, infinite, homogeneous and perfectly smooth with a permittivity contrast (Fig. 2). The signals from Tx to Rx undergo reflections on the floor and ceiling, except in the case of the direct path. An analytical computation of all these rays can be performed using some geometrical considerations.

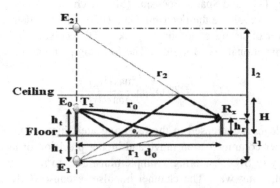

Fig. 2. Ray channel model

The general expression for the equivalent impulse response is given by Eq. 8 [1]:

$$heq_{MISO}(t) = \sum_{i=1}^{N_t} \sum_{m=0}^{N-1} \alpha_{mi}^2 \Phi_{si}(t) \tag{8}$$

Where Nt is the number of transmit antennas and $\Phi_{si}(t) = \int_0^\infty s_i(t - t_{mi})s_i$ $(t + \tau - t_{mi})dt$

The expression of FG is given by Eq. 9 [1]

$$FG_{[dB]} = 10Log_{10} \left[\frac{\sum_{i=1}^{N_t} \sum_{m=0}^{N-1} \alpha_{mi}^2}{\sum_{i=1}^{N_t} \alpha_{0i}^2} \right] \tag{9}$$

Table 1 represents the focusing gain in the case of MISO 3 × 1. This focusing gain is evaluated using successively 2, 4, 6 and 10 paths. We note that the focusing gain increases with the complexity of the channel (and the number of transmitters [1]). Indeed, from 2 to 10 paths, the focusing gain increases from 9.2 dB to 16.5 dB.

Table 1. FG Using 2, 4, 6 and 10 paths

Ray model	2 paths	4 paths	6 paths	10 paths
$FG[dB]$	9.2	14.0	15.9	16.5

4   Experimental Validation

The purpose of this experimental validation is to assess the impact of environmental complexity on performance related to temporal/spatial focusing and positioning error, and to compare these conclusions to our preceding simulation results.

4.1   Experimental Setup

An Arbitrary Waveform Generator (AWG) associated with a fast sampling oscilloscope (TDS) is used. These equipment have different available ports that can be used to respectively generate and acquire signals. The pulses generated by the AWG are radiated using wideband horn antennas. Similar antennas are used for receiving; their outputs are connected to the TDS ports through low noise amplifiers (LNA). We consider an anechoic chamber with metallic reflectors in order to create, different configurations of multipath. In each type of environment, MISO 3 × 2 configuration is used. The dimension of the anechoic chamber we used is $7 \times 7 \times 3$ m, it is operating from 100 MHz to 10 GHz. Three cases are considered: the anechoic chamber without addition of metal reflectors; two reflector plates; four reflectors plates. Figure 3 presents a view corresponding to configuration 2.

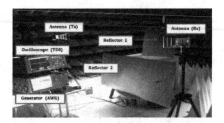

Fig. 3. Implementation of third configuration (presence of two reflector plates)

4.2   TR Focusing Effect Experimental Evaluation

In this section, we experimentally evaluate the TR focusing effect before measuring its impact in terms of positioning errors. Our objective is to evaluate the FG, as the complexity of the propagation channel increases, MISO 3×1 configuration corresponds to the addition of a three transmitting antenna using a distance of 4 m between Tx3 and Rx. In a first step, a pulse is transmitted using the AWG; the received signal is acquired by the TDS, and then returned temporally. In the cases of MISO 3×1, each Tx re-emits its corresponding reversed in time signal. We calculate the FG obtained in each case. The overall results are grouped in Table 2. We obtain that the FG increases with the number of reflector introduced. These results confirm the benefit of a higher complexity of the propagation environment when using TR.

Table 2. Focusing Gain (FG) according to the number of reflector plates inserted in the propagation environment

Configuration	$FG_{[dB]}$
without reflector	*1.7*
2 reflector plates	*8.2*
4 reflector plates	*12.8*

To evaluate SF, we consider the scenario using two reflector plates. The receiver is moved by 10 cm from its initial position. The results are summarized in Table 3. By making a comparison between, the three considered reflector cases SF values increase with the number of reflectors. This confirms, the results obtained in simulation.

Table 3. Spatial focusing (SF) according to the number of reflector plates inserted in the propagation environment

Configuration	$SF_{[dB]}$
without reflector	*3.1*
2 reflector plate	*11.1*
4 reflector plates	*16.4*

5 Conclusion

In this paper, we studied a new system for railway track-to-train. This new system associates the UWB technology and time reversal technique. Simulation study of TR characteristics and error localization is analyzed. Measurements were also performed in an anechoic chamber using an added set of metallic reflectors. The results show, on the one hand, time reversal has major assets to ultra wide band radio in terms of spatio-temporal focusing, and, on the other hand, that this advantage is transferred on the application to the localization.

References

1. Fall, B., Elbahhar, M.F., Heddebaut, M., Rivenq, A.: Time-reversal UWB positioning beacon for railway Application. In: IEEE Proceeding, IPIN, Sydney (Australia), pp. 18 (2012)
2. Ke-Lin, D., Swamy, M.N.: Wireless Communication Systems, pp. 1020, 15 April 2010, ISBN-13: 978-0- 521-11403-5
3. Pavon, J.D.P., et al.: The MBOA-WiMedia specification for ultra wideband distributed networks. IEEE Commun. Mag. **44**(6), 128–134 (2006)
4. Brutin, E.: ERTMS: Global dimensions, global challenges. Signal. Telecommun. Suppl., Eur. Railway Rev. **18**(3) 2012
5. Maaref, N., Millot, P., Ferriéres, X., Pichot, C., Picon, O.: Electromagnetic imaging methode based on time reversal processing applied to through the wall target localization. Prog. Electromagnet. Res. **1**, 59–67 (2008)
6. Liu, X., Wang, B.-Z., Xiao, S., Deng, J.: Performance of impulse radio UWB communication based on time reversal technique. Prog. Electromagnet. Res., PIER **79**(11), 401–413 (2008)

Special Session on Cyberspace Security

The Terrorist Threat
to the Critical Information
Infrastructure in South East Europe

Metodi Hadji-Janev[(⊠)] and Mitko Bogdanoski

Military Academy "General Mihailo Apostolski", Goce Delcev University,
Vasko Karangelevski bb, 1000 Skopje, Macedonia
{metodi.hadzi-janev,mitko.bogdanoski}@ugd.edu.mk

Abstract. The rise of ICT (Information and Communication Technologies) in
the age of globalization significantly affects SEE (South Eastern European)
security. Although these technologies help the region of SEE to become more
interconnected, interrelated and thus, boost the SEE countries' commodity,
prosperity and competitiveness put in security context, these technologies have
increased unpredictability, complexity and the threats to the SEE security. In this
line, as to the rest of the world, modern terrorism represents an inevitable burden
of the SEE governments' security. Today, it is more than clear that modern
terrorist groups and individuals exploit cyberspace to achieve strategic advantage against the mightier enemies. Therefore, based on the recent experience the
article explains how and in which way terrorist use of a cyberspace could affect
CII (critical information infrastructure) in the region of SEE. Giving the specific
dynamics in the region, article first explains how terrorists' use of modern ICT
and cyberspace serves to accomplish their strategic agenda. Then it explains
how terrorist could affect CIIs in the region of SEE and thus affect the overall
SEE regions' security.

Keywords: Critical information infrastructure · Terrorism · Cyberspace ·
South East Europe

1 Introduction

The ICT and the use of a cyberspace are important elements for the prosperity of the
region of South Eastern Europe (SEE). As to the rest of the world, these technologies
along with the cyberspace enhance social, economic and political activities in all SEE
countries. In this line business efficiency among others, urge SEE countries to introduce
supervisory controlled and data acquisition systems (known as SCADA) that run
critical infrastructure to the internet. So far, however, little focus has been placed on
security on these systems.

At the same time, the terrorists' use of cyberspace raises serious concerns about the
safety of SCADA systems and with that security on CII in SEE. Given that terrorists'
agenda is violent, abstract and apocalyptic, protection of the critical information
infrastructure has become one of the main concerns of the UN, EU, NATO and its
allies [1]. The article, based on the recent experience of the regional experts,

© Institute for Computer Sciences, Social Informatics and Telecommunications Engineering 2015
V. Atanasovski, L.-G. Alberto (Eds.): Fabulous 2015, LNICST 159, pp. 191–196, 2015.
DOI: 10.1007/978-3-319-27072-2_24

will explain the possibility of terrorists and terrorist organizations to attack vulnerable cyberspace and especially the critical information infrastructure in the region of SEE. In that context, the article is organized as following: Sect. 2 is giving general explanation of the threats of terrorism to the cyberspace in the SEE region. Moreover, the Sect. 3 explain how terrorist could affect critical information infrastructures in the region of SEE and thus affect the overall SEE regions' security. Finally, Sect. 4 concludes the work in this paper.

2   The Threat of Terrorism to the Region of South East European's Cyberspace

Several studies have shown that to achieve strategic advantage and gain global support while confronting mightier adversaries the core cadre of AQAM (Al Qaeda and its Associated Movements) heavily abuse modern information and communication technology (ICT). For example, according to the UN study, terrorists are using the internet to promote and support terrorist activities through six different and overlapping categories [2]. The terrorist use of internet according to the UN study is for: propaganda (including recruitment, radicalization and incitement to terrorism); financing; training; planning (including through secret communication and open-source information); execution; and cyber attacks. John Rollins in his study points that the decentralized nature of the Internet as a medium and the associated difficulty in responding to emerging threats match the franchised nature of terrorist organizations and operations [3]. On the other hand, Gabriel Wimann explains how internet boosts the learning capabilities of the terrorists [4]. London Bombing attacks are a clear example of how powerful this can be [5]. Committing cyber crime activities to fund their decentralized terrorist operations is another abuse of internet. According to press reports, Indonesian police officials believe the 2002 terrorist bombings in Bali were partially financed through online credit card fraud [6]. Additionally, during the 2007, UK trial for 2005 London terrorists' bombing accused revealed that 72 stolen credit cards were used to register over 180 Internet web domains at 95 different web hosting companies [7]. Other well supported evidence about the modern terrorists' intent to use internet for direct attack of the critical infrastructures and cause severe consequences clearly attest about the danger that modern terrorism poses to our security.

Although these dynamics are global, not SEE based specifically, there are evidences that speak about abuses of the SEE cyberspace. NATO has experienced the first ever organized cyber attacks during the Kosovo campaign, for example [8]. According to the local SEE and the world news, recent reports and studies, many SEE countries are facing experienced cyber activists, but the awareness of these threats is not promising. The news reports, back in May of 2013, informed that three Romanian nationals were caught taking part in a multimillion dollar cyber fraud ring that specifically targeted U.S. consumers and the trio ended up making off with more than $2 million [9]. A young hacker from Macedonia back in 2012 was detained due to the cyber crime allegations (i.e. attempting to penetrate illegally several security websites in the US) [10]. Reports about working in a network with hackers from different countries also indicate the threat in the SEE Cyberspace. Individuals from Britain, the US, Bosnia and Herzegovina, Croatia, Macedonia, New Zealand and Peru were arrested in an operation carried out with the assistance of Facebook and international law enforcement agencies [11]. Giving all of these and many other facts the lack of awareness about the threat from cyberspace in SEE is alarming [12].

At the same time, many arguments show that the SEE cyberspace has become a platform for committing various types of illegal activities including terrorist activities through cyberspace. Former is especially important in the light of the recent trend to connect control systems that run critical infrastructure to the internet.

Establishing such market among the SEE countries where SCADA systems will play crucial role is a major development that this region needs. It is well established fact that implementing SCADA will help to improve system reliability, and therefore support integrated system operation, reducing potential negative spillover effects between countries [13]. Some SEE country based studies confirm these findings [14]. Hence, knowing these facts it is logical to asses how terrorists can affect SEE CII.

3 Assessing the Threat to the South Eastern European Critical Information Infrastructure

According to the existing findings, direct threat to the SEE CII at the moment when this article was written is not alarming. However, giving the rapid development of ICT technology these doubts will soon become reality. Hence, we will explain how terrorist use of a cyberspace could cause serious threat to the security of SEE.

3.1 Dissemination of Propaganda

According to the official UN Study on the Use of the Internet for Terrorist purposes *"...propaganda generally takes the form of multimedia communications, providing ideological or practical instruction, explanations, justifications or promotion of terrorist activities"*. Practice shows that designing the propaganda materials is a carefully prepared process that articulates the existing challenges that create burden to the all societies. Like other parts and regions of the World, SEE have its own specifics. Usually propaganda in SEE has the following patterns. First, there is a misinterpretation of the general social challenges (unemployment or severe social conditions). Then, they bring these challenges in the context of ethnic challenges. Inconsistencies and social inequalities in the SEE societies are usually emphasized with specific graphic material acceptable to the target audience and always with religious prefix. The religion is offered as relief and hope. Thus, the final product is ideological material ready to be shared online or through SEE cyberspace.[1]

---

[1] See the following sites for example: Websites such as the "Way of the Believer" (*putvjernika.com*), Way of Islam (*stazomislama.com*), *Ensarije Serijata* ("Partisans of Sharia" http://www.geocities. ws/ensarije_seriata/index-2.html), and "News of the Community" (*vijestiummeta.com*), and the Sandžak Wahhabi website *kelimetul-haqq.org*.

There are some sites that spread religious intolerance, violence, including suicide attacks and anti-democratic messages. Some analyses explain that there are dozens of videos and Facebook pages that advocate extremism in the SEE cyberspace [15]. Balkan Insight published a story about Lavderim Muhaxheri who called on Muslims to join the fight to establish an Islamic state based on *Sharia law via YouTube* [16]. The problem with this is that these reports are not isolated incidents anymore [17].

3.2   The Threat to SEE CII Through Instigation, Recruitment, Radicalization and Communication

The Use of the Internet on Terrorist purposes, *"recruitment, radicalization and incitement to terrorism may be viewed as points along a continuum"* [2]. The process of "radicalization" refers primarily to the process of indoctrination that often accompanies the transformation of recruits into individuals determined to act with violence based on extremist ideologies. The process of radicalization, involves *"the use of propaganda, whether communicated in person or via the Internet, over time"* [2]. The length of time and the effectiveness of the propaganda and other persuasive means employed vary depending on individual circumstances and relationships. These circumstances are specific to the region of SEE.

According to some views, the Internet may be used as a way of communication. Terrorist develop relationships with, and solicit support from, those most responsive to targeted propaganda [18].

Online instigation, recruitment, radicalization and communication processes in the SEE consider demographic factors, such as age or gender, as well as social or economic circumstances. Hence, the Internet is a particularly effective medium for the recruitment of minors, who comprise a high proportion of users. According to the EU Commission, the process of online instigation, recruitment and radicalization in the region of SEE commonly capitalizes on an individual sentiment of injustice, exclusion or humiliation [19]. Clear example of how these activities could create dangerous practice in the physical world and thus, affect SEE CII is the case of Arid Uka [20].

3.3   Terrorists' Funding via SEE Cyberspace

There is no officially processed case of terrorist financing via Internet in the region of SEE. However, the Balkans are suspected of harboring Hezbollah network, with infrastructure, operational and financial resources readily available for use [21]. Others claim that SEE cyberspace has been used to support terrorist financing by some charitable organizations. Charitable organizations, such as the Benevolence International Foundation, Global Relief Foundation and some others are listed as a potential online supporters using SEE cyberspace in many studies including in the above-mentioned UN study. This is not to say that these organizations have not been confirmed as real supporters of terrorist organizations by funding their activities, but that there is no evidence that this has happened via SEE cyberspace.

Even though the terrorists' use of a cyberspace includes planning, training along with committing cyber crime activities, there are no evidences that these types of activities have happened through SEE cyberspace. Thus, the real threat from terrorist use of Cyberspace to SEE region comes from the use of the internet and ICT for propaganda, instigation, recruitment, radicalization and communication. Some reports indicate that there are potential online terrorist financing activities, nevertheless so far, this has not been proved. Hence, since the SCADA systems are still not massively exploited in the SEE region, the most threaten information infrastructure in the region is the internet itself. However, considering the fact that many industries from the region follow the world trends and they are in phase of integration of these systems within their companies, it is just question of time when the SCADA controlled CII will become one of the main targets of the terrorists, who will make and attempt to attack these systems for deferent purposes. Moreover, most of the countries in the region started with development and some of them with implementation of the eGovernment services, which are based on the usage of the same vulnerable technologies and Internet, so we should expect these services will also be often attacked by terrorists and terrorist organizations. Furthermore, the new promising technologies as WSNs (Wireless Sensor Networks) as well as the integration of WSN with RFID (Radio-Frequency IDentification) technologies, which are already implemented in some of the crucial sectors (i.e. Medical and Healthcare Sector), should be considered as a potential target of the terrorists and terrorists organizations.

4 Conclusion

Direct threat to SEE critical information infrastructure in terms of causing an attack that could result in loss of lives and material cost is almost impossible. At this point, the biggest threat in SEE is the "Internet itself".

Modernization, efficiency and market competitiveness urge SEE countries to introduce sophisticated SCADA systems. Hence, concerns about direct threat to CII in the region of SEE for now are not realistic. However, giving that Internet itself could be considered as the most vulnerable information infrastructure, other indirect methods of terrorists' use of a cyberspace urge SEE countries to undertake serious measures to identify and assess, mitigate and counter cyber-based threat vectors that modern terrorist pose to their security.

References

1. Bogdanoski, M., Petreski, D.: Cyber terrorism-global security threat. Contemp. Maced. Defense-Int. Sci. Defense, Secur. Peace J. **13**(24), 59–73 (2013)
2. The United Nations Office on Drugs and Crime, The Use of the Internet for Terrorist Purposes, The United Nations New York (2012)
3. Rollins, J.: Al Qaeda and Affiliates: Historical Perspective, Global Presence, and Implications for U.S. Policy, CRS Report R41070 (2011)

4. Weimann, G.: How modern terrorism uses the Internet. United states institute of peace. Accessed 22 March 2015 (2004). http://www.terror.net, http://www.usip.org/pubs/special reports/srl16.pdf

5. House of Commons Intelligence and Security Committee. Report into the London Terrorist Attacks on 7 July 2005, May 2006

6. Sipress, A.: An Indonesian's Prison Memoir Takes Holy War into Cyberspace. Washington Post, New York (2004). http://www.washingtonpost.com/wp-dyn/articles/A62095-2004Dec13.html. Accessed 14 December 2004

7. Krebs, B.: Three Worked the Web to Help Terrorists, p. D01. Washington Post, New York (2007)

8. Aaronson, M., Diessen, A., de Kermabon, Y., Long, M.B., Miklaucic, M.: NATO countering the hybrid threat. Prism 2(4), 111–124 (2012)

9. Amaruso, J.: Romania Global Center for Cyber Crime in USA, USA Toaday, 14 January 2014. http://guardianlv.com/2014/01/romania-global-center-for-cybercrime-in-u-s/. Accessed 22 March 2014

10. FBI Arrested Young Hacker from Struga, Press 24, November 20 2012. http://star.press24.mk/story/poznato/foto-fbi-uapsi-mlad-haker-od-struga-sin-na-poznata-struzhanka. Accessed 22 September 2013

11. 10 arrested in cyber-crime probe, Express UK, 13 December 2012. http://www.express.co.uk/news/world/364435/10-arrested-in-cyber-crime-probe. Accessed 24 March 2014

12. Maja, D., Bojan, D.: Perception of cyber crime in slovenia. J. Crim. Justice Secur. 12(4), 378–396 (2010)

13. Oklopčić, Z., Brestovec, B., Dalibor, S., Njavro, B.: IT solution for gas supply management in open gas market conditions. http://www.koncar-ket.hr/docs/koncarketHR/documents/158/1_0/Original.pdf. Accessed 17 April 2014

14. Kennedy, D., Besant-Jones, J.: World Bank Framework for Development of Regional Energy Trade in South East Europe, Energy and Mining Sector Board Discussion Paper, No.12, March 2004

15. Likmeta, B.: Al Qaeda Using Sical Media to find new Recruits, Global Post, 24 January 2014). http://www.globalpost.com/dispatch/news/regions/europe/140123/albania-isis-al-qaeda-social-media-europe. Accessed 22 April 2014

16. Albanian Jihadists Recruit Fighters for Syria on Facebook, BalkanInsight. http://www.balkaninsight.com/en/article/albanian-jihadist-use-internet-to-recruit-fighters. Accessed 15 January 2014

17. Theohary, C.A., Rollins, J.: Terrrorist Use of Internet: Information operations in Cyberspace, CRS Report, R41674 (2001)

18. Gerwehr, S., Daly, S.: Al-Qaida: terrorist selection and recruitment. In: Kamien, D., (ed.) The McGraw-Hill Homeland Security Handbook, McGraw-Hill. New York (2006)

19. European Commission, Expert Group on Violent Radicalisation, Radicalisation processes leading to acts of terrorism (2008). www.clingendael.nl/publications/2008/20080500_cscp_report_vries.pdf

20. Associated press, Kosovan Albanian admits killing two US airmen in Frankfurt terror attack. http://www.theguardian.com/world/2011/aug/31/kosovan-albanian-admits-killing-airmen. Accessed 31 August 2011

21. Tereshchenko, N.: Financing Terrorism: The European Nexus. In: Research Institute for European and American Studies, 25 March 2013. http://www.rieas.gr/research-areas/editorial/1939-financing-terrorism-the-european-nexus-.html. Accessed 23 April 2014

Simulation Analysis of DoS, MITM and CDP Security Attacks and Countermeasures

Biljana Tanceska[1], Mitko Bogdanoski[2], and Aleksandar Risteski[1(✉)]

[1] Faculty of Electrical Engineering and Information Technologies,
Saints Cyril and Methodius University,
Rugjer Boshkovik 18, 1000 Skopje, Macedonia
bibe_tancevska@hotmail.com, acerist@feit.ukim.edu.mk
[2] Military Academy "General Mihailo Apostolski", Goce Delcev University,
Vasko Karangelevski bb, 1000 Skopje, Macedonia
mitko.bogdanoski@ugd.edu.mk

Abstract. In this paper, an analysis of security attacks on network elements along with the appropriate countermeasures is presented. The network topology that has been attacked is designed in GNS3 software tool installed on Windows operating system, while the attacks are performed in Kali Linux operating system. Three groups of security attacks (Denial of Service, Man in the Middle, and Control Plane attacks) are observed in simulation scenarios with a detailed analysis on each of them, followed by a presentation of practical performance and ways of prevention (protection) against the attacks.

Keywords: GNS3 software tool · Kali linux OS · Network topology · Attacks · Denial of service · Man in the middle · Control plane · Prevention

1 Introduction

Internet security is a fundamental component in every network, whether we are talking about a local area network, metropolitan or a backbone network. The extremely significant benefits of the Internet are very well known, but when it comes to knowing how to cost-effectively protect the cyber infrastructure and the information that flows throught it, we are all in uncharted territory. Malicious users are constantly looking for weaknesses and ways to disrupt the normal functioning of a given network, thereby causing damage by stealing or modifying information or by making a service unavailable to its legitimate users. These are the reasons why the main questions in every organization are: How can we protect from a security violation? How can we be one step ahead of the attacker?

The main objective of this paper is to analyze some of the attacks that individuals or corporations are dealing with on a daily basis. In order the analysis to recognize all the specifics and opportunities of the analyzed attack, GNS3-based network topology is implemented. The paper is organized as follows: Sect. 2 gives detailed theoretical analysis of all security attacks covered in the paper; Sect. 3 complements the theoretical analysis with Kali Linux – based practical analysis which gives answers how the attacks are performed by the malicious users and which vulnerabilities each of the

© Institute for Computer Sciences, Social Informatics and Telecommunications Engineering 2015
V. Atanasovski, L.-G. Alberto (Eds.): Fabulous 2015, LNICST 159, pp. 197–203, 2015.
DOI: 10.1007/978-3-319-27072-2_25

considered attacks exploit; the prevention of the network from the previously analyzed attacks is explained in Sect. 4; finally, Sect. 5 concludes the work of this paper.

2 Theoretical Analysis of the Security Attacks

The paper will consider several attacks which are divided into three different groups: Denial of Service (DoS) attacks, Man In The Middle (MITM) attacks and Control plane attacks.

DoS Attack is any type of the attack where the attacker (hacker) attempt to prevent legitimate users from accessing the service [1]. The DoS attack may be initiated from a single machine, but typically many computers are used to carry out the attack - Distributed Denial of Service (DDoS) attack [2, 3]. The DoS attack analyzed in this paper is **DHCP Starvation attack**.

MITM is type of security attack where a malicious actor inserts himself into a conversation between two parties, impersonates both parties and gain access to information that the two parties were trying to send to each other [5]. The paper presents the **ARP Poisoning attack**.

Control Plane Attack targets the control plane of a network device (router). Local events can have nearly global impact on the control plane. This disruption can lead to network instability, resulting in a loss of connectivity and data [6]. The paper analyzes **Cisco Discovery Protocol (CDP) Flooding attack.**

DHCP Starvation Attack. DHCP Starvation attack is a method used to exhaust the IP address pool from the DHCP server. A DHCP Starvation attack works by broadcasting the DHCP requests with spoofed MAC addresses. The attacker sends numerous DHCP request to the DHCP server from different spoofed MAC addresses. The DHCP server tries to respond to all DHCP requests. If enough requests are sent, the network attacker can exhaust the DHCP server's address space available, for a period of time. In this period of time, if a legitimate user has sent a request, the request will be dropped since the DHCP server cannot response because it is too busy responding to the attacker. Then the network attacker can set up a rogue DHCP server on their system and respond to the new DHCP requests from the clients [4].

ARP Poisoning Attack. ARP Poisoning attack works by modifying the ARP tables in target machines by exploiting fundamental weaknesses in the way network drivers handle ARP traffic. The attack begins with the attacker sending unsolicited ARP reply packet to the target machine. These ARP packets contain the IP address of a network resource and its spoofed MAC address (in this case, the attacker puts the MAC address of his hardware). The victim receiving this forged packet will accept the reply, and load the MAC/IP pair contained in the packet into the victim's ARP table. In this way, the attacker places himself in the middle of the connection between the victim and the network resource.

CDP Flooding Attack. CDP Flooding attack is a control plane attack and it can be only performed on a Cisco network device. The CDP Flood attack works by sending a large number of CDP messages from fake CDP neighbors to the router. The attacker will cause maximum utilization of the CPU of the router, and also clogging the memory with all the neighbor entries. Thus, the performance of the router will slow down, and the router cannot route legitimate packet from other users.

3   Practical Analysis of the Security Attacks

The network topology on which the attacks are performed is shown in Fig. 1. It is composed of two parts: emulated part consists of a pre-configured router and a router configured as a DHCP server; and physical part consists of a pre-configured switch and two users connected to the switch. One of them is the malicious user who executes the attacks.

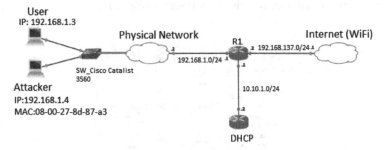

Fig. 1. Illustration of the analyzed network topology.

3.1   Rogue Server with DHCP Starvation and Rogue Rounting

Before launching the attack, we discuss how it affects the analyzed topology (Fig. 2).

The following steps allow practical execution of DHCP Starvation attack with Rogue server, using the Kali Linux OS.

1. Create a network sub-interface on the Kali machine to be used as the default gateway to route our rogue DHCP clients through.
2. Set the IP address on the new eth0:1 interface to another currently unused IP address.

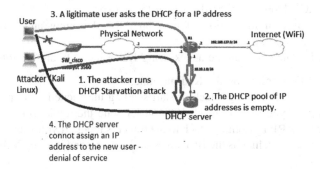

Fig. 2. Illustration of DHCP server with rogue server attack.

3. Allow IP forwarding on your Kali machine.
4. Set the default gateway and default route on the eth0:1 sub-interface.
5. Show the route Table.
6. In another terminal open new Metasploit console.
7. Launch the DHCP module and show the optional and required options that have to be set in order to run the rogue DHCP server.
8. Set the options.
9. In another terminal window launch the DHCP Starvation attack.
10. Start the rogue DHCP server from the Metasploit console [7].

After that, a new user is connected on the network, and the IP address he gets is assigned from the rogue DHCP server. Now, the default gateway is actually the IP address of the running Kali machine. The attacker is now in the middle of the communication between the user and the DHCP server (Fig. 3).

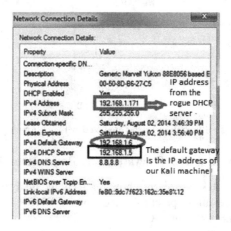

Fig. 3. The man in the middle attack is realised after successful DoS DHCP starvation attack.

3.2   ARP Poisoning Attack

Before starting to perform an ARP Poisoning attack, the malicious user should know the IP and MAC addresses of the devices in the network.

Figure 4 shows an illustration of how an ARP Poisoning attack performs on designed network topology.

The steps for launching an the attack using Kali Linux OS are the following:

1. Enabling IP Forwarding on the Kali machine.
2. Launch the ARP Poisoning attack or start sending unsolicited reply packets to the user saying: "If you want to reach 192.168.1.1 send the traffic to me."
3. Activating the ARP Poisoning attack to the router, saying "If you want to sent traffic to the 192.168.1.3, which is the IP address of the user, send it to my MAC address".

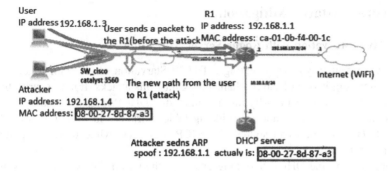

Fig. 4. Illustration of ARP Poisoning attack.

The results of the attack are shown in the Fig. 5, where can be clearly seen that the IP/MAC entry on the ARP table of the user is changed, so now every packet sent to the IP address of the router is going to the attacker.

```
Interface: 192.168.1.3 --- 0xc
    Internet Address       Physical Address        Type
    192.168.1.1            08-00-27-8d-87-a3       dynamic
    192.168.1.2            4X-5b-39-4h-W7-49       dynamic
    192.168.1.4            08-00-27-8d-87-a3       dynamic
    192.168.1.5            00-1e-33-11-1d-33       dynamic
```

Fig. 5. The ARP Poisoning attack is successful.

3.3 CDP Flooding Attack

Before launching the CDP Flooding attack, the Fig. 6 shows how it affects our topology.

The CPU utilisation of the switch before the attack is 5 %. The steps in Kali Linux OS that should be performed during the CDP attack are the following:

1. Start Yersinia from the terminal window on the Kali machine.
2. Go to Launch attack → CDP → Flooding CDP Table → OK.

After launching the attack and running for a few minutes, the CPU utilisation of the switch is increased to 58 %. If the attack is running a little bit longer the switch will start to drop packets because it will be become too busy.

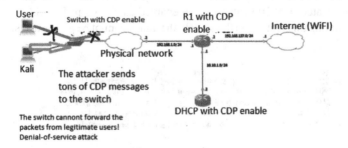

Fig. 6. Illustration of CDP Flooding attack on our topology

4 Security Attacks Mitigation

4.1 DHCP Starvation with Rogue Server Mitigation

There are several ways of preventing a DHCP Starvation attack with rogue server. **DHCP Snooping** is one of the mechanisms against this attacks. It is a security feature that provides network security by filtering untrusted DHCP messages and by building and maintaining a DHCP snooping binding table. Ports are identified as trusted and untrusted. Trusted ports can source all DHCP messages, while untrusted ports can source requests only.

After enabling the DHCP Snooping option in the Cisco Catalyst switch using the commands: **ip dhcp snooping** and **ip dhcp snooping vlan1**, the attack cannot be performed successfully (Fig. 7).

```
SW1#
03:31:38: %SYS-5-CONFIG_I: Configured from console by console
SW1#sh interface g
SW1#sh interface gigabitEthernet0/2
GigabitEthernet0/2 is down, line protocol is down (err-disabled)
  Hardware is Gigabit Ethernet, address is 0022.56a6.d102 (bia 0022.56a6.d102)
  MTU 1500 bytes, BW 10000 Kbit, DLY 1000 usec,
    reliability 255/255, txload 1/255, rxload 1/255
  Encapsulation ARPA, loopback not set
  Keepalive set (10 sec)
  Auto-duplex, Auto-speed, media type is 10/100/1000BaseTX
```

Fig. 7. Unsucessful DHCP Starvation attack

4.2 ARP Poisoning Mitigation

The most effective way to prevent an ARP Poisoning attack is by enabling DHCP Snooping or by enabling DAI (Dynamic ARP Inspection).

DAI is a secure feature that helps in prevention of ARP poisoning and other ARP-based attacks by intercepting all ARP requests and responses, and by verifying their authenticity before updating the switch's local ARP cache or forwarding the packets to the intended destinations. ARP Inspection creates a special IP to MAC address binding table in the switch. This table is dynamically populated based on the DHCP snooping database content.

When the switch receives an ARP packet on an untrusted port, it inspects the packet content. Based on the IP to MAC address binding table information in the packet, the switch permits the packet only if it matches the ARP Inspection table. The DAI feature on the Cisco Catalyst 3560 switch can be enabled as shown in Fig. 8.

After enabling this feature on the switch, the attack cannot be performed successfully.

```
SW1(config)# ip arp inspection vlan 1
SW1(config)# ip arp inspection log-buffer entries 1024
SW1(config)# ip arp inspection log-buffer logs 1024 interval 10
SW1(config)#interface gigabitEthernet0/1
SW1(config-if)#ip dhcp snooping trust
SW1(config-if)#ip arp inspection trust
```

Fig. 8. Enabling DAI

4.3   CDP Flooding Mitigation

There is only one easy step to prevent from a CDP Flooding attack and that is to **disable CDP** feature on all the ports that does not need it. The command of dissabling CDP is *no cdp enable*.

5   Conclusion

The paper gives a theoretical and practical analysis of several attacks: DHCP starvation with rogue server attack, ARP poisoning attack and CDP Flooding attack, as well as the effective mitigation techniques against these attacks.

From the analyses performed in this paper, it can be concluded that the internet users can easily become victims to these attacks, but there are mitigation techniques which are very easy to perform. Potential victims can efficiently defend themself from security attacks if they know how their network topology functions. However, achieving the desired security level is not without costs. It requires continuous investment in the area of security and upgrades of the security mechanisms which is the only way in preventing the network and systems from the advanced security attacks.

References

1. Stojanoski, P., Bogdanoski, M., Risteski, A.: Wireless local area network behavior under RTS flood DoS attack. In: 20th Telecommunications Forum TELFOR 2012. IEEE (2012)
2. Bogdanoski, M., Risteski, A.: Wireless network behavior under ICMP ping flood DoS attack and mitigation techniques. Int. J. Commun. Netw. Inf. Secur. (IJCNIS) 3(1), 2 (2011)
3. Bogdanoski, M., Suminoski, T., Risteski, A.: Analysis of the SYN flood DoS attack. Int. J. Comput. Netw. Inf. Secur. (IJCNIS) 5(8), 1–11 (2013)
4. Preimesburger, C.: DDoS Attack Volume Escalates as New Methods Emerge, 28 May 2014
5. TELELINK, Access Networking Threats, IT Threats (2013)
6. TELELINK, Corporate WAN Threats, IT Threats – Control Plane attack (2013)
7. Straatsma, P.: Rogue DHCP Server with DHCP Starvation and Rogue Routing, November 2013

An Analysis of the Impact of the AuthRF and AssRF Attacks on IEEE 802.11e Standard

Mitko Bogdanoski[1]([✉]), Pero Latkoski[2], and Aleksandar Risteski[2]

[1] Military Academy "General Mihailo Apostolski", Goce Delcev University,
Vasko Karangelevski bb, 1000 Skopje, Macedonia
mitko.bogdanoski@ugd.edu.mk
[2] Faculty of Electrical Engineering and Information Technologies,
Saints Cyril and Methodius University, Rugjer Boshkovik bb,
PO Box 574, 1000 Skopje, Macedonia
{pero,acerist}@feit.ukim.edu.mk

Abstract. The paper shows detailed analysis of the effects of the AuthRF (Authentication Request Flooding) and AssRF (Association Request Flooding) MAC Layer DoS (Denial of Service) attacks on 802.11e wireless standard based on a proposed queuing model. More specific, the paper analyzes the Access Point (AP) behavior under AuthRF DoS attacks with different frequency of the requests arrival, i.e. Low Level (LL), Medium Level (ML) and High Level (HL), at the same time considering different traffic priorities. The proposed queuing model and the developed analytical approach can be also used on each protocol layer, especially if the attacks are seen in terms of the flooding influence over AP with too many requests (ICMP, TCP SYN, UDP etc.).

Keywords: Denial of service · Flooding attack · MAC layer · Queuing model · AuthRF · AssRF · 802.11e

1 Introduction

The rapid development of wireless networks significantly fosters the need for flexibility of communications requiring anytime and anywhere connectivity. At the same time, the fast development of IEEE 802.11-based networks has become the main target of the attackers, who attack for various reasons, ranging from simple entertainment, to the attacks conducted with the main purpose of inflicting major damages (including the cyber terrorist attacks) [1] or making profit. This is possible primarily due to the wireless transmission media, which proved to be much more vulnerable target compared to the traditional wired networks.

Among many different types of wireless and wired attacks, the DoS attacks are most commonly used. Their basic goal is to disable access to a legitimate network or to specific network resources. DoS attacks can be conducted against all protocol layers separately, depending on the main goal of the attacker. The major DoS attacks disrupting the MAC sublayer are the attacks with huge amount of authentication and association requests, as well as the attacks with huge amount of deauthentication and disassociation requests [2]. Although the introduction of the 802.11w standard by

© Institute for Computer Sciences, Social Informatics and Telecommunications Engineering 2015
V. Atanasovski, L.-G. Alberto (Eds.): Fabulous 2015, LNICST 159, pp. 204–211, 2015.
DOI: 10.1007/978-3-319-27072-2_26

the IEEE in November 2009 puts a greater emphasis on mitigation of the deauthentication/disassociation attacks, still this standard does not give an appropriate protection against this kind of attacks, especially in the case when a huge number of deauthentication and disassociation messages attack the network [3]. Furthermore, the effects of the standard implementation against the authentication and association request flooding are still minor.

The aim of this paper is to develop an analytical model for 802.11e AP behavior, which will consider the effects of the DoS attacks with different number of authentication and association frames.

2   Queuing Model Analysis on the AuthRF and AssRF DoS Attacks on IEEE 802.11e WLAN

Extending the IEEE 802.11 queuing model presented in [4, 5], for the case when there are different traffic priorities, the paper presents a mathematical analysis of DoS attacks' impact on the 802.11e access points performance. It is clear that IEEE 802.11e-based AP will have different classes with different QoS (priority), which will lead to a more complex analysis and queuing model. In that sense, the presented model provides an upgrade of the queuing model proposed in [4] and its details of operation are shown in Fig. 1.

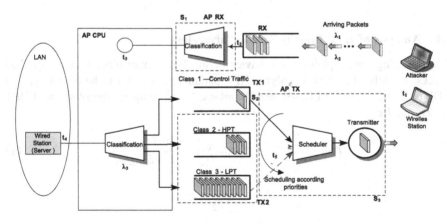

Fig. 1. Queuing model of the 802.11e AP.

The variables involved in the queuing model, similar as in [4], are grouped in four categories (see [4] for more details). According to Fig. 1, the queuing model of the AP consists of five elements. (1) Wireless station (legitimate user or attacker) sends and receives 802.11 frames to and from AP. This includes data, voice/video, management and control frames. (2) AP RX is responsible for acceptance of the 802.11e frames by the AP. A RX queue is connected to the RX serving center of the AP [5, 6]. (3) AP TX is responsible for sending 802.11 frames. As it can be seen in Fig. 1, there are two queues in the AP, TX1 and TX2. TX1 is responsible for serving management and control traffic, and TX2 is subdivided in two queues, HPT (High Priority Traffic) responsible for voice/video traffic, and LPT (Low Priority Traffic) responsible for the other data and background traffic. This part of the model represents the major extension proposed by the paper towards priority traffic modeling of IEEE 802.11e station. (4) AP CPU covers a group of internal modules. The processing time in CPU is very low and it is not considered during our analysis. (5) The wired station (or server) using LAN exchange data with the wireless station.

As it can be seen in the Fig. 1, despite the TX1 queue, which is planned to serve the control traffic, there are two additional queues (TX2). One is used to serve prioritized payload (one of higher QoS class, i.e. voice or video), considered as a HPT, and one to serve low prioritized payload (i.e. data traffic), considered as LPT. This model is a modification of the general queuing model, and the priorities are defined in accordance with 802.11e standard.

According to the 802.11 standard, control traffic is always served first, while voice/video traffic is second and data traffic has lowest priority (in our case the background traffic is not considered, because if the AP is under DoS attack this traffic will not have any priority). It should be noted that unlike in [4], the paper considers different types of attack (Low Level/LL, Medium Level/ML and High Level/HL) comparing the situation of HPT and LPT. Accordingly, the values and expressions for Tr and Ta for both types of traffic will be different. Tr refers to the time required for transmitting the data frames queued during an attack in the TX2 queue, while Ta refers to the time available for transmitting queued data frames in the TX2 queue before the next attack.

2.1 Analysis of High Priority Traffic Parameters

The following part explains the behavior of the HPT under different level of DoS attacks. Namely, the section analyzes HPT parameters, which can be of any type of UDP based traffic, under LL, ML and HL attack. If one compares the situation of HPT the Tr and Ta:

$$Tr_{HPT} = S_2 \sum_{i-1}^{\infty} (\lambda_{3HPT} S_3)^i = \frac{S_2 S_3 \lambda_{3HPT}}{1 - S_3 \lambda_{3HPT}} \tag{1}$$

$$Ta_{HPT} = \frac{1}{\lambda_2} - S_2 \tag{2}$$

Since HPT is UDP traffic, where the data frames should be served in almost real time or should be rejected, it is obtained that the HPT throughput (T_{HPT}) in different DoS modes will be:

$$T_{HPT} = \lambda_{3HPT}(LL) \tag{3}$$

$$T_{HPT} = \lambda_{3HPT} \frac{Ta_{HPT}}{Tr_{HPT}} = \lambda_{3PHT} \left(\left(\frac{1}{\lambda_2} - S_2 \right)(1 - S_3\lambda_{3HPT}) \right) \Big/ S_2 S_3 \lambda_{3HPT}(ML) \tag{4}$$

$$= (1/\lambda_2 - S_2)(1 - S_3\lambda_{3HPT})/S_2 S_3 \lambda_{3HPT}$$

$$T_{HPT} = 0(HL) \tag{5}$$

From the previous three expressions can be concluded that the HPT traffic throughput during different level of DoS attack is different. Namely, in the case of LL attack the HPT throughput will not be affected at all. During the ML attack, the throughput will depend on the ratio of the T, considering the HPT. In the case of HL attack, due to the fast transmission of the fake authentication requests, which are with highest priority, there will not be available time T at all for HPT to be served, so the HPT throughput in this case is 0.

2.2 Analysis of Low Priority Traffic Parameters

In this section the behavior of the LPT parameters under different levels of AuthRF DoS attack are considered. While HPT have the highest traffic priority after the control traffic, the LPT will be considered only after HPT traffic is served, so the case of LPT will differ then the previous one (Fig. 2).

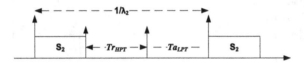

Fig. 2. *Ta* in LPT for LL DoS.

If we consider LPT we will notice that in this case there is a slightly different situation (Fig. 2).

The available time for transmitting the queued data frames for the LPT can be calculated using the following equations:

$$Ta_{LPT} = 1/\lambda_2 - S_2 - Tr_{HPT} \tag{6}$$

$$Ta_{LPT} = 1/\lambda_2 - S_2 - \frac{S_2 S_3 \lambda_{3HPT}}{(1 - S_3 \lambda_{3HPT})} \tag{7}$$

On the other hand, the required time Tr_{LPT} for transmitting the data frames queued during the attack for the case of LPT is obtained as:

$$
\begin{aligned}
Tr_{LPT} &= Tr_{LPT}{}^0 + Tr_{LPT}{}^1 + \cdots + Tr_{LPT}{}^{i-1} \\
&= (S_2 + Tr_{HPT})S_3\lambda_{3LPT} + (S_2 + Tr_{HPT})S_3{}^2\lambda_{3LPT}{}^2 + \cdots \\
&+ (S_2 + Tr_{HPT})\, S_3{}^i\lambda_{3LPT}{}^i = (S_2 + Tr_{HPT})\, S_3\lambda_{3LPT}/(1 - S_3\lambda_{3LPT})
\end{aligned}
\tag{8}
$$

$$Tr_{LPT} = \left(S_2 + \frac{S_2 S_3 \lambda_{3HPT}}{1 - S_3 \lambda_{3HPT}} \right) S_3 \lambda_{3LPT}/(1 - S_3 \lambda_{3LPT}) \tag{9}$$

According to previous expressions, it can be seen that in some point different conditions for HPT and LPT will be fulfilled. For LL DoS attack, $0 < Tr < Ta$, TX2 queue *has enough* resources to process queued data frames. In case of ML DoS attack, $Tr > Ta > 0$, TX2 queue *does not have enough* resources to process queued data frames. Finally, for HL DoS attack, $Ta = 0$, *and* TX2 queue *has no* resources to process queued data frames. For example, HPT may be still in LL, while LPT can be switched in ML mode. The mode for both, HPT and LPT, depends on λ_2 and λ_3.

Figure 3 shows the λ_3 dependence, taking that $\lambda_{3HPT} = \lambda_{3LPT} = \lambda_3$. The results in the figure are obtained for the following parameters' values: $S_2 = 50$ ms and $S_3 = 10$ ms, λ_3 is independent variable, while $\lambda_2 = 5$fps. The actual values for S_3 are lower, but the value of 10 ms in the analysis clearly shows clearly the transitions form one mode to another, without loss of generality.

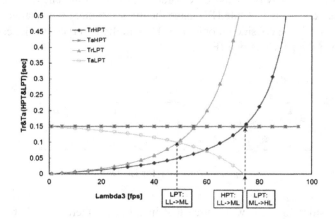

Fig. 3. Operation modes in HPT and LPT.

The Fig. 3 shows that the transition HPT: LL→ML causes simultaneous transition LPT: ML→HL.

If it is assumed that the LPT, as well as HPT, are UDP–based traffic that apply analogous relations as (3), (4), (5), the throughputs under different conditions of DoS attack can be compared. If it is considered that LPT is TCP traffic, where each frame is waiting for proper acknowledge message (ACK), then further analysis is needed to calculate the throughput, which can be realized in terms of DoS (LL, ML, HL) (Fig. 4).

- *Low Priority Traffic – Low Level (LPT – LL)*

The relations (3) to (10) in [4] apply for RTT for the considered model, but an additional correction to the relation (11) in [4] is needed. For this purpose the paper use the relation (5) from [6], where Y_1 and Y_2 present the complete waiting time in the case when the data frame arrives during the time when TX1 is empty and the complete waiting time in the case when the data frame arrives during the time TX1 is not empty, respectively. Unlike in [6], in our case Y_1 and Y_2 are calculated as:

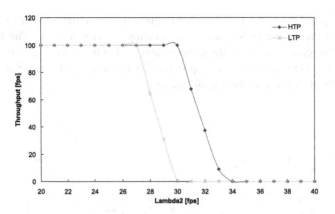

Fig. 4. Throughput (HPT, LPT) as a function of attacking rate (the following values are considered as constants: $S_2 = 0.03$ s, $S_3 = 0.001$ s and $\lambda_3 = 100$fps).

$$Y_1 = \lambda_2 \sum_{j=1}^{N} \{S_2 + Tr_{HPT} + (j-1)(S_3 - 1/\lambda_{3LPT})\} \tag{10}$$

where:

$$N = (S_2 + Tr_{HTP})\lambda_{3LPT} \tag{11}$$

Finally, the equation for Y_1 is:

$$Y_1 = \lambda_2/2(S_3(S_2 + Tr_{HTP})^2\lambda_{3LPT}^2 + (S_2 + Tr_{HTP})^2\lambda_{3LPT} + (S_2 + Tr_{HTP}) \\ - S_3(S_2 + Tr_{HTP})\lambda_{3LPT}) \tag{12}$$

while equation for Y_2 is:

$$Y_2 = \lambda_{3LPT}(1 - S_2\lambda_2 - Tr_{HTP}) \times \left[\left(\frac{S_3}{1 - \lambda_{3LPT}S_3}\right) - S_3\right] \tag{13}$$

The throughput can be calculated according the following relation:

$$Throughput(LPT) = 1/RTL_{LPT} \tag{14}$$

Where RTTLPT is calculated as [4],

$$RTT = t_2 + t_5 + T_0 - S_1 - S_3 \tag{15}$$

with necessary changes introduced according (12) and (13) of our mathematical model.

The graph is obtained using the following values: $S_1 = 0.0002$; $S_2 = 0.030$; $S_3 = 0.001$; $\lambda_{3LPT} = 100$; $\lambda_1 = 10$; $\lambda_{3HPT} = 10, 100$ and 200; $T_0 = 0.010$

According to Fig. 5, it is easy to come to the conclusion that the LPT throughput in LL decreases during the DoS attack intensification (λ_2 is increased). The HTP intensifying is also reason for lower throughput (this is also the reason for LPT ML to be reached faster). Here it should be emphasized that, according to the relation (3), the HTP throughput is constant during all this time.

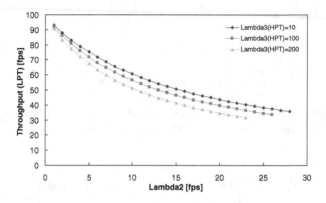

Fig. 5. Throughput of LPT in LL at different HPT and DoS conditions.

- ***Low Priority Traffic – Medium Level (LPT – ML)***

Unlike [3], where a single DoS attack is assumed with limited duration of $D = 5$ s, the paper considers that $D \rightarrow$ Inf.

In such conditions, the LPT ML throughput can be calculated as:

$$Throughput(LPT_{ML}) = N/(1/\lambda_2) = \lambda_2 Ta_{LPT}/(t_1 + t_2 + t_3 + t_4 + S) \qquad (16)$$

- ***Low Priority Traffic – High Level (LPT HL)***

If the conditions are considered in terms of D, which we previously accepted for HL DoS mode, it is obvious that the LPT throughput in this case is always zero.

Using this analytical model, the differences between 802.11 [4] and 802.11e when they operate in same mode can be seen, i.e. when both of them are attacked by the same number of authentication frames. This primarily occurs due to different priorities of different types of traffic in 802.11e.

3   Conclusion

The primary emphasis in the analysis of this paper is placed on the AuthRF (Authentication Request Flooding) and AssRF (Association Request Flooding) DoS attacks. Due to the lack of effective authentication mechanisms in wireless networks, which should be used to check the control and management frames, it is very easy to use one of the many possible DoS attacks against MAC sublayer and cause a significant loss, and even a complete interruption of the legitimate traffic. Therefore, the paper presents the weaknesses of the MAC sublayer and possible DoS attacks, as well as a new queuing model of 802.11e AP for complete traffic analysis in the case when there is not attack and when the AP is attacked by low, medium and high rate of infiltrating false authentication frames. Based on the proposed model and using an analytical approach, results of the effects of the attacks are obtained, which are graphically depicted and explained.

References

1. Bogdanoski, M., Petreski, D.: Cyber terrorism-global security threat. Contemp. Maced. Defense-Int. Sci. Defense, Secur. Peace J. **13**(24), 59–73 (2013)
2. Cisco Systems, Inc., Cisco Wireless Control System Configuration Guide, Software Re- lease 7.0.172.0 (2011)
3. IEEE Standard for Information Technology – Telecommunications and information exchange between systems – Local and metropolitan area networks – Specific requirements. Wireless LAN Medium Access Control (MAC) and Physical Layer (PHY) Specifications. Amendment 4: Protected Management Frames. IEEE Std. 802.11w-2009 (2009)
4. Liu C., Yu J., Brewster G.: Empirical studies and queuing modeling of denial of service attacks against 802.11 WLANs. In: IEEE International Symposium on World of Wireless Mobile and Multimedia Networks (WoWMoM), Montreal, Canada (2010)
5. Liu, C., Yu, J.: A solution to WLAN authentication and association DoS attacks. IAENG Int. J. Comput. Sci. **34**, 31 (2007)
6. Liu, C., Yu, J.: Detail derivations of Tr, Ta, t_2, and t_5 (2009)

Radio Capacity Planning in the Case of Major Incidents for Public Safety Agencies

Zoran Nusev[1(✉)] and Aleksandar Risteski[2]

[1] Government Mobile Communications Branch, Government of Ontario,
Osprey Blvd, Mississauga 6196, Canada
nusev@hotmail.com
[2] Faculty of Electrical Engineering and Information Technologies,
Saints Cyril and Methodius University,
Ruger Boskovic 18, 1000 Skopje, Macedonia
acerist@feit.ukim.edu.mk

Abstract. Public Safety Agencies deal with emergency events on a regular basis. They require reliable, highly available and secure network to provide services to the public. Furthermore, the demand for new features, such as video and audio streaming, transmission of still pictures, short messages and access to database applications, is on the rise. It is up to the design engineers to plan and support all current and future requirements. This paper will simulate emergency scenario where Public Safety agencies are called upon and analyze the network impact from the capacity point of view.

Keywords: Erlang · Interoperability · Public safety agencies · Radio capacity · Land mobile radio · Traffic requirements

1 Introduction

The idea to have one uniform and fully integrated and interoperable communication system between the public safety agencies is as old as the agencies themselves. But more than often, this is not the case. Because of budget restrictions, multi-layer government structures, even social and cultural differences, the result is multiple communications systems operating on different frequency bands and different technologies.

In cases of the emergency events and in day-to-day operations, public safety agencies rely heavily on the ability to communicate via their established private land mobile radio (LMR) systems, such as P25 and TETRA. There is a requirement to secure radio spectrum to plan for the unknown and to accommodate communication requirements. To accomplish such a task, we have to start taking actions such as making priority spectrum available and developing associated spectrum policies, processes and technical standards. These can be accomplished by defining the regional radio spectrum plan [1].

The issue of radio interoperability is a broad and complex matter [2, 3]. The issue is even more challenging based on the variety of vendor proprietary technologies, different levels of security [4], spectrums used, functionalities, standard operating procedures, etc. Developing associated spectrum policies, processes and technical

© Institute for Computer Sciences, Social Informatics and Telecommunications Engineering 2015
V. Atanasovski, L.-G. Alberto (Eds.): Fabulous 2015, LNICST 159, pp. 212–218, 2015.
DOI: 10.1007/978-3-319-27072-2_27

standards greatly improves the communication compatibility. Optimizing the network design, based upon the user and environmental requirements, provides the final step in highly accessible and reliable networks.

In this paper we implement simulation framework using OPNET Modeler and quantify the effect of increased traffic. Results will show the need of proper channel and capacity design in order to accommodate Public Safety agencies requirements.

The paper is organized as follows. Section 2 discusses the background and scenario which is used for the analysis. Section 3 summarizes the scenario and our simulation results related to the effects of the increased traffic load during the major incidents. Finally, we conclude our work in Sect. 4.

2 Background and Scenario

Technology is developing rapidly. This is more accurate for the commercial users but the public safety agencies are demanding some of those services, too. This is a high pace environment which demands changing the communication requirements. The need of sending and receiving short messages (SMS), videos, alerts, status updates, GPS coordinates, etc. is already embedded into the public safety agencies strategic plans to provide services to the public. For the time being, public safety agencies will use whatever mean of communications to provide services to the public, even if that means using commercial networks.

The technologies used as communication infrastructure in Public Service networks include security mechanisms needed to meet the requirements for secure communications among users. Typical algorithms are deployed for data encryption, data integrity, authentication, etc. Radio interfaces (wireless links) are more vulnerable and specially designed mechanisms provide the necessary security level (e.g. over the air re-keying). Besides the protection of data over the radio interfaces, additional cryptographic mechanisms are used to provide end-to-end security for various applications at application level. However, as any other communication network, these networks are still vulnerable and open to various types of security threats and attacks which may corrupt, compromise or even disable the normal network operation. Therefore, special care should be taken in order to provide the necessary security level for the critical information infrastructure used by Public Safety Agencies.

Public Safety users have higher demand of availability and reliability as compared to the commercial users. This is known as QoS (Quality of Service) or GoS (Grade of Service) term mostly used for the private networks. GoS mechanism controls the performance, reliability and usability of a telecommunications service. The grade of service standard is the acceptable level of traffic that the network can lose. GoS is calculated from the Erlang-B formula, as a function of the number of channels required for the offered traffic intensity.

GoS for the public safety agencies is defined by the clients and it is usually 1 %, 97 % of the time and 97 % terrain coverage availability and DAQ (Delivered Audio Quality) of 3.4.

In comparison with the Public Safety requirements, commercial (cellular) circuit groups usually demand GoS of 2 %, 50 % time and 50 % coverage availability and DAQ of 3. These facts will have direct impact on the network design.

Technologies for the Land Mobile Radio Networks [5–8], such as TETRA and P25 are trying to integrate some of these clients' requirements for additional data traffic in their product lines. IV&D (Integrated Voice and Data) infrastructure has been introduced. The capacity and throughput are not comparable to the new commercially available technologies such as LTE and LTE-A [9], but it is a good step forward. In addition, integrating LTE into LMR design is on the roadmap too and it will provide even more capabilities for the public safety agencies.

In order to plan the radio capacity, first we have to define some of the scenarios. As we previously said, there will be unknown scenarios, but based on experience, we can predict the worst-case scenarios and plan accordingly. The definition of the worst case scenarios is the situation were the affected area is geographically bigger, number of involved people is greater and maximum number of public safety agencies are put in service. Some of the scenarios defined in the crisis management center of the Republic of Macedonia [10, 11] are:

- Fire
- Flood
- Earthquakes
- Ecologic catastrophes
- Others (explosion in the major oil refinery, major incident on the main traffic arteries and celebrations or protests).

The common element for all of these scenarios is the involvement of all public safety agencies (police, fire and ambulance) and broader public safety agencies (crisis management center, tow track services, clean-up crews, etc.).

The first step is to define the number of radio channels (in this simulation TETRA technology has been used) that will always be available for the public safety agencies for inter and intra operability during the crisis. It is imperative to understand that any of the subjects coming to the scene have multi-layered structures. This further complicates the interoperability capacity requirements during the Major Incidents (MI).

To calculate the maximum number of communication paths and the number of interoperability radio channels to accommodate the communication requirements, the following formula can be used [12]:

$$Q = \frac{A * x\left(t_{(s)} + t_d\right)}{3600} * \frac{c(c-1)}{2} \tag{1}$$

Where:

Q is the number of interoperability channels
A is the number of users
x is the number of calls per user
$t_{(s)}$ time duration in seconds
t_d system time delay in seconds (network access and hang time)
C is the number of Agencies at the scene.

The formula calculates the traffic capacity and the maximum communications paths based on the number of agencies on the scene. The formula calculated for the worst case scenario expected in the predicted emergency/major incident, as described in section B. Using the Erlang's table [13], Q can be converted into the number of radio channels including the control channels.

In order to maximize the use of the dedicated radio spectrum, Public Safety Agencies and the Crisis Management Centre have to define and implement standard operating procedures. This will include the hierarchy (priority users), and when and how the capacity will be used. In some cases, these challenges can be great, where additional training will have to be provided, cultural and linguistic barriers have to be overcome, etc.

The scenario analyzed in this paper is the explosion in the oil refinery. It is assumed that a large explosion occurs at a 50,000 m^2 oil production plant in the industrial area of a suburb of the capitol of Macedonia, Skopje. The blast shatters windows of buildings in the immediate vicinity. There are a significant number of casualties both from within the oil plant and outside. Multiple sensors detect and report the incident to the Police, Fire and Emergency Medical Services dispatch center. Within minutes, the dispatch centers are also flooded with calls from motorists, pedestrians, and residents. Soon, commercial cellular networks become overloaded. Air quality sensors around the area detect hazardous substances emanating from the site of the accident. The wind speed and direction reported from environmental monitoring stations indicate that the fumes will drift over a residential area with an elementary school, a high school, a library, a hospital, and numerous retail businesses. As it drifts over the major highway Skopje - Kumanovo, car accidents ensue and some motorists abandon their cars to escape the scene on foot. Debris expelled by the explosion damages a nearby electrical sub-station, causing a localized power failure.

Expected effects of the scenario are: since the accident is between two major cities, emergency calls will be directed to both dispatch centers; dispatchers will assign immediately neighboring Fire Department, Police and Emergency Medical Services; Fire department will be deployed to extinguish the fire; Police will be there to secure the site and the first responders; initially, no one would have the accurate information what caused the explosion, multiple teams from the Police and Crisis Management will be responding.

3   Analysis and Results

The topology for the analyzed scenario is presented in Fig. 1. There are two Dispatch Centers presented (Skopje and Kumanovo), day to day users, extension 1, add on users from SK (Skopje), KU (Kumanovo) and VE (Veles). For the backhaul we have used MW links and fiber over the PSTN network. In the center of the screen is Okta, the place where the Major Incident (MI) takes place, based on the scenario. For the simulation, Core Server has only the users included into the MI to analyze only the traffic occurred during the normal day to day operation and the MI.

The suburb of the capitol of Republic of Macedonia, Skopje, has been used as location where the predicted MI scenario could take place. The results will present normal day to day operation and when the major incident occurs.

Parameters used into the analysis are:

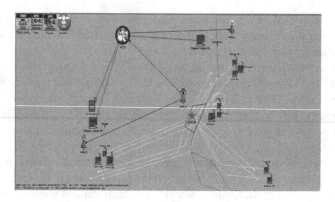

Fig. 1. MI simulation topology

For TDMA Analysis
Utility   TDMA Configuration
Users   TDMA mobile nodes

Increased based on the scene arrival
All users have created trajectories for roaming and access to and from the MI.
Traffic generation

Start - Normal day to day use	Erlang 0.1 is used
During - during the MI	Erlang 2 is used
After the MI – back to regular operation	Erlang 0.1 is used

Work conducted regarding presentation of the traffic analysis is based on OPNET Modeler 14.5. The simulation has been run over 2 days but the focus was and extract taken for the period of 6 h from the beginning of the MI. Traffic after the MI will be back to the regular day to day levels and it is not part of this analysis.

For TETRA/TDMA analysis, parameters that have been used into the calculations are:

- All the nodes are mobile;
- All mobiles have predefined trajectories for in/out of the scene;
- Capacity is defined for the start/during/after the MI as presented above;
- TETRA and P25 TDMA (formerly Phase II) have been used to generate the simulation.

The results are shown as follows: Light blue line presents the normal day to day traffic use at the scene. The results show average traffic load of 42Kbps with load of 0.1 erlangs. This traffic would include regular police highway patrols and EMS units on standby in the region, as per their plan of coverage during and off rush hours (Fig.2).

Green line presents the beginning of the MI, the immediate arrival of the units from Skopje and added traffic to the network. First at the scene would be Police units for

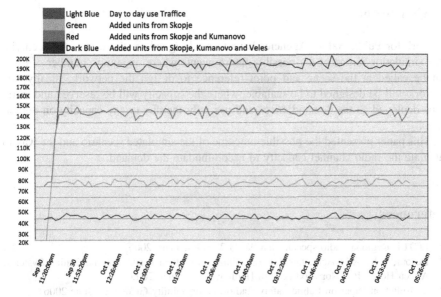

Light Blue	Day to day use Traffice
Green	Added units from Skopje
Red	Added units from Skopje and Kumanovo
Dark Blue	Added units from Skopje, Kumanovo and Veles

Fig. 2. MI simulation traffic results

securing the area, plus additional EMS and Fire units deployed for rapid response. The results show average traffic load of 75Kbps with load of 0.1 erlangs.

Because the MI is on the major highway and the area is covered by 2 dispatcher centers, units from the neighboring Kumanovo have been dispatch. Red line presents the arrival of the additional EMS, Fire and Special Police units at the MI scene. The traffic load rises to average of 140 Kbps with load of 2 erlangs.

Dark blue line presents the final number of units deployed to the MI. These numbers include Police (HWY patrols, special investigation units and local police), Fire and Emergency Medical Services (including the rapid deployment units). Traffic load for the simulated scenario averages 195 Kbps with load of 2 erlangs.

The results based on the predicted and simulated scenario shows the exponential increase of the traffic load by introducing more users at the scene of the MI.

Based on the number of users, which can be added into the analysis and their pre-requirements for accessing applications and voice communication, historical records of capacity utilization, radio and data channel capacity can be design to accommodate Public Safety user requirements. As previously mentioned, dedicated voice only, voice and data and data only channels will be assigned to accommodate the traffic.

After collecting the results from the simulation, formula (1) can be utilized to calculate the maximum number of communication paths and the number of interoperability radio channels. The results should be used for network design and optimization.

The analysis were conducted for this one scenario but can be used for multiple planned and/or unplanned events, where first responders are called upon. Historical reports of traffic accidents, natural disasters can be utilized to properly plan for these events.

4 Conclusion

Network for Public Safety Agencies have to be designed for the worst case scenario. This simulation is one of the possible future events where maximum number of users can be called at the scene and point reference to design the network. Ideally, the network will be designed to be scalable, where the capacity will be reserved and ready to be deployed as the demand arises and use only the day to day capacity on regular bases.

This paper presented the possible outcome of the simulated scenario and the way to calculate the radio channel capacity to accommodate the demand.

References

1. ECTEL Regional radio spectar plan 06 03 23, 17 January 2006
2. Desourdis Jr., R.I.: Achieving Interoperability in Critical It and Communication Systems. Artech House Inc, Norwood (2009). Hardcover - 30 June 2009
3. Consultation Paper on Public Safety Radio Interoperability Guidelines, June 2006
4. Information security for the clasified informations, Government of the Republic of Macedonia, March 2005; Uredbata za informati ~ ka bezbednost na klasificirani informacii, Mart 2005
5. Motorola: ASTRO25 Digital Trunking Solution. www.motorolasolutions.com. Accessed March 2014
6. Evolution of TETRA – White Paper P3 Communications GmbH, 22 November 2011
7. Cassidian: Product specs and network solutions for TETRA and TETRAPOL. www.cassidian.com. Accessed March 2014
8. ICOM: Product specs IC F70/80 and network solutions. www.icomcanada.com. Accessed March 2014
9. Furht, B., Ahson, S.A.: Long Term Evolution: 3GPP LTE Radio and Cellular Technology, 23 April 2009
10. Preparation plan for health system responding in the case of embergency, Republic of Macedonia, June 2009; Plan za Podgotovka I odgovor na zdravstveniot system pri vonredni/krizni sostojbi ve Republika Makedonija, Juni 2009
11. Crisis Management Center, Government of Republic of Macedonia. www.cuk.gov.mk. Accessed March 2014
12. Nusev, Z., Risteski, A.: Design issues of interoperable communication system for public safety - planning for the unplanned. In: CICSyN2014, May 2014
13. Erlang's Table. http://www.pitt.edu/~dtipper/2110/erlang-table.pdf. Accessed January 2015

Addressing Communication Security Issues in BAN Medical System: SIARS

Goce Stevanoski[1], Jugoslav Achkoski[1], Saso Koceski[2],
Ana Madevska Bogdanova[3], and Mitko Bogdanoski[1(✉)]

[1] Military Academy "General Mihailo Apostolski", Goce Delcev University,
Vasko Karangelevski bb, 1000 Skopje, Macedonia
gstevanos@gmail.com, {jugoslav.ackoski,
mitko.bogdanoski}@ugd.edu.mk
[2] Faculty of Computer Science, Goce Delcev University,
Krste Misirkov 10-A, P.O 201, Stip 2000, Republic of Macedonia
saso.koceski@ugd.edu.mk
[3] Faculty of Computer Science and Engineering,
Saints Cyril and Methodius University, Rugjer Boshkovikj 16,
P.O. Box 393, 1000 Skopje, Macedonia
ana.madevska.bogdanova@finki.ukim.mk

Abstract. Considerations for implementing system that will record medical condition of participants on the battlefield always follow a path for best data gathering, data analyzing and fast implementation of medical procedures for saving lives. Smart I (eye) Advisory Rescue System (SIARS) has aim to process and transmit medical data of injured or wounded person which will allow saving more injured patients and lessen the death-rate on the battlefield. The dataflow in the system has a military significance during the military missions and communication security must be on an appropriate level. This paper presents review for communication and authentication security challenges in the process of SIARS development. The overarching goal for security issue about the system is to determine the factors that are influencing the secure communication and authentication between endpoints. Furthermore, the paper presents the best practices for achieving secure communication and authentication by using existing solutions. The focal points in this paper are security gaps in Bluetooth Smart communication with data collectors and security issues in VHF radio and 4G communications for data transport to database elements.

Keywords: BAN security · Bluetooth security issues · 4G security challenges

1 Introduction

The rapid development of e-health hardware and software in recent years, provide opportunities to deploy e-health systems on the battlefields as a reliable tool to the first responders. The Smart I (eye) Advisory Rescue System (SIARS) project has a goal to develop a telemedical information system that will allow saving more injured patients and lessen the death-rate on the battle fields. This article is about identifying security vulnerabilities in information flow between different SIARS elements.

© Institute for Computer Sciences, Social Informatics and Telecommunications Engineering 2015
V. Atanasovski, L.-G. Alberto (Eds.): Fabulous 2015, LNICST 159, pp. 219–225, 2015.
DOI: 10.1007/978-3-319-27072-2_28

The article starts (see Sect. 2) with brief description of SIARS network architecture, the security requirements and main security threats/risks for SIARS. The Sect. 3 addresses the security vulnerabilities in SIARS wireless communication links. The section discus security challenges in data flow between data collectors in Bluetooth Smart. Section 4 of the article deals with security challenges in information flow from data collectors to the main database servers. Here, the paper considers the Fourth generation Long Term Evolution (4G LTE) and Very High Frequency (VHF) radio communication vulnerabilities. The article ends up with concluding remarks.

2 The Reference Network Architecture

According to the defined model, the SIARS will have internal network (intranet) that is going to be deployed by a combination of Body Area Network (BAN) and project specific Wide Area Network (WAN) (See Fig. 1). The BAN is part of the network that uses Bluetooth Smart technology for data transfer and combines all body sensors (nodes) and tablet (hub).

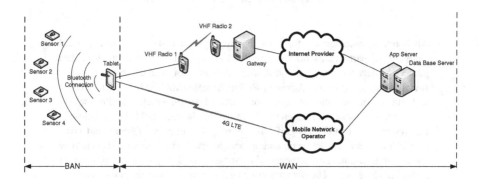

Fig. 1. SIARS reference network architecture with different data communication links from data collectors to data base server

The WAN part of the network architecture is the part where the collected data from body sensors are transmitted to the main database server using 4G LTE or VHF radio communication. Because the information flow is done over wireless channels communication security should be enforced. For providing end to end security the SIARS architecture development should be focused on 8 security dimensions [1] as: Access control, Authentication, Non-repudiation, Data Confidentiality, Communication security, Data integrity, Availability and Privacy.

3 Data Collectors' Communication Link

All data collectors in SIARS system are needed to be capable of transferring data over Bluetooth Smart/IEEE 802.15.6 communication channels. This technology is an integral part of the Bluetooth Core Specification from Bluetooth v4.0 and gives unique abilities in power consumption and data transfer.

From security point of view IEEE 802.15.6 has predefined communication levels for achieving secure communication and authentication. These levels are [2]:

- Level 0 - Unsecured Communication. This level has no build in mechanisms for data authentication and integrity, confidentiality, or privacy protection.
- Level 1 - Authentication Level. This level has secure authentication but doesn't have encryption. Therefore this level does not support confidentiality or privacy.
- Level 2 - Authentication and Encryption. This level has secure authentication and employs encryption. It's the most secure level from all three.

During the association process, one of the security levels above is selected.

The security protocol in Bluetooth Smart/IEEE 802.15.6 is generally based on the asymmetric cryptography, which employs the elliptic curve public key cryptography. The association and disassociation processes it is made by using private keys. According to the standard, a Master Key (MK) is activated for secure communication. The MK may be pre-shared or established using unauthenticated association. After that, for single session a Pairwise Temporal Key (PTK) is created and for multicast secured communication, a Group Temporal Key (GTK) is shared with the corresponding group using the unicast method (See Fig. 2).

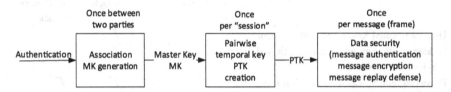

Fig. 2. Process of activating MK and establishing PK for building secure communication link.

All the frames can be transferred in both secured and unsecured communication modes.

3.1 Security Vulnerabilities in Bluetooth Smart/IEEE 802.15.6

Recent researches [2, 3] done on Bluetooth Smart/IEEE 802.15.6 standard showed that, although this technology is developed for secure and reliable data transfer, there are still vulnerabilities that can have serious impact on the communication process.

Implementing technology with low power gives limited range of connectivity and good starting point for physical security, but does not provide highest protection on information flow. The following identified vulnerabilities in Bluetooth Smart/IEEE 802.15.6 showed that the impact on information flow in SIARS system can be significant.

1. In Bluetooth Smart, all communication is done over Radio Frequency (RF) spectrum which gives very good opportunities for intercepting and interfering in to radio traffic. Even though the frequency hopping is employed there are noted vulnerabilities which potential attacker can use to compromise the information flow [3].

By using this vulnerability the attacker can exceed the (physical) PHY layer of the connection and receives all the packets which are transmitted over the RF spectrum. This gives to the attacker an opportunity to launch an eavesdropping attack as an active or passive eavesdropper.

2. Although the Bluetooth Smart/IEEE 802.15.6 is generally based on the Diffie-Hellman key exchange, which employs the elliptic curve public key cryptography [4], there are vulnerabilities that are affecting data confidentiality in the process of data transmitting. These vulnerabilities are noticed at the first stage of key exchange process [2], during the process of establishing MK between node and the hub. The mathematical analysis, which is given in [2], showed that none of the four different protocols defined for generating MK [4] can guaranty secure data flow [2]. Beside the confirmed vulnerabilities, the work done in [2] showed that none of the four protocols has forward secrecy. The result of the math analysis is given in the Table 1.

Table 1. List of protocols in the process of establishing MK and their vulnerability to specific attacks

Protocol	Impersonation attack	KCI attack	Offline dictionary attack
Unauthenticated key agreement protocol	$\checkmark$	$\checkmark$	
Hidden public key transfer authenticated key agreement protocol		$\checkmark$	
Password authenticated association procedure	$\checkmark$	$\checkmark$	$\checkmark$
Display authenticated association procedure	$\checkmark$	$\checkmark$	

3. Despite the aforementioned vulnerabilities in Bluetooth Smart/IEEE 802.15.6 the work done in [3] also showed that Bluetooth Smart/802.15.6 has a potential to be vulnerable to packet injection. This vulnerability incises the chances for future attacks on crypto system and Bluetooth stack on different devices [3].

All aforementioned vulnerabilities, identified in Bluetooth Smart/IEEE 802.15.6, are affecting different security dimensions as: access control, authentication, communication security and availability. In addition, by identifying these vulnerabilities we can conclude that full-protected environment for SIARS cannot be accomplished by the current security mechanisms in the standard [2].

4 Database Communication Links in SIARS

According to the network architecture of SIARS system the mobile device is going to have a role of hub in Bluetooth Smart connection with others nodes (data collectors). All the data should be transmitted to the main database on SIARS servers.

The processing of data to data server is planned to be accomplished by one of these two different technologies:

- 4G LTE; and
- VHF Radio communication

Both of these technologies have their own advantages and disadvantages.

The 4G LTE has a broad international coverage, reliable communicational infrastructure and excellent speed, over 300 Mbps in downlink and over 75 Mbps in uplink. However, it has some disadvantages for military use as: the whole connection is outsourced to commercial Mobile Network Operators (MNO) and it is not always accessible in non-urban areas.

On the other hand, the VHF radio communication has great and reliable communication in all areas and the accessibility of the communication does not depend on commercial providers. The VHF-based radio networks can be created from current military radio infrastructure. Main disadvantage in this type of communication is the data rate, which in VHF radio communication goes up to 5 Mbps [5].

4.1 Security Vulnerabilities in 4G LTE

The 4G LTE standard is packet switching technology (based on its All-IP Core Network). The voice communication is transformed in data packets and transmitted over the 4G LTE network. Although the 3rd Generation Partnership Project (3GPP) in core security requirements for 4G LTE regulated strong cryptographic techniques and authentication between LTE elements [6, 7], the change to All-IP Core Network opened a very big door for potential security threats on different levels in 4G LTE net architecture.

This 4G LTE All-IP Core Network has a range of risks beginning from end user equipment up to LTE service network.

- The end user equipment is out of the MNO (Mobile Network Operator) control and it represents the weakest point in 4G LTE infrastructure. This provides opportunities to the attacker to conduct attacks like physical attacks, application layer attacks (virus, malware) etc. [6].
- The security risks are not only end user equipment concern; the 4G LTE access points Evolved Node B (eNode B) are next part of the 4G LTE that has security weakness. The potential attacker on this part of the network can compromise the network by gaining physical access to eNode B's, creating rogue eNode B, Man in the middle attack's (MitM) [6], jamming the eNode B [8] or if the MNO did not implemented encryption to user plane form eNode B to Evolved Packet Core (EPC) [9].
- The EPC is part of the LTE network that manages user authentication, access authorization and accounting (AAA), IP address allocation, mobility related signaling, charging, QoS and security. Main security threats on this part of 4G LTE are the unauthorized access on the network by an intruder during data roam, Denial of Service (DoS) and Distributed Denial of Service Attack (DDoS) attacks on Mobility Management Entity (MME) and Overbilling attacks (IP address hijacking, IP spoofing) [6].

- Different vulnerabilities are part of the 4G LTE Service network infrastructure. As a way of distributing the multimedia content the IP multimedia subsystem (IMS) faces various security challenges. The key threats in this part of the network are unauthorized access to IMS, Service abuse attacks, theft of service, network snoop, session hijacking [6].

All of these threats in 4G LTE can compromise the entire communication and lead to corruption or modification of information, theft or loss of information, disclosure of information and interruption of services [1]. By using the 4G LTE for data transfer to main data base, the SIARS will have to take in consideration all security threats known for 4G LTE network. Many of aforementioned threats should be mitigated by MNO, but a system like SIARS will have to have system specific security mechanisms.

Due to security vulnerabilities in 4G LTE main aspect of implemented security actions in SIARS would be data confidentiality and data integrity. The data availability or possible interruption of services is part of the MNO costumer care. Therefore, SIARS will need to have its own:

- Secure Virtual Private Network (VPN) tunnel to the main data base server – a Secure Sockets Layer (SSL) tunneling protocol that will encrypt the data flow and will authenticate the system equipment;
- User authentication – process of authentication SAIRS users by user access levels to different parts of the system (management or regular user).

By implementing SIARS system specific security mechanisms the overall data protection and end user equipment security will be upgraded.

4.2   Security Vulnerabilities in VHF Radio Link

According to the SIARS Network Diagram, Fig. 1, the second way of data transfer to SIARS database server is by VHF radio communication.

This communication as a part of military tactical radio communications provides secure data transfer on short distances. Because of the nature of radio waves propagation, one big security vulnerability is that all data transfer is broadcasted over the air. This gives to the potential attacker excellent opportunities to disclose or interrupt the data transfer. To mitigate the attacks on military VHF radio networks, military organizations deploy VHF radio nets with predefined user members, radio parameters and radio procedures. The security of radio communications is divided in two parts: Communication security (COMSEC) and Transmission security (TRANSEC) [10].

COMSEC has a role to protect the data confidentiality and integrity by enforcing data encryption.

TRANSEC has a role to protect the data availability by employing number of techniques to signal detection and jamming of the transmission path. Because the SIARS is developed as a military project, the VHF radio communication is going to be based on military procedures for securing VHF radio communications from end user equipment to the radio gateway.

The data transfer from radio gateway to SIARS database server should be protected by system specific security mechanisms, described in Sect. 4.1.

5   Conclusion

Incorporating security mechanisms to SIARS has big significance in protecting information flow between SIARS elements. By addressing the security threats in different parts of SIARS communication infrastructure, we noticed that different types of communication have different vulnerabilities. This vulnerability mainly affects data confidentiality and data integrity in SIARS system.

To mitigate potential risks on data exchange, the SIARS must adopt their own specific security mechanisms that will harden the encryption protection and improve end user access control.

Acknowledgement. This work was supported by the NATO Science for Peace and Security Program Project ISEG.IAP.SFPP 984753.

References

1. ITU-T Recommendation X.805 Recommendation A.8: Security architecture for systems providing end-to-end communications, 29 October 2003
2. Toorani, M.: On vulnerabilities of the security association in the IEEE 802.15.6 standard. In: Brenner, M., Christin, N., Johnson, B., Rohloff, K. (eds.) FC 2015 Workshops. LNCS, vol. 8976, pp. 245–260. Springer, Heidelberg (2015)
3. Ryan, M.: Bluetooth Smart: The Good, the Bad, the Ugly, and the Fix! BlackHat USA, Las Vegas, USA (2013)
4. Association, T.I.S.: IEEE P802.15.6-2012 Standard for Wireless Body Area Networks (2012). http://standards.ieee.org/findstds/standard/802.15.6-2012.html
5. Harris Corporation, Tactical Radio and Networking, RF7800M – MP. http://rf.harris.com/capabilities/tactical-radios-networking/rf-7800m/default.asp
6. Bhasker, D.: 4G LTE security for mobile network operators. Cyber Secur. Inf. Sys. Inf. Anal. Cent. (CSIAC) 1(4), 20–29 (2013). https://www.csiac.org/journal_article/4g-lte-security-mobile-network-operators
7. 3rd Generation Partnership Project: TS 33.401: System Architecture Evolution (SAE); Security architecture. Network, ver.12.14.0, release 12, 3GPP, April 2015
8. The National Telecommunications and Information Administration (NTIA) US Department of Commerce. http://www.ntia.doc.gov/files/ntia/va_tech_response.pdf
9. Donegn, P.: The security vulnerabilities of LTE: Opportunity & Risks for Operators, Heavy Reading, October 2013
10. Harris Corporation: Radio Communication in the Digital Age. vol. 1, edn. 2 (2005)

Performance Analysis of Wireless Sensor Networks Under DDoS Attack

Marija Bubinska and Aleksandar Risteski[(⊠)]

Faculty of Electrical Engineering and Information Technologies,
Saints Cyril and Methodius University, Ruger Boskovic 18,
1000 Skopje, Republic of Macedonia
bubinskamarija@yahoo.com, acerist@feit.ukim.edu.mk

Abstract. Security is a major issue in networks these days. Network attacks are widely explored topic when it comes to network security and protection. In this paper two types of DDoS attacks are explored considering the mesh Wireless Sensor Network topology. That is, a path based attack on the PAN Coordinator and a path based attack on the ZigBee router. Several performance parameters which are analyzed show severe deterioration of performance of the network under attack.

Keywords: WSN · Ddos · Performance analysis · Simulation

1 Introduction

A wireless sensor network (WSN) is a wireless network consisting of spatially distributed autonomous devices using sensors to monitor physical or environmental conditions [1]. A WSN system incorporates a gateway that provides wireless connectivity back to the wired world and distributed nodes. Each such sensor network node has typically several parts: a radio transceiver with an internal antenna or connection to an external antenna, a microcontroller, an electronic circuit for interfacing with the sensors and an energy source, usually a battery or an embedded form of energy harvesting.

In WSNs, the topology is a crucial element which plays an important role in minimizing various constraints like limited energy, latency, computational resource crisis and quality of communication. The energy consumption in these networks depends upon the number of sent and received packets. The transmission energy consumption depends upon the distance between sender and receiver nodes. On the other hand, the packet size also plays vital role in this. This can be handled through the use of more efficient routing algorithms, but the topology of the network sets the initial stage for it. The sensor networks may be deployed in the remote areas which makes the probability of failure of nodes and data loss very common. Thus, an efficient topology selection ensures that neighbor nodes are at a minimal distance and reduces the probability of message being lost between sensors. Basic topologies that are used in WSNs which can be modified by the requirements of the application for which this technology will be used. The following topologies are frequently used in WSNs: star topology, mesh topology, hybrid topology and tree topology (Fig. 1).

© Institute for Computer Sciences, Social Informatics and Telecommunications Engineering 2015
V. Atanasovski, L.-G. Alberto (Eds.): Fabulous 2015, LNICST 159, pp. 226–232, 2015.
DOI: 10.1007/978-3-319-27072-2_29

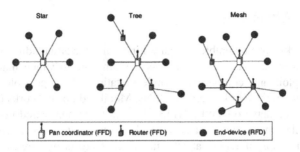

Fig. 1. Types of topologies in a wireless sensor network

Three types of routing protocols are used in WSNs: proactive (Table driven routing protocols), reactive (on demand) routing protocols and hybrid routing protocols. The routing protocol that is used in the analyzed scenarios in this paper is AODV (Ad-Hoc On demand Distance Vector). AODV is a reactive routing protocol. This protocol is based on two mechanisms i.e. route discovery and maintenance. AODV nodes use four types of messages to communicate among each other. Route Request (RREQ) and Route Reply (RREP) messages are used for route discovery. Route Error (RERR) messages and HELLO messages are used for route maintenance. Reactive routing protocol always uses the current status of the network hence the traffic is generated in bursty manner, which may create congestion during high activities. The significant delay may occur as a result of route discovery. But it saves energy and bandwidth during inactivity period. It is good choice for low traffic [2].

A DDoS (Distributed Denial of Service) attack is a type of web attack that seeks to disrupt the normal function of the targeted computer network. This is any type of attack that attempts to make the computer resource unavailable to its users. A DDoS attack is simply a combined effort to prevent communication/computer systems from working as well as they should, typically from a remote location over the internet. A number of compromised systems attack a single target, thereby causing denial of service for users of the targeted system. The flood of incoming messages to the target system essentially forces it to shut down, thereby denying service to the system to legitimate users. The most common method of attack is to send a mass saturation of incessant requests for external communication to the target. These systems are flooded with requests for information from non-users, and often non-visitors to the website. WSN has several issues like energy, computation, communication capabilities, deployment, storage, power consumption, longevity etc. that makes it prone to various attacks. DDoS is one of them [1].

In this paper two types of DDoS attacks are explored considering the mesh WSN topology. That is, a path based attack on the PAN (Personal Area Network) Coordinator and a path based attack on the ZigBee router.

The remaining parts of this paper are ordered in the following manner: the types of attacks are discussed in Sect. 2, in Sect. 3 a few similar projects and related work are described. Then, in Sect. 4 the simulation scenario is introduced and the results are discussed.

2 Types of Attacks

Wireless networks are vulnerable to many kinds of attacks including DDoS attacks. Their main vulnerability is shared wireless medium due to which many attacks are possible to exploit and compromise wireless stations. It is possible in almost all variations of wireless networks such as WSNs, Mobile ad hoc networks (MANET) and Wireless local area networks (WLAN) [3]. Like in traditional wired networks, DDoS attacks on wireless networks are also possible in different layers of communication. Some common forms of DDoS attacks in different layers of wireless networks are indicated in Table 1.

Table 1. Types of DDOS attacks at different layers in the protocol stack

Layer	Attack
Physical Layer	Jamming Attack Node Tampering Attack
Link /MAC Layer	Interrogation Attack Collision Attack
Network Layer	Black Hole Attack HELLO Flood Attack
Transport Layer	SYN Flooding Attack
Application Layer	Overwhelming Attack DoS Attack (Path- based)

Since this paper focuses on the application level attacks in WSN, two of them will be described in this section.

At the application layer, an attacker might attempt to overwhelm network nodes with sensor data, causing the network to forward large volumes of traffic to a base station. This attack consumes network bandwidth and drains node energy. However, it is effective only when particular sensor readings (such as motion detection or heat signatures) trigger communications–not when sensor readings are sent at fixed intervals [4].

Another application-layer attack involves injecting spurious or replayed packets into the network at leaf nodes in a path-based DoS attack. As the packet is forwarded to its destination, nodes along the path to the base station waste bandwidth and energy transmitting the traffic. This attack can starve the network of legitimate traffic, because it consumes resources on the path to the base station, thus preventing other nodes from sending data to the base station.

3 Related Work

Part of the related work done in exploring the DDoS attack on WSNs that includes performance analysis is described in this section. A similar study has been conducted in [5]. This paper provides a survey of attacks on WSN, discusses the various DoS attacks, and the impact of DoS on the performance of the system. The authors present three scenarios of a DoS attack on WSN with a tree topology. An attack on the coordinator, on the router and on the end devices and the simulation is done in OPNET 16. The simulation results show that the impact of DoS attacks on performance of WSN can be more severe, if carried out on coordinator or router, instead of just targeting the end devices. Other effort by Anthony D. Wood and John A. Stankovic explores the DoS attack taxonomy to identify the attacker, his capabilities, the target of the attack, vulnerabilities used, and the end result. They survey vulnerabilities in WSNs and give possible defenses [6].

In [7], authors assess the security issues of wireless sensor networks with respect to medical applications and find out the possibility of a scenario when a distributed denial of service (DDoS) attack may be injected in the system using wormhole attack. They also propose schemes for detecting those attacks and provide solutions for its mitigation.

As oppose to [5] this paper provides a performance analysis on a different type of WSN topology, i.e. a mesh topology. The other thing that is different in the scenarios in this paper is that the network includes a larger number of nodes.

4 Simulation Scenario and Result Analysis

This paper focuses on the application level attacks. Particularly, on the combination of a path based attack and a node overwhelming attack. There are two scenarios observed. Both simulation scenarios try to present attack towards a different network node. The first one represents a DDoS attack on the PAN coordinator and the second one represents an attack on one of the routers. The variations of the scenarios show an attack to the mentioned nodes conducted by different number of adversaries in the network (from 1 to 5 adversaries) and the case when there is no attack. The result is a product of an averaging over 100 experiments for each variation of the two scenarios (i.e. a Monte Carlo simulation). A comparison is made for the results for both scenarios.

The scenarios are designed in Qualnet v5.2 [8], which is a simulation tool designed for research in the area of wireless and mobile networks.

The scenarios consists of a mash Wireless Sensor Network with 50 sensor nodes, 5 ZigBee routers and 1 PAN coordinator. They span over an area of 200 m^2. The routing protocol that is used on the interfaces is AODV. Node 56 is the gateway, which means the sensor information is meant to arrive there. Each transmitting node sends packets with a size of 512 Bytes (and with a packet fragmentation unit of 70 Bytes) at the server node. In the scenario without an attack, 10 sensor nodes are actively transmitting towards the gateway. The simulation time is 30 min. Figure 2 presents a view of the simulation scenario.

The results were observed during an attack from 1 to 5 adversary nodes and the calculated parameters are: the average throughput (on the server side- node 56), the average jitter, average end-to-end delay and the number of established sessions per experiment. These metrics are all calculated in dependence of the number of adversaries in the scenario. The average throughput is defined as the average ratio between the aggregate throughput and the number of successful sessions per experiment. The average jitter and end-to-end delay follow the same Eq. (1) respectively, like in the case

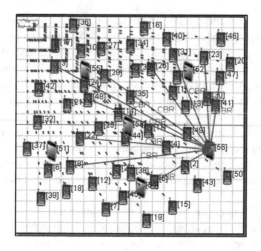

Fig. 2. The scenario setup

with the average throughput. In (1), N represents the number of sessions and T_i is the throughput in every established session. N_E is the number of established sessions per experiment.

$$T_{AVG} = \frac{\sum_{i=1}^{N} Ti}{N_E}, 1 \leq N \leq 10 \tag{1}$$

The throughput achieved in this simulation is the average throughput at the server node. It is quite smaller than it should be and this is due to the small packet fragmentation unit of 70 Bytes. The clients are the sensors that usually send information to that node. In Fig. 3 it is fairly understandable that the throughput achieved when the router is under attack is slightly larger since the PAN coordinator does play a higher role in the network (i.e. binds the network together).

The average end-to-end delay, as presented in Fig. 4 above, has higher values when the router is attacked. The reason is that since the node attacked is relatively close to the gateway, the routing protocol will try to set its route through that node. Then, when it will not be able to pass its traffic through it, it will look for an alternative route, which causes the increase in the end-to-end delay and with it, the delay variance, i.e. the jitter (Fig. 5).

As shown in the Fig. 6, which is considering the number of established sessions, the number decreases slightly more in the case of the attack on the router. In this case, it is intuitive to say that the delay plays a great role in here, as it is greater in the case of the attack on the router. This is because delay is caused by a congestion in the network and the more the network is congested, the more the packet needs hops to get to its destination. As a result of this, the Time to Live (TTL) field may drop to zero even during the establishment of the session and the setup of the group session key.

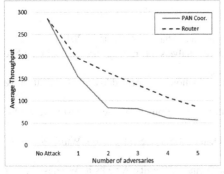

Fig. 3. The average throughput

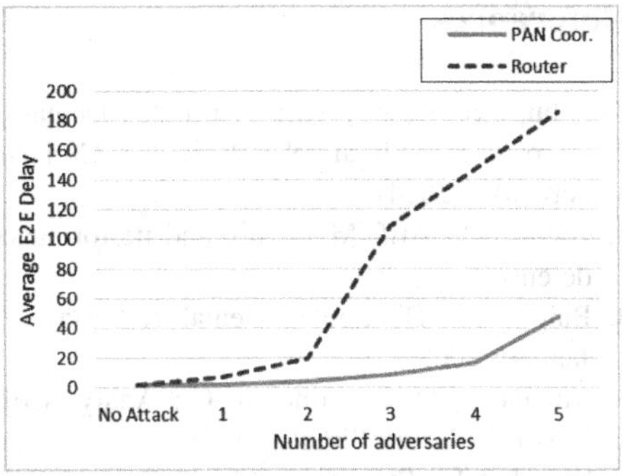

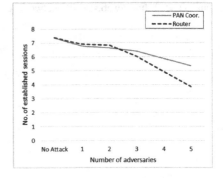

Fig. 4. The average end-to-end delay

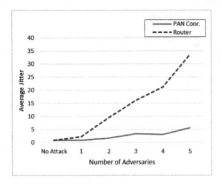

Fig. 5. The average Jitter

Fig. 6. The number of established sessions

5 Conclusion

By examining the application level DDoS attacks in mesh WSN with simulation, it can be concluded that the attack does affect the average throughput at the gateway. The difference in the performance of the network during the attacks on one of the routers vs. during the attack on the PAN Coordinator concerning the throughput is not as great as it is seen to be in the analysis of the tree topology mentioned in the related work section.

The average end-to-end delay and the average jitter both increase with the increase of the number of adversaries. Both are definitely larger in the scenario with the attack on the router. The number of established sessions is variably decreasing with the increase of the adversary nodes in both scenarios. Finally, it can be generally concluded that the performance of a ZigBee network is fairly different in case of DDoS attacks on different types of network devices.

References

1. Sahu, S.S., Pandey, M.: Distributed Denial of Service Attacks: A Review (2014)
2. Sharma, K., Mittal, N., Rathi, P.: Comparative analysis of routing protocols in ad-hoc networks (2014)
3. Aamir, M., Arif, M.: Study and performance evaluation on recent ddos trends of attack & defense
4. Baig, Z.A.: Distributed Denial of Service Attack Detection in Wireless Sensor Networks, January 2008
5. Chaitanya, D.K., Arindam, G.: Analysis of Denial-of-Service attacks on Wireless Sensor Networks Using Simulation
6. Wood, A.D., Stankovic, J.A.: A Taxonomy for Denial-of-Service Attacks in Wireless Sensor Networks
7. Farooq, N., Zahoor, I., Mandal, S., Gulzar, T.: Systematic Analysis of DoS Attacks in Wireless Sensor Networks with Wormhole Injection
8. Qualnet v5.2. http://web.scalable-networks.com/content/qualnet

Demo Session:
Student Innovation Corner

CHEST (COPD E-Health Sensor Solution)

Ivana Todorovska, Maja Janeva, Sinisha Pecov, Kristina Darkoska,
Tomche Mitrov, Sofija Shutarova, Katerina Darkoska, Hristina Chingoska,
Konstantin Chomu, Valentin Rakovic[✉], and Liljana Gavrilovska

Faculty of Electrical Engineering and Information Technologies,
Saints Cyril and Methodius University, Skopje, Macedonia
ivana.todorovska@ymail.com, maja_janeva@hotmail.com,
{nine_pec,darkoska.kristina,tomce_mitrov,sofija.shutarova}@yahoo.com,
kdarkoska@gmail.com,
{cingoska,konstantin.chomu,valentin,liljana}@feit.ukim.edu.mk

Abstract. The CHEST demo platform facilitates a solution that can
help patients suffering from COPD to adjust the conditions in their home
environment and everyday life. The developed demo offers a simple and
user-friendly solution, which consists of a sensor network that measures
the relevant COPD parameters (number of steps; indoor temperature;
level of carbon dioxide; air humidity; temperature), a developed cloud
solution for data management, and a graphical user interface (GUI) that
displays daily measured parameters, parameters' statistics and interacts
with the patients via specific notifications.

Keywords: Sensors · e-health · COPD

1 Introduction

Chronic Obstructive Pulmonary Disease (COPD) is a term referring to two lung
diseases, chronic bronchitis and emphysema. Both conditions cause obstruction
of airflow that interferes with normal breathing. Some ongoing studies have suggested that COPD will become the third leading cause of death by the year 2020 [1].
However, COPD is a medical disease that can be preventable and treatable [2].
While lung damage as a result of COPD is irreversible, there are treatments that
can improve a patient's quality of life, such as long-term administration of oxygen
(>15 h per day). Oxygen concentrators that are used throughout the day usually
control the administration of oxygen. There are two types: a home oxygen concentrator that is plugged in the patient's home and a portable oxygen concentrators
that is used when the patient leaves his home. The introduction of portable oxygen concentrators has allowed many patients with chronic lung disease to travel
and maintain active lifestyles [3]. The COPD patients benefit from pulmonary
rehabilitation that focuses on supervised exercise training to help the patients
manage their disease. These activities play an important part in supporting the
patients to maximize their ability to perform daily activities [1]. Moreover, the

© Institute for Computer Sciences, Social Informatics and Telecommunications Engineering 2015
V. Atanasovski, L.-G. Alberto (Eds.): Fabulous 2015, LNICST 159, pp. 235–238, 2015.
DOI: 10.1007/978-3-319-27072-2_30

COPD patients have strict requirements regarding the quality of living. It is often recommended that the room where they stay is well ventilated and the temperature is constantly monitored and controlled. In order to monitor the previously stated parameters, we developed a system that observes the environment, collects and processes data and visualizes the results.

2   Demo Architecture

The generic layout of the demo architecture is shown in Fig. 1.

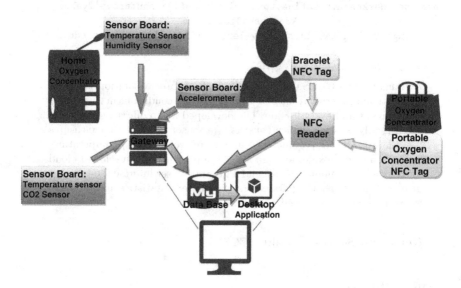

Fig. 1. A simple preview of the architecture of the demo

The demo is consisted of three main functional entities:

● *Wireless Sensor Network.* The wireless sensor network consists of several distinct sensory devices that gather the required COPD parameters. The sensor demo platform is build of:

- SunSPOT sensor board with a humidity sensor and a temperature sensor
- SunSPOT sensor board with an accelerometer
- SunSPOT sensor board with a CO_2 sensor and a temperature sensor
- SunSPOT gateway that accepts the sensor's data
- NFC reader with two NFC tags.

The sensors and the NFC reader send data to the gateway. The gateway sends the data to the cloud component utilizing http post messages. The code for the sensor devices and the NFC is developed in Java using the SunSPOT Programmers Manual [4] and Application Programming Interface V2.03 Manual [5].

- *Cloud Component.* The cloud component is the main storage and processing entity responsible for managing the actuated COPD parameters. It is consisted of a database and processing libraries (developed in MySQL) [6] and it is hosted on an Apache server. The cloud component: (*i*) accepts the information sent by the wireless sensor network, (*ii*) stores them in the data base and (*iii*) reasons upon them based on predefined thresholds that reflect the COPD patient's preferences and needs. Moreover, the cloud component is responsible for sending all required information towards the GUI.
- *Graphical User Interface.* The graphical user interface is a desktop application that utilizes the data from the cloud in order to adjust all alarms, display the patient statistics and monitor the current state of all the measured parameters. The graphical user interface is developed in the Java Programming environment [7].

3   Demo Setup and Demo Flow

The specific parameters and thresholds used in the demo are related to the specific COPD medical requirements. The values of the parameters are delineated in Table 1.

Table 1. Demo parameters and ranges

Parameter	Threshold value/range
Number of steps (daily)	2000
Indoor temperature range	$20^oC \div 25^oC$
Level of carbon dioxide (CO_2)	< 1000 ppm
Air humidity (nasal cannula monitoring)	$> 80\%$
Temperature (nasal cannula monitoring)	$> 36^oC$

When active, the demo monitors in real-time the parameters presented in Table 1. If a specific parameter violates the predefined thresholds, the system triggers a notification that will inform the patient regarding the detected abnormalities in his home environment. The demo targets four distinct use cases for monitoring and notification:

- *Nasal Cannula Monitoring.* During the night the nasal cannula of the home oxygen concentrator may fall off the COPD patient. The demo utilizes a combination of two sensors to monitor the status of the cannula: a humidity sensor and a temperature sensor, Table 1. If the humidity sensor measures humidity less than 80 and the temperature sensor measures temperature lower than 36^oC, the system will decide that the cannula has fallen off and notify the patient with an alarm. The alarm will wake up the patient and remind him to put the cannula back in the nose.

- *Oxygen Concentrator Reminder.* If a COPD patient leaves its home, it has to take its portable oxygen concentrator with him. The proposed demo incorporates a NFC (Near Field Communication) reader and two NFC tags to monitor this process and remind the patient if he leaves the home without the oxygen concentrator. The NFC reader is set on the patient's home entry door. The patient wears one tag as a bracelet and the other one is put on the portable oxygen concentrator. If the patient goes out without his portable oxygen concentrator (only the patient's tag is read by the NFC) an alarm goes off in order to remind the patient to take its portable oxygen concentrator.

- *Step Count Monitoring.* The proposed demo also incorporates a sensor with an accelerometer that counts the patient's steps and measures its daily physical activity. The patient wears the sensor in his pocket during the day. If the patient has not moved enough or has moved too much during the day, a notification is sent that reminds the patient to either perform some additional walking or refrain from lengthy walks.

- *Home Environment Monitoring.* Since the COPD patients have strict requirements regarding the air quality and the indoor temperature, the CHEST demo monitors the environmental temperature and home air quality by a temperature sensor and CO_2 sensor. These sensors are positioned in the patient's living room. The demo triggers an alarm informing the patient regarding the deviation in his home temperature or air quality if any of the parameters are under or above the predefined thresholds.

4   Conclusions

This demo shows that a smart and user-friendly solution can be incorporated in COPD patients' everyday life. Our system consists of sensors, cloud and GUI that measures the parameters, processes them and notifies the users for the required actions. In the future the platform can be upgraded with additional sensors that would measure other significant parameters. This would improve the uses experience and life quality.

References

1. Brown, R.E., Miller, B., Taylor, W.R., et al.: Health care expenditures for tuberculosis in the U.S. Arch. Intern. Med. **155**(15), 1595–1600 (1995)
2. American lung association. http://www.lung.org/
3. The National Coalition for Elimination of Tuberculosis. Tuberculosis Elimination: The Federal Funding Gap. http://www.lung.org/
4. Sun SPOT Programmers Manual. https://www.java.net/
5. Application Programming Interface V2.03 Manual. http://www.acs.com.hk/
6. MySQL 5.1 Reference Manual. http://dev.mysql.com/
7. Java Programming Tutorial-Programming Graphical User Interface (GUI). https://www3.ntu.edu.sg/home/ehchua/programming/java/J4a_GUI.html

Regular Session

Evaluating Scalability Performance in Azure

Marjan Gusev[1], Sasko Ristov[1]([✉]), and Kristina Kolic[2]

[1] FCSE, University Saints Cyril and Methodius, Rugjer Boshkovikj 16,
1000 Skopje, Macedonia
{marjan.gushev,sashko.ristov}@finki.ukim.mk
[2] Haybrooke Associates from 2013, 10 Pelham Street, Leicester LE2 4DJ, UK

Abstract. The main research goal of this paper is to find out if scaled resources offer scaled performance in case of a demo e-Business application hosted on Windows Azure. The results prove that scaled resources can give even better performance than the expected the scaling factor, usually expressed as ratio between the number of used cores in rented virtual machines. A superlinear region is observed when the performance is higher than the scaling factor of the used resources.

Keywords: Cloud computing · Scaling · Performance · Windows Azure · Load testing

1 Introduction

In this article we evaluate the scalability performance of an e-Business application. The research goal is to find if the scaled resource configurations can offer the scaled performance.

Our previous study [1] has analyzed the performance with goal to find an optimal configuration for a given load and in this paper we would like to find out if scaling the resources will give the customer scaled performance and also to measure if this increased performance is proportional to the scaling factor. This is very important, since the price models of cloud providers are based on a linear scaled pricing for scaled resources and the customers would like to know if they get performance equal to the performance of the default configuration multiplied by the scaling factor.

We have performed a research on modeling the speedup for scalable web services in [2]. For related work and state-of-the-art, an interested user can check [3–7] and the references specified in our paper on Windows Azure resource organization performance analysis [8]. However, most of these results are towards finding an optimal configuration for a given application and load, and do not analyze what happens in case of scaling.

The paper is organized as follows. The testing methodology is given in Sect. 2 and the results are evaluated in Sect. 3. Section 4 discusses the results and gives explanation about superlinear speedup. Finally, conclusions and directions for future work are given in Sect. 5.

© Institute for Computer Sciences, Social Informatics and Telecommunications Engineering 2015
V. Atanasovski, L.-G. Alberto (Eds.): Fabulous 2015, LNICST 159, pp. 241–247, 2015.
DOI: 10.1007/978-3-319-27072-2_31

2   Testing Methodology

The testing environment, as described in [1] is using at most 20 cores in Azure cloud datacentre placed in South Central US. Each configuration is denoted by v At, where v presents the number of VMs, which can be 1, 2, ..., and t is the VM type. Particularly, using the latest Azure offer in 2015 [10], A1 means a VM with one core and 1.75 GB RAM, A2 a VM with 2 cores and 3.5 GB RAM, and A3 an Azure VM with 4 cores and 7 GB RAM.

The SaaS solution [9,11] is used as a typical e-Business application, realized as a transactional ASP.NET web application that processes documents related to the e-Business ordering, invoicing and financial clearing processes. It uses Microsoft SQL Server database management system.

To realize valuable results we have performed two experiments, explained in more details in [1]. The first test case (TC1) presents the lighter case, when a list of the orders has to be selected under a certain user load, and realizes 3 HTTP requests per each user. The second test case (TC2) is more complex, since it realizes 6 HTTP requests per user, a case when a user inserts a new offer under a certain user load.

The load for both test cases is simulated by various number of users: starting from 1, 5, 10, 50, 100, and increasing by 50 up to 1000 users.

In this paper we analyze the scaling behavior, based on calculation of performance. Let's define by T_R the average response time for executing the HTTP requests on a given test case, measured in 5 test executions. The performance P to process N user requests in a given response time is calculated by $P = N/T_R$.

Let's analyze a default resource configuration by x and the scaled configuration by y that uses n times more resources (in our case processors). The scaling speedup S_{xy} compares the performance behavior of the scaled with the default configuration divided by the scaling factor n, by calculating $S_{xy} = P_y/(n \times P_x)$.

According to the Gustafson's Law [12], one would expect that the scaled configuration will have at most the performance of the default configuration multiplied by the scaling factor. Values $S_{xy} \geq 1$ should be interpreted as a superlinear effect, where the scaled configuration offers a performance which is greater than the scaling factor.

3   Analysis of Results

In this section we will analyze if the scaling strategy that increases the number of cores of the VMs makes the system perform proportionally better with the number of cores. The scaling speedup S_{xy} is used to evaluate its scaling behavior. The experiment contains the test cases with scaling factor n equal to: 2, 3, 4, 5, 6, 8 and 10, analyzed as average value in 5 test executions for each user load.

Figure 1 shows the measured performance curves for TC1 and TC2 starting from 1 user load. y-axis represents the relative performance compared to the initial load of 1 user, and x-axis the number of users. Note that due to clarity of presentation, we present only the most representative curves instead of presenting all measured results. For TC1 we can conclude that almost every configuration reaches better performance $S > 1$ in a certain region of user loads until they saturate, when the performance is not proportional to the user load. Most configurations in TC2 have lower performance for more than 200 users.

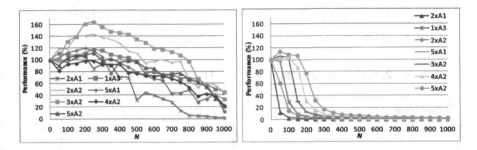

Fig. 1. Measured performance curves: (a) TC1 left and (b) TC2 right.

Depending on the processing demands, each measurement shows similar performance behavior, where the processing speed does not change with user load up to a certain saturation level, then it decreases and slows down to the zero value. The user load when the processing speed enters in the saturation region is dependent on the number of requests to be processed by the given configuration. For example, this is evident for smaller configurations with total number of 1, 2 or 3 cores for TC1, and for all configurations for TC2. The conclusion is that the saturation point depends on the number of cores in configurations, the more cores, the higher the value of the saturation point is.

Figures 2, 3, 4, 5, 6 and 7 present the scaling speedup (y-axis) for various user loads (x-axis) increasing the number of cores of the first configuration by a certain scaling factor. Note that we present only the most representative scaling combinations to reach clarity of charts.

The scaling speedup for $n = 2$ presented in Fig. 2(a) shows that just certain scaling combinations for TC1 reached the state when the scaling iwill speed up the system. Scaling the configuration 3xA1 to 3xA2 for almost each user load has speedup, while the scaling 2xA1 to 2xA2, 2xA1 to 1xA3, 1xA2 to 1xA3, 4xA1 to 2xA3 and 4xA1 to 4xA2 reaches speedup for load of 700 users and above. The rest of the combinations do not reach speedup.

Most of the scaling combinations for TC2 (in Fig. 2b) reach scaling speedup starting at load of 50 users until 400 users, when these configurations get into saturation.

Figure 3(a) presents the scaling speedup of the TC1 configurations for $n = 3$. Only some scaling combinations get speedup greater than or equal n, such as scaling the 2xA1 to 6xA1 for more than 900 users.

Figure 3(b) presents the scaling speedup for $n = 3$ of the TC2. Similar to the previous case, some configurations achieve scaling speedup, such as scaling 2xA1 to 3xA2 and 4xA1 to 3xA3 in the interval of 50 to 350 users.

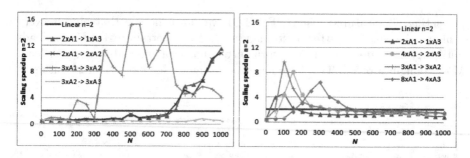

Fig. 2. Scaling speedup for $n = 2$: (a) TC1 left and (b) TC2 right.

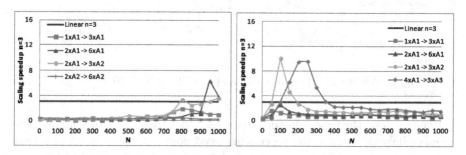

Fig. 3. Scaling speedup for $n = 3$: (a) TC1 left and (b) TC2 right.

The scaling speedup for TC1 for $n = 4$ is presented in Fig. 4(a). Most of the scaling combinations perform better than n for more than 450 users and the saturation appears for more than 1000 users. The more powerful configurations do not enter in the region when this effect occurs.

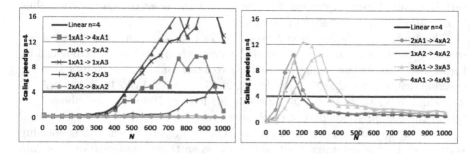

Fig. 4. Scaling speedup for $n = 4$: (a) TC1 left and (b) TC2 right.

The chart for the scaling speedup for $n = 4$ of the TC2 configurations is shown on Fig. 4(b). The trends are the same to the previous cases: the configurations get speedup at small user load, and afterwards at higher load they get into saturation. The highest speedup is achieved when a configuration that has VMs of smaller type (A1) is scaled to a configuration that has large VMs (A3).

The performance behavior for TC1 configurations for $n = 5$ or 10 is presented on Fig. 5(a). The identified trend is also present for TC2 in Fig. 5(b), that is a region is detected when the scaling configuration performs better than the original configuration, such as scaling the 1xA1 to 5xA1. However, this effect is not obtained for $n = 10$ for TC1 and for TC2 this region is very small compared to previous cases.

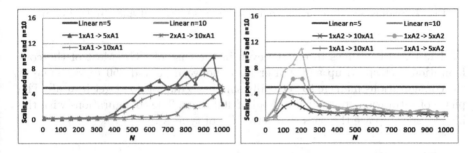

Fig. 5. Scaling speedup for $n = 5$ or 10: (a) TC1 left and (b) TC2 right.

In Fig. 6(a) and (b) we can observe the performance behavior for $n = 6$ or 8 correspondingly for TC1 and TC2. There are two batches of scaling combinations for TC1, one that achieve scaling speedup greater than n in certain user load region smaller than 1000 users, such as scaling the 1xA1 to 3xA2 and another that achieves speedup at higher user loads. The performance behavior of most scaling combinations for TC2 achieve scaling speedup greater than n for loads in range between 50 and 350 users.

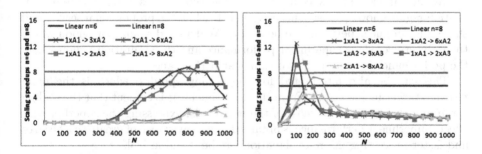

Fig. 6. Scaling speedup for $n = 6$ or 8: (a) TC1 left and (b) TC2 right.

Figure 7 shows the case of horizontal scaling the configurations for only one VM of the same type that they have. Only two configurations for TC1 achieve speedup that greater than 1, 3xA1 to 4xA1 and 1xA1 to 2xA1.

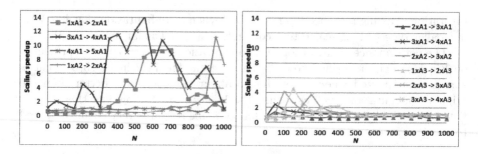

Fig. 7. Scaling speedup for horizontal scaling: (a) TC1 left and (b) TC2 right.

The trend continues to emerge even in the case of TC2. Most of the configurations get speed up at the user loads between 50 and 350 users. Some of the configurations manage to get really small speedup or don't get it at all. The phase of saturation starts at user load of 400 users. The configurations with the highest speedup are the ones that have VM of type A3.

4 Discussion

All experiments have proven that the scaled resources offer scaling performance, except in the case of underutilization. However, this is expected, since, one would prefer scaling, only if the resource configuration is saturated and nobody would pay more if the current resource configuration satisfies the requirements and offers sufficient quality of service.

The obtained results are tightly connected to the performance saturation point of the analyzed resource configuration. If the saturation points of the current and scaled configuration are far, then we achieve better scaling speedup of the analyzed configurations.

We have modeled the speedup for scalable web services in [2]. The underutilization region shows performance less than 1, while the proportional server load shows the sublinear performance behavior. We detected a superior region where the web services show superlinear performance and the saturation region where the performance is degrading into sublinear performance.

This can be also interpreted for the scaling speedup which is the main research target in this paper. From this experiment, it is evident that the scaling speedup factor $S_{xy} > 1$ for most of the user loads, expressing the superlinearity effect. Superlinear performance is obtained due to existence of greater cache sizes and faster processing. More explanation can be found in [13].

5 Conclusion

Our experiments on the performance of a typical e-Business SaaS solution have showed that scaling the resources results in scaled performance. This means that the customers will get performance proportional to the scaled resources.

In addition, we have observed a superlinear effect, meaning that the scaled configuration offered performance higher than the performance of the default configuration multiplied for the scaling factor, mostly due to increased use of caches and available memory.

As future work we will analyze details on superlinear effect offered in web services using scaled resources.

References

1. Kolic, K., Gusev, M., Ristov, S.: Performance analysis of a new cloud e-Business solution. In: 2015 Proceedings of the 35th International Convention on MIPRO, pp. 276–281. IEEE Conference Publications, Opatija, Croatia (2015)
2. Ristov, S., Gusev, M., Velkoski, G.: Modeling the speedup for scalable web services. In: Bogdanova, A.M., Gjorgjevikj, D. (eds.) ICT Innovations 2014. AISC, vol. 311, pp. 177–186. Springer, Heidelberg (2015)
3. Brebner, P., Liu, A.: Performance and cost assessment of cloud services. In: Maximilien, E.M., Rossi, G., Yuan, S.-T., Ludwig, H., Fantinato, M. (eds.) ICSOC 2010. LNCS, vol. 6568, pp. 39–50. Springer, Heidelberg (2011)
4. Hill, Z., Li, J., Mao, M., Ruiz-Alvarez, A., Humphrey, M.: Early observations on the performance of Windows Azure. In: Proceedings of the 19th ACM International Symposium on High Performance Distributed Computing, HPDC 2010, pp. 367–376 (2010)
5. Xiong, K., Perros, H.: Service performance and analysis in cloud computing. In: 2009 World Conference on Services-I, pp. 693–700. IEEE (2009)
6. Iosup, A., Ostermann, S., Yigitbasi, M.N., Prodan, R., Fahringer, T., Epema, D.H.: Performance analysis of cloud computing services for many-tasks scientific computing. IEEE Trans. Parallel Distrib. Syst. **22**(6), 931–945 (2011)
7. Khanghahi, N., Ravanmehr, R.: Cloud computing performance evaluation: issues and challenges. Comput. **5**(1), 29–41 (2013)
8. Gusev, M., Ristov, S., Koteska, B., Velkoski, G.: Windows Azure: resource organization performance analysis. In: Villari, M., Zimmermann, W., Lau, K.-K. (eds.) ESOCC 2014. LNCS, vol. 8745, pp. 17–31. Springer, Heidelberg (2014)
9. Kolic, K., Ristov, S., Gusev, M.: A model of SaaS e-Business solution. In: Proceedings of the 22nd International TELFOR Forum, pp. 1146–1149. IEEE Conference Publications (2014)
10. Microsoft: Windows Azure, June 2015. http://www.windowsazure.com/pricing/
11. Kolic, K., Gusev, M., Ristov, S.: A new e-Business solution with ticket management. In: Proceedings of i-Society 2014, pp. 203–208. IEEE Conference Publications (2014)
12. Gustafson, J.L.: Reevaluating Amdahl's law. Commun. ACM **31**(5), 532–533 (1988)
13. Gusev, M., Ristov, S.: A superlinear speedup region for matrix multiplication. Concurrency Comput.: Pract. Exp. **26**(11), 1847–1868 (2014)

An Overview of Cloud Portability

Magdalena Kostoska, Marjan Gusev, and Sasko Ristov (✉)

FCSE, University Saints Cyril and Methodius, Rugjer Boshkovikj 16,
1000 Skopje, Macedonia
{magdalena.kostoska,marjan.gushev,sashko.ristov}@finki.ukim.mk

Abstract. The application cannot be moved to other cloud vendor on
the same cloud service layer easily since it depends on the lower cloud
services, as well as on the target vendor's application and data structure. In general case the cloud applications are neither interoperable,
nor portable. This paper overviews the cloud portability and its application on various service models. It analyzes and categorizes all aspects
of cloud computing portability, puts perspective on each defined process
and describes the current development stage for each perspective.

Keywords: Cloud computing · Interoperability · Portability ·
Performance

1 Introduction

The cloud market is rapidly growing recently. The outsourcing of computing
infrastructure reduces not only the CAPEX (Capital Expenditure) and OPEX
(Operational Expenditure), but also the costs for human resources and management [1]. The increased army of cloud service providers (CSP), as well as the
improved and user friendly open source cloud frameworks, push the potential
cloud clients and consumers to migrate their services, data and applications to
the cloud. However, the CSPs are doing everything (even unfair issues some-
times) to lock the clients into their clouds. This trap of vendor-lock-in should
be considered very carefully because it can provide even greater costs than the
savings that the cloud provides.

Therefore, two main features must be considered by the CSPs and cloud
clients, i.e. the *interoperability* and *portability*. Both these features are familiar
to the computing industry, but in the cloud environment they become even
more important. The former allows the ability of at least two heterogeneous
cloud applications to communicate between each other, as well as to use the
exchanged information. The latter allows the client to migrate an application
from one cloud platform or / and infrastructure to another with less or even
without efforts. The final benefit of the cloud portability is to avoid customer
lock-in by the CSPs into their environment forcing them to use only the services
they provide. Cloud computing is about opening the gates to all clients allowing
them to interoperate with services of other CSPs or to move freely to other CSPs
whenever they are not satisfied with the service level. This will probably reduce

© Institute for Computer Sciences, Social Informatics and Telecommunications Engineering 2015
V. Atanasovski, L.-G. Alberto (Eds.): Fabulous 2015, LNICST 159, pp. 248–254, 2015.
DOI: 10.1007/978-3-319-27072-2_32

the number of CSPs' clients, which will be compensated with new potential clients due to the CSP's openness.

This paper observes both of these important cloud features and inspects how they can be considered as a service model.

The rest of the paper is organized in several sections. The basic concepts of portability in cloud computing are presented in Sect. 2. Section 3 discusses the portability as a service model, that is, portability of data, applications and platforms. The discussion of state-of-the-art solutions are discussed in Sect. 4. Finally, Sect. 5 concludes the paper.

2   Background

According to NIST, *cloud computing* is *"a model for enabling ubiquitous, convenient, on-demand network access to a shared pool of configurable computing resources (e.g., networks, servers, storage, applications, and services) that can be rapidly provisioned and released with minimal management effort or service provider interaction."* [2].

This cloud computing model is composed of five essential characteristics: *on-demand self-service, broad network access, resource pooling, rapid elasticity,* and *measured service.*

Services in cloud are available in three major ways: *Infrastructure as a Service (IaaS), Platform as a Service (PaaS),* and *Software as a Service (SaaS)* [2]. Additionally, other layers have been proposed, such as *Data Storage as a Service (DaaS), Communication as a Service (CaaS)* [3], etc.

According to definitions in NIST [2], there are four essential deployment models: *public cloud, private cloud, hybrid cloud,* and *community cloud.*

Portability is referred as ability to move software on different runtime platforms with reasonable effort (i.e. without having to rewrite it partly or fully) [4]. Three types of portability are considered: Binary, Source and Intermediate-Level Portability [5,6].

Binary Portability is referred to porting the executable form of the software unit and it is possible only across similar environments.

Source Portability is referred to porting the source language representation of the software unit, but assumes availability of source code. This type of porting is considered to be most commonly used.

Intermediate-Level Portability is referred to porting software representation which is between source and binary code.

Cloud computing interoperability allows different services on different clouds to process data with a common specification as well as allows simple exchange and reuse of data among different infrastructures on cloud.

On the other hand, *cloud computing portability* allows simple data and service use from one cloud to another for two or more cloud infrastructures [2]. We have proposed a new cloud portability service platform [7].

Interoperability and portability in cloud computing are not unambiguous and depend on the context in which they are considered, and therefore they require further definition according to the application.

3   Cloud Portability

According to Petcu and Vasilakos [8] the Cloud Portability Taxonomy can be analyzed in three different perspectives:

- Implementation perspective - implementation-specific requirements or restrictions
- Ecosystem perspective - application specific dependencies
- Business perspective - business relevant, non-functional and abstract constraints

We will further discuss the implementation perspective categories: portability of data, applications, and platforms, which depend upon ecosystem perspective properties.

Data portability may be considered as data reuse:

- in different cloud applications (SaaS), in other words, as a quick and easy transfer and reuse of data from one application to another, or
- as quick and easy transfer and reuse of data among different cloud storages (DaaS).

Application portability may be considered as an easier reuse of applications among:

- different platforms (PaaS); in other words, an application developed on one platform should be easily transferrable and reusable on another platform, or
- different infrastructures in cloud; in other words, an application set on one infrastructure (IaaS) and cloud system should be easily transferrable and reusable on another infrastructure or different cloud system

Platform portability may be considered as an easier reuse of platforms by:

- transfer of platform components and their reuse on another infrastructure (IaaS), or
- complete transfer (image) of platform on another infrastructure (IaaS) in cloud.

A proper PaaS taxonomy should be established in order to perform Platform portability. An initial step in this direction is presented by Kolb et al. [9]. They classify a general taxonomy, shown in Fig. 1 based on 68 PaaS offerings. Two general categories are defined: ecosystem and business, each with subcategories and further refinements.

4   Discussion

Reasons why a standard may not be interoperable can include Incompleteness; Inadequate interfaces; Poor handling of options; Lack of clarity; Poor maintenance; Lack of system overview; Using standards beyond their original purposes; and Varying quality [10].

Ecosystem

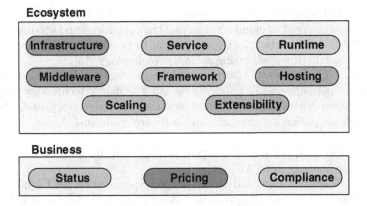

Business

Fig. 1. PaaS taxonomy [9]

Table 1. Development status of each aspect of interoperability and portability of cloud computing

Activitiy	Context	Layer	Developing standards
Interoperability	Management	IaaS	OCCI, CIMI, UCI
	Platform	PaaS	Stub
	Application	SaaS	mOSAIC
Portability	Platform	IaaS (components)	Stub
		IaaS (image)	OVF
	Application	PaaS	CAMP
		IaaS	OVF, TOSCA, mOSAIC
	Data	SaaS	OData
		DaaS	CDMI

In previous section we have described various aspects of the cloud portability. For most categories the current state in the areas is either in research and development or stub definition. Very few commonly adopted solutions exist. In this section we will describe the ongoing standardization efforts and possible solutions. We will present only the standards that have published at least initial documentation and we will omit the standardization efforts.

Marjan - Table moved to magazine paper Table 1 presents the current development stage for each of the perspectives (i.e. categories).

It is noticeable, given Table 1, that certain aspects are more developed than other (i.e. interoperable management of virtual machines and application portability). We can also notice that the Platform context is least developed.

Large number of developing standards has arisen during the past few years:

- OCCI - The Open Cloud Computing Interface standard represents protocol and API for all kinds of IaaS management tasks [11]

- CIMI - Cloud Infrastructure Management Interface standard represents an interface for management of cloud services and the operations and attributes [12]
- UCI - Unified Cloud Interface concept aim to provide a unified interface for entire infrastructure stack using semantic technology [13]
- mOSAIC - The mOSAIC platform and engine enables deployment, configuration and management of applications using semantic technology [14]
- OVF - Open Virtualization Format standard provides open and platform-independent packaging format for software solutions based on virtual systems [15]
- CAMP - Cloud Application Management for Platforms aims to standardizing cloud PaaS management API [16]
- TOSCA - The Topology and Orchestration Specification for Cloud Applications aims to standardize application description in order to provide portability and management [17]. We introduced the extension - P-TOSCA, which handles several TOSCA weaknesses and ambiguities [18]. The demo applications for automated portability with P-TOSCA are developed for porting a SOA application [19] and an N-tier application [20].
- OData - The Open Data Protocol enables service creation to publish, share and edit resources via HTTP [21]
- CDMI - The Cloud Data Management Interface standard defines interface for creation, retrieval, update and deletion of data elements from the Cloud [22]

Unfortunately none of the standards is widely adopted. In general the cloud computing providers resist adopting open standards and thus disable clients to switch provider easily. This is especially important for the standards regarding the IaaS layer, the lowest level in the cloud computing stack, since it is not possible to build and adopt fully functional standard for the other layers missing standardization on the lowest level.

A lot of research is done towards autonomous porting of cloud applications. We have also reviewed these approaches [23] and analyze the corresponding state-of-the-art. Interestingly, there are a lot of world initiatives and EU research projects, such as REMICS, Cloud4SOA, OPTIMIS, CONTRAIL, ARTIST, PaaSage, MODAClouds, RighScale or CloudFoundry. We have classified them in two approaches [23], the first that realizes a direct engine to support TOSCA implementation, and the second that translates TOSCA based application specification onto a specification used existing cloud management tools, such as CAMP, Brooklyn, Chef, Puppet, etc.

Several research papers [8,9,24] cover more details about who stands behind each standard and what is the market positioning and potential of each standard. We can conclude that most of the big players support the TOSCA approach, including Cisco, Citrix, EMC, Fujitsu, Hewlett-Packard, Huawei, IBM, SAP, VMWare, etc.

5 Conclusion

Although the interoperability and portability are similar, they differ among each other. Nevertheless, they are very important issues for both the CSPs and clients.

The overall benefit of the cloud portability is the possibility to freely migrate part or all services to other CSPs, increase their agility and reliability by hosting on several providers and allow the services to interoperate among each other.

This paper overviews the cloud application portability as data, application and platform portability.

Most common method to provide cloud portability is standardization and accepting de-facto standards. We have analyzed every aspect (as category) and suggested methods. Further on, we have appropriately mapped most relevant standardization efforts to these categories. We have identified aspect and gaps that require further development, as well as aspects that are prevalent in the research areas. We can conclude that the landscape of cloud computing is too diverse to accept any standard unanimously at this moment, and still it remains a hot research topic, especially towards automated porting of applications. This is especially important for customers, since they prefer the freedom to choose the cloud provider which will satisfy the user requirements in the best possible way.

Still there are a lot of open issues and the standardization waits for further solutions. The highest importance is the fact that most of the cloud providers do not support porting since they prefer lock-in situations, and already have a sufficient market share. Next open issue is the fact that several solutions do not support change of the virtual machine (image) and have limited applicability. The third on the list are those proposals that have not been widely adopted and are only supported by the cloud providers themselves. The future of these proposals with limited applicability is limited unless they adopt to the current trends and extend their applicability domain.

Besides the open issues, there are several challenges about obstacles that prevent easy porting. The highest obstacle is the variety of cloud management tools, that prevents an application to be ported using the conventional batch files or those that translate management commands from one environment to another. The next obstacle is the application topology, since it may be rather complex and prevent easy sequential execution of cloud management operations.

References

1. Rana, O.: The costs of cloud migration. Cloud Comput. IEEE 1(1), 62–65 (2014)
2. National Institute of Standards and Technology: Nist cloud computing standards roadmap, July 2013. http://www.nist.gov/itl/cloud/upload/NIST_SP-500-291_Version-2_2013_June1_FINAL.pdf
3. Hu, F., Qiu, M., Li, J., Grant, T., Taylor, D., McCaleb, S., Butler, L., Hamner, R.: A review on cloud computing: Design challenges in architecture and security. J. Comput. Inf. Technol. CIT 19(1), 25–55 (2011)
4. Brown, P.J.: Software portability. In: Encyclopedia of Computer Science. John Wiley and Sons Ltd., Chichester, pp. 1633–1634 (2003)
5. Mooney, J.D.: Issues in the specification and measurement of software portability. Technical report TR 93-6, West Virginia University (1993)
6. Mooney, J.D.: Developing portable software. In: Reis, R. (ed.) Information Technology. IFIP International Federation for Information Processing, vol. 157, pp. 55–84. Springer, US (2004)

7. Kostoska, M., Gusev, M., Ristov, S.: A new cloud services portability platform. Procedia Eng. **69**, 1268–1275 (2014)
8. Petcu, D., Vasilakos, A.: Portability in clouds: approaches and research opportunities. Scalable Comput.: Pract. Exp. **15**(3), 251–270 (2014)
9. Kolb, S., Wirtz, G.: Towards application portability in platform as a service. In: 2014 IEEE 8th International Symposium on Service Oriented System Engineering (SOSE), pp. 218–229, April 2014
10. van der Veer, H., Wiles, A.: Achieving Technical Interoperability. European Telecommunications Standards Institute, New York (2008)
11. Open Grid Forum: OCCI, Open Cloud Computing Interface (2011). http://occi-wg.org/
12. Distributed Management Task Force: Cloud infrastructure management interface (cimi) model and restful http-based protocol, March 2015. http://dmtf.org/sites/default/files/standards/documents/DSP0263_2.0.0c.pdf
13. Google: Unified cloud (2010). http://code.google.com/p/unifiedcloud/wiki/UCI_Architecture
14. Moscato, F., Aversa, R., Di Martino, B., Fortis, T., Munteanu, V.: An analysis of mosaic ontology for cloud resources annotation. In: 2011 Federated Conference on Computer Science and Information Systems (FedCSIS), pp. 973–980, September 2011
15. Distributed Management Task Force: Open virtualization format specification version 2.1.0, January 2014. http://www.dmtf.org/sites/default/files/standards/documents/DSP0265_1.0.0.pdf
16. Carlson, M., Chapman, M., Heneveld, A., Hinkelman, S., Johnston-Watt, D., Karmarkar, A., Kunze, T., Malhotra, A., Mischkinsky, J., Otto, A., et al.: Cloud application management for platforms (2012). http://cloudspecs.org/camp/CAMP-v1.0.pdf
17. Han, R., Ghanem, M.M., Guo, Y.: Elastic-TOSCA: Supporting elasticity of cloud application in TOSCA. In: The Fourth International Conference on Cloud Computing, GRIDs, and Virtualization, CLOUD COMPUTING 2013, pp. 93–100 (2013)
18. Gusev, M., Kostoska, M., Ristov, S., Donevski, A.: Autonomous portability of cloud applications. In: Proceedings of 5th International Conference on Cloud Computing and Service Science (CLOSER), pp. 71–78 (2015)
19. Ristov, S., Kostoska, M., Gusev, M.: P-TOSCA portability demo case. In: 2014 IEEE 3rd International Conference on Cloud Networking (IEEE CLOUDNET), pp. 269–271 (2014)
20. Gusev, M., Kostoska, M., Ristov, S.: Cloud P-TOSCA porting of N-tier applications. In: Proceedings of the 22nd International TELFOR Forum, pp. 935–938. IEEE Conference Publications (2014)
21. OASIS: Open Data Protocol (OData) 4.0., Febuary 2014. http://docs.oasis-open.org/
22. SNIA: Cloud Data Management Interface (CDMI) v1.1.1., March 2015. http://www.snia.org/sites/default/files/CDMI_Spec_v1.1.1.pdf
23. Gusev, M., Kostoska, M., Ristov, S.: Autonomous porting of cloud applications. Technical report LiiT:15/2015, University Ss Cyril and Methodius, FCSE (2015)
24. Di Martino, B., Cretella, G., Esposito, A.: Methodologies for cloud portability and interoperability. In: Di Martino, B., Cretella, G., Esposito, A. (eds.) Cloud Portability and Interoperability. SpringerBriefs in Computer Science, pp. 15–44. Springer, Heidelberg (2015)

Basic Internet Foundation

George Suciu$^{(\boxtimes)}$, Alin Geaba, Cristina Butca, Victor Suciu,
and Octavian Fratu

University Politehnica of Bucharest,
Splaiul Independentei 313, Bucharest, Romania
{george,alin.geaba,cristina.butca}@beia.ro

Abstract. Basic Internet foundation is an institute that aims to ensure optimized content delivery for capacity-limited networks. In this paper we describe the foundation's initiative in offering free access to low capacity Internet to people in areas with low admission and economic problems and/or no Internet coverage. The main contribution of this paper consists in pointing out solutions that this foundation proposes, as well as what other programs or companies have found encouraging their development.

Keywords: Basic internet foundation · Capacity-limited networks · Free internet

1 Introduction

There is a constant need for evolution and the only way humanity has gotten to the point it is today is by using the collective knowledge of different individuals. Because of that desire to form a connection with others the Internet has been developed as the solution for sharing and receiving data by linking billions of devices worldwide and thus becoming a global system of interconnected computer networks.

The origins of the Internet date back to the 1960 s, when the United States government developed a research program that aimed to build robust, fault-tolerant communication via computer networks [1]. The Internet consists of a multitude of networks local to global scope, private or public connected to a broad array of networking technologies [2]. As of December 2014, nearly 37.9 percent of the world's human population has already used the services of the Internet [3]. On the other hand two thirds of the geographical populated areas don't have Internet infrastructure.

The Internet Protocol (IP) represents the main communications protocol for relaying datagrams across the Internet [4]. The IP is the main heart of Internet technologies because of its routing function that enables internetworking.

The definition for Wi-Fi given by the Wi-Fi Alliance is that of any "wireless local area network" (WLAN) product based on the Institute of Electrical and Electronics Engineers' (IEEE) 802.11 standards.

The Internet can be used for multiple purposes, one of them is to promote teacher training. In the case of rural areas, the internet has an important role in giving teachers some pointers to a better educational experience as well as offering them materials for

© Institute for Computer Sciences, Social Informatics and Telecommunications Engineering 2015
V. Atanasovski, L.-G. Alberto (Eds.): Fabulous 2015, LNICST 159, pp. 255–262, 2015.
DOI: 10.1007/978-3-319-27072-2_33

the same task [5]. By using a network-based training system, teachers can keep in touch with each other or receive support from some of the best universities.

The Basic Internet foundation does not plan on offering its services unless the situation requires it. Based on factors such as social conditions, markets or economy the foundation determines if its interventions are necessary, and once those factors have evolved satisfactorily, the foundation can terminate its involvement in the region. Afterwards it may then decide to sell or to transfer those assets, rights and obligations onto the selected commercial operators.

The paper is organized as follows: Sect. 2 presents solutions proposed by other companies with similar goals, while Sect. 3 describes the involvement of the Ministry of Communications and Information Society (MCSI) in Romania. Section 4 presents the results of basic Internet and Sect. 5 concludes the paper.

2 Related Work

In this section we provide an overview of existing solutions for Internet distribution in areas with economic issues and present the main challenges.

2.1 Nextelco

Nextelco Foundation is a nonprofit company founded in 2013 by Guy Kamanda and aims at providing Internet to Africa [6]. The main goal is to provide free information access which the company considers to be a human right.

The United Nations' Human Rights Council has unanimously backed the notion of equal rights for every person to be allowed to connect to and express themselves freely on the Internet, approving it in a resolution on the fifth of July 2012.

The company is using the new concept of user involved service and that of the infrastructure provision. What the real challenge that Nextelco recognized is that in emerging economies like Congo the Internet is only accessible for the well-established people, but the main purpose is for it to soon become a consumer product in Africa for people of all ages and economical standards.

2.2 WaveTek

WaveTek Nigeria Limited is an innovative company that provides information and communications technology (ICT) solutions that offers customers cutting-edge infrastructure and devices independent of their social area [7]. The virtual fiber solution the company has come up with for reducing the cost as an alternative for the fiber circuits is a high-capacity wireless. The way to do that is by transmitting data over microwave or millimeter wave frequencies at gigabit speeds, approximately 2 Gigabits per second (Gbps), with the possibility to upgrade it in the future up to 10 Gbps. The reason for its efficiency it that has multiple advantages such as: add/drop data ports and optional wire-speed with an Advanced Encryption Standard (AES) encryption built-in thus making existing fiber network redundant.

2.3   Multi-Tier Architecture for the Internet of Internets (MTAII)

The Next Generation Internet (NGI) consists of a multitude of projects that have the objective of improving Internet performance as well as content quality in different regions [8]. Nowadays, when we talk about NGI we focus on the research regarding the design, protocols, engineering, and operation regarding the new signal processing techniques in 3G/4G/LTE/B4G [9]. Other important researches are that of the Ad Hoc Network and Wireless Mesh Network [10], channel allocation [11], Internet of things (IoT) [12], cloud computing [13], and some other fields.

Specific Internet Protocol (SIP) isolates IPv4 on hosts from wide area network (WAN) infrastructures while delivering IPv4 traffic through WANs between hosts. Multi-Tier Internet Protocol (MTIP) provides a tree-like topology and is used for delivering SIP traffic. The exhaustion of the IPv4 address space was foreseen, so many resolutions had been suggested but the problem was that none of them was accepted as a solution so they were all combined into another Internet protocol IPv6 [14]. One of the main functions that the IPv4 should have is to run on hosts independently from the WAN infrastructures and that its traffic between two hosts should be delivered directly by WAN protocols.

2.4   The Common Object Request Broker Architecture (CORBA)

In the U.S. Army there are many computer platforms, which are running different applications, using CORBA to facilitate the communication of systems that are deployed on diverse platforms. It enables the collaboration between devices that are on different operating systems, programming languages, and computing hardware.

The CORBA standard brings forth a solution to some of the problems in achieving interoperability across platforms and applications in a Transmission Control Protocol TCP/IP based client-server network [15]. CORBA has several methods to achieve the interoperability on the Internet addressing what is needed for greater efficiency in using channels designated for communications. The role of the bit-packer is to transform the data from the CORBA message to a bit-packed message. The message is then presented to the receiver as a set of linked lists of records [16].

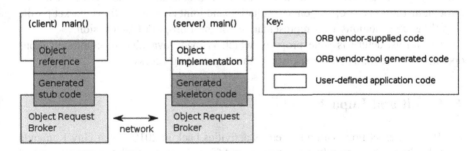

Fig. 1. Illustration of the auto generation of the infrastructure code from an interface defined using the CORBA interface definition language (IDL)

The implementation of a bit-efficient variable format messages and a description of how the generated code is used within the CORBA infrastructure can be observed in Fig. 1.

3 MCSI Involvement

The Ministry of Communications and Information Society (MCSI) in Romania has distributed in 2010 over 300 hotspots in public areas throughout the country [17]. The measure was intended to further the transition process to a modern, information-centric society, based on the increasing number of areas with free Internet access.

The Minister of Communications said that the institution he leads will present a study on the advantages and disadvantages of open-source programs. Valerian Vreme has plans to open-source software similar to those used by the local government of France. Local governments can use open-source systems (free and can be improved by users) in the near future, instead of those that require a license [18].

The RO-NET project consists of building a national broadband infrastructure in deprived areas, by using structural funds [19].

The Cisco Broadband Quality Research Study 2010, conducted by the Universities of Oxford and Oviedo, in terms of quality Internet connection, Romania is relatively well in this respect, ranking 10th in the world according to the report regarding the connection quality and the Internet access.

The Romanian Government launched the National Broadband Strategy in order to increase the penetration rate in households of the broadband connection. The broadband coverage remains limited, especially in rural areas among households and companies.

In 2009 the "Government strategy of developing broadband electronic communications in Romania for the period 2009–2015" was adopted. Starting from the provisions of this Strategy, correlated with those of the European Structural Funds Regulations and with the specific state aid, the Ministry of Communications and Information Society has developed a Model for Implementation of projects aimed at developing broadband infrastructure in disadvantaged areas.

The use of Structural Funds available for infrastructure development was decided after analyzing patterns of implementation of broadband infrastructure, achieved through institutional cooperation, consultation and joint communications market profile as well as consultations with representatives of the European Commission.

The infrastructure is state property which is made available to communications operators on a commercial basis, and without restricting access.

4 Result and Impact

The Basic Internet Foundation started its activities back in 2010, when Guy Kamanda needed help in developing Internet Access in Africa. A series of pilots were established in 2011, and the company worked together on a workshop with the University of Lisala in April 2012. The project Basic Internet access was the steppingstone of the infrastructure for free access to basic information via Internet.

Nowadays the foundation joined forces with the Norwegian Agency for Development Cooperation (NORAD) for the Vision 2030 improving their efficiency in achieving their main goal to ensure optimized content delivery for capacity-limited networks in low-developed countries [20].

In certain areas where it is almost impossible to provide Internet services, data can be sent through a bandwidth limited link. Some examples of such low-availability links are satellite links and congested mobile networks. Basic Internet provides solutions for optimizing the stream of information in such a way that a high amount of information can be provided despite the unfavorable conditions mentioned earlier.

The Basic Internet Core Network is the one responsible for the information optimization and its partners are the ones that make it possible.

Opera Mini is one of the best examples of a browser designed primarily for mobile phones, smartphones and personal digital assistants that can provide a maximum of information, even though it has limited capacity in the network [21].

A cost-effective Internet distribution worldwide is possible due to state of the art architectures that offer free basic access requiring 4.5 megabytes per user a month.

A high-bandwidth local distribution network represented by a server fully loaded with information freely available for everyone is presented in Fig. 2.

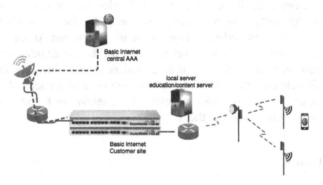

Fig. 2. The basic internet central AAA and the basic internet customer equipment

The Basic Internet foundation offers full business access through the sales of vouchers giving full access to the Internet, thus promoting individual development.

When we are talking about the distribution of the Basic Internet, we need to refer to the method of using two satellite modems: one that includes Router Board and the other that has an external one. The Router Boards are preconfigured with an IP address, so by connecting to the satellite the connection to the billing center at Kjeller is done automatically. In its complete form the configuration contains: a satellite dish, a satellite modem, a distribution network, and a Wi-Fi unit.

The Basic Internet software was developed by making integrations and by adapting certain devices to its needs. Considering the previous affirmation, the foundation decided to make the mobile networks possible with the use of the BRCK (pronounced "brick") [22]. The name was given because it has the shape similar to that of a brick and it helps people better relate to it as a necessity. The BRCK is a connectivity device that fit the needs of networking, where electricity and Internet connections are a big problem both in urban and rural areas. It is used as a backup generator for the Internet, but one of the important features is that the BRCK comes included with a backup battery. It also has an external omnidirectional antenna and a solar panel, helping it to adapt to the application areas.

Another option for having Internet access through mobile networks is by combining a USB modem and USB capable MikroTik router [23].

Following the principle of the Basic Internet of a low-bandwidth information provision, the focus is mainly on the applications specifically developed for distributing a large amount of collective information without high requirements, like Wikipedia and other information pages that can work with a minimum bandwidth.

An important development projects is the one referring to health applications that provide information based on the feedback given by the sensor or user. The main idea is to transmit the data about a person's health over the low-bandwidth link and to get reliable personalized information back to the user for treatment.

Referring to the business innovations the core idea is to foster business innovation in developing economies, by receiving up-to-date information about: customers, partners, markets and innovations that can be implemented.

Google Inc. dedicated its resources to the development of running wireless networks in emerging markets for connecting more people to the Internet [24]. The main areas targeted are the ones underdeveloped such as sub-Saharan Africa and Southeast Asia. The plan is for Google to develop the networks by teaming up with local telecommunications firms and equipment providers in the emerging markets. The contribution Google can make to these countries are on a larger scale than imagined, since the company could use airwaves reserved for television broadcasts as well as create business models to support them.

5 Conclusions

In this paper we have presented the development as well as the principles which the Basic Internet Foundation is based on. The core of the initiative is to help provide free Internet to underdeveloped areas with economic issues by using a cost efficient way of networking.

The main problem is convincing people to trust in this initiative. Since most of the people living in areas mentioned before don't see the benefits that come with such projects, the approach must be one of offering assistance and demonstrations, and not of imposing an idea without their acceptance.

Other initiatives, programs and companies that support the same ideas as well as their results are also presented and many solutions for future work envisioned for the purpose of life improvement were reviewed. The development of such programs will enable strong impact in many areas by making enhancements regarding: data transfer, health, economy, knowledge, business, entertainment and others.

Acknowledgments. The work has been funded by the Sectoral Operational Programme Human Resources Development 2007-2013 of the Ministry of European Funds through the Financial Agreement POSDRU/159/1.5/S/134398 and supported by UEFISCDI Romania under grants no. 20/2012 "Scalable Radio Transceiver for Instrumental Wireless Sensor Networks - SaRaT-IWSN", TELE-GREEN, NMSDMON, CarbaDetect and CommCenter projects, grant no. 262EU/2013 "eWALL" support project, grant no. 337E/2014 "Accelerate" project and by European Commission by FP7 IP project no. 610658/2013 "eWALL for Active Long Living - eWALL".

References

1. IPTO – Information Processing Techniques Office. In: Stewart, B., (ed.)The Living Internet, January 2000
2. RFC 1122, Requirements for Internet Hosts – Communication Layers, 1.1.2 Architectural Assumptions (1989)
3. The Open Market Internet Index. Treese.org. 1995-11-11. Accessed 15 June 2013
4. Huston, G.: APNIC, "Network Service Models and the Internet". Internet Protoc. J. 16(2), (2013)
5. Feenberg, A.: Building a global network: the WBSI experience. In: Harasim, L. (ed.) Global Networks: Computers and International Communication, pp. 186–197. The MIT Press, (1993)
6. Burch, B.: Nextel co-founders' firm buys back push-to-talk spectrum from sprint. Kansas City Bus. J. (2014)
7. Nurudeen, N.A.: Virtual fibre solutions will enhance connectivity, says WaveTek, The Nation Publication For Monday 1 June 2015
8. Liu, Y., Wu, J., Wu, Q.: Recent progress in the study of the next generation Internet in China. Philos. Trans. R. Soc. A (2015)
9. Duan, L., Huang, J., Walrand, J.: Economic analysis of 4G network upgrade. In: Proceedings of the IEEE INFOCOM, pp. 1070–1078 (2013)
10. Song, L., Zhao, C., Zheng, C.: Analysis and optimization model of cognitive wireless mesh networks. In: Proceedings of the International Conference on Industrial Control and Electronics Engineering (ICICEE 2012), pp. 1426–1429, August 2012
11. Ohatkar, S.N., Bormane, D.S.: Channel allocation technique with genetic algorithm for interference reduction in cellular network. In: (INDICON 2013), pp. 1–6, December 2013
12. Nastic, S., Sehic, S., Vogler, M., Truong, H.L., Dustdar, S.: PatRICIA—a novel programming model for IoT applications on cloud platforms. In: Proceedings of the 2013 IEEE 6th International Conference on Service-Oriented Computing and Applications (SOCA 2013), pp. 53–60, December 2013
13. Bourguiba, M., Haddadou, K., Korbi, I.E., Pujolle, G.: Improving network I/O virtualization for cloud computing. IEEE Trans. Parallel Distrib. Syst. 25(3), 673–681 (2014)
14. Deering, S., Hinden, R.: Internet Protocol, Version 6 (IPv6) Specification. Internet RFC 2460, December 1998
15. Stowers, J., Westby-Gibson, D.; Marsic, I.: Interoperability over low data rate channels using CORBA. In: MILCOM 97 Proceedings, vol. 1, no., pp. 455–459, 2–5 November 1997
16. Blow, J.: Packing Integers, The Inner Product, May 2002
17. Sandu, L.: Poftiți la internet gratuit!, Market Watch, [Nr. 116], 01 Iulie 2009
18. Vântu, R.: Adevarul, Ministrul Comunicatiilor: Softurile gratuite pot fi implementate, 16 November 2010

19. Oprea, M., de Europa, B.: Internet pentru 400.000 de români, cu bani europeni, Nr. 54, p. 4, November 2014
20. Maalim, M.I.: Kenya's vision for an equitable, rights-based health system. Africa Policy J. (2014)
21. Duncan, G.: (24 January 2006). Opera Mini Officially Brings Web to Mobiles. Digital Trends News, 18 October 2007
22. Vogt, H.: Africa's challenges are tech startups' opportunities. Wall Street J. (2014)
23. Langobardi, F.: BoulSat Project: Radio network implementation by low cost technology, Master's Thesis, Politecnico di Torino, p. 78 (2007)
24. Efrati, A.: Google to fund, develop wireless networks in emerging markets. Wall Street J. (2013)

From Global Bellies to Global Minds: The Bread Platform for Geo-Cultural Integration

Remo Pareschi[1(✉)] and Maria Felicia Santilli[2]

[1] Department of Bioscience and Territory, University of Molise, Pesche, IS, Italy
remo.pareschi@unimol.it
[2] Bread Team Leader, Cultural Anthropologist, Rome, Italy
mariafsantilli@gmail.com

Abstract. As demonstrated by numerous ethno-anthropological studies, food can be a powerful basis for the integration of different ethnic groups and populations. The Bread project uses this integration capability, rooted in the convivial atmosphere of the experience of eating together, to address the pressing issue of the integration of migrant communities and host communities in the face of the recent migration flows that cross the world and that in Mediterranean Europe find one of their focal hubs. As part of the Bread philosophy, food is the Trojan horse for full-spectrum cultural integration, so we can actually say that the goal is to go from "global bellies" to "global minds". To this end, a platform was developed that merge this ancestral capacity of food with the potential offered by the Internet, Web 2.0 and technologies and advanced solutions for social networking and for the dynamic acquisition and sharing of content. But Bread is a concept replicable on a global scale as well as adaptable to local needs and features, and the implementation referred to here is indeed adapted to the specific context of the city of Rome.

Keywords: Geo-cultural integration · Social networks · Blogs · Content analysis · Management

1 Introduction

All human history can be viewed as an effort of mankind towards globalization, and this in turn has triggered various efforts of integration such as: the integration of trade routes through which goods can travel; the integration of roads on which armies can march; the integration of local institutions like provinces and regions into larger institutions like national states, empires and federations; the international integration of local financial regulations, so as to extend the scope of financial and economic exchanges. Migration flows have been in the past and are in the present, and everything suggests they will continue to be in the future, one major factor of ethnic-cultural integration. Unlike other cases of integration, they happen as a bottom-up spontaneous

Bread project received financial support from the European Commission, via the FI-PPP Project ICT-632868 FI-ADOPT Call 1.

© Institute for Computer Sciences, Social Informatics and Telecommunications Engineering 2015
V. Atanasovski, L.-G. Alberto (Eds.): Fabulous 2015, LNICST 159, pp. 263–269, 2015.
DOI: 10.1007/978-3-319-27072-2_34

action rather than through top-down planning, and can be considered both an effect and a cause of globalization. Like all unplanned activities involving a multiplicity of actors with mostly contrasting interests, they bring with them a considerable potential for conflict, and in the past have been the basis for a series of momentous changes occurring in a manner anything but painless. The conditions for epochal migration are being repeated now, mainly in consequence of two combined factors: the north / south geopolitical dichotomy, such as Central / Northern America and South / North of the Mediterranean sea; and the global mobility of diverse communities, made possible by globalization as such and propelled by a variety of reasons like seizing opportunities, economic improvement, political exodus etc. These more recent migrations mostly occur in a peaceful manner, and in no way can be considered as hostile. Thus, facilitating the integration processes that follow them is crucial in order to ensure that they are immediately bearers of economic prosperity and social harmony, both for the host population and for the new comers [1, 2]. This is the purpose of the "Bread" project, that aims to integrate visitors and emigrants by combining a very old form of dialogue and contact between people, namely the sharing of the food experience as a primary form of conviviality, [3, 4]with the very latest possibilities offered by the social networks and the blogosphere.

The idea behind Bread is to define a concept that can be implemented and rooted in specific local/urban contexts, with their own migrant and hosting communities. Each implementation of Bread defines its own ecosystem, and this will be in turn open to federate with other instances of Bread in a broader ecosystem. The first implementation of Bread, used here as a case study, is being carried out in the territory of the city of Rome, which is a particularly stimulating one for several evident reasons. Rome, capital of Italy, and formerly of the Roman Empire, the seat of the Vatican, is one of the largest cities of Mediterranean Europe, whose age-old cultural heritage includes a rich culinary tradition. It is also receptacle of a wide, varied and layered migrant community, which carries its own ethnic and cultural traditions, including the culinary ones, that often are also a primary source of income [5, 6]. In this context Bread, that started operations in April 2015, uses food as a "Trojan horse" to facilitate integration and mutual understanding, coherently with the assumption that integration is not a one-way process (migrant-> host) but mutual (migrant <-> hosting) [7]. The potential pool of users and the consequent potential for integration is enormous: just in Rome, there are around 200 communities of migrants that cover nearly the whole range of nationalities. Migrants registered to the city registry are 381.101 (52.4% are female) and represent the 13,1 % of the total residents (as at January 2013). This percentage is steadily increasing and does not take into account a significant number of illegal migrants.

Thus the Bread concept addresses in a simple and effective way a complex reality, and requires the support of an adequate IT architecture for its implementation, which involves the use of systems of creation, management, classification and recommendation of content, as well as of geo-referenced management of the points of interest involved (which can be either in the city of residence, ie in this case Roma, or in the territories of origin of migrants), as well as of social networking and e-commerce. The goal of this article is to describe the adopted criteria of design and use of the current Bread implementation, and is for the rest structured as follows. Section 2 describes the socio-cultural context of use of the Bread implementation in Rome. Section 3 describes the Bread architecture and the various components it relies on, and exemplifies typical cases of use focused on the aspect of dynamic recommendation of content aimed at fostering geo-cultural integration. Section 4 concludes the article.

2 The User Basis for BREAD in Rome

Who will be the Bread users in Rome then? From the point of view of migrants, they consist primarily of those who work in catering and restaurants, and those who work in families. Those who work in restaurants are typically from the first and second generations, such as the Chinese (the wealthiest, and the most present in the area as owners of restaurants and bars) and the North Africans (mostly Egyptians for pizzerias), but also South Americans for meeting places and clubs. What do they find in Bread? A place where to advertise their restaurants and shops, take reservations, advertise events, and where to learn more about our eating habits (ie pizza courses for the Egyptians). Bread will thus be a place where they can raise awareness of their idea of cuisine and culture, and where there is space to exchange experiences. Those who work in families are for the most part Filipinos and east Europeans, especially in the first generation, and mainly women, employed as domestics, caregivers or nannies. What do they find in Bread? A place where they can learn about our idea of cuisine, useful so as to find out how and what to cook in a typical Italian family, to the children, to the elderly. A place where to find simple recipes, video clarifiers and "tips" on where you buy better. Bread will thus be a useful ally, a tool to not make mistakes, to fit best in a household environment. And they too will find a space where to exchange experiences. The Italian user can be anyone. In virtue of this mutual process the Italian will learn more about the culture of migrants by going through their recipes and getting access to events and news. For instance, from Chinese caramelized pork ribs one can get an idea about Chinese food aversions and about Chinese holidays, can link to those restaurants that prepare them better, and perhaps plan a travel to China, and so on.

3 The Bread Architecture

In the definition of an architecture to fulfil the objectives of BREAD we have therefore kept in view the following three main requirements:

(a) the specific theme of food requires the creation and constant feeding of dedicated content, of informative and educational nature, by a team of editors and journalists with expertise in the field;
(b) at the same time, the main aim should be pursued through the routing and the facilitation of bottom-up participation so as to promote the integration process through the development of an inter-ethnic community of hosts and migrants;
(c) to be fully effective, such a process of integration must go beyond the initial context of food, and cover the wider spectrum of the cultures of origin of hosts and migrants.

In order to fulfill the indications above, Bread is built from one main component, given by a social network. The social network itself is partitioned in two areas. One area is assigned to registered users in order to fill it with their content. Thus each user has a profile page which she can update freely. The other area corresponds to the news feed, which each user receives arranged according to her own preferences by exploiting a powerful methodology for the classification and recommendation of contents. The news feed not only contains user-generated content but also content generated by the editorial team of Bread through a structured process of content generation, covering a variety of themes that appear relevant for the Bread user communities. For the purpose of best conveying to users such wealth of contents the news feed is partitioned according to categories and topic areas, in the style of a blog. Content generated by the editorial team is manually inserted into the appropriate topic areas, while user generated content is assigned in a semi-automated fashion to topic areas through the use of a classification engine. Furthermore, a Web crawler constantly collects and updates also contents residing outside of Bread that nevertheless may be relevant for Bread users, particularly those contents that reach from food into wider domains and thus contribute crucially to the objective of geo-cultural integration.

In this way the Bread architecture encompasses in a simple and effective way three successful paradigms of Web 2.0, namely social networks, blogs and content crawling. Further elements that support an even more immersive and effective user experience are geo-referenced searches through points-of-interest and augmented reality.

This architecture has been implemented by leveraging a number of enabling components (enablers), some of which were developed in-house, such as the Web crawler, while others were taken and adapted from the open-source world on the basis of such criteria as their established reliability and quality, as well as their adaptability to the methodologies specifically defined and adopted by the development team of Bread. The support for journalistic content creation is given by Wordpress www.wordpress. org, the content management system that has become the standard infrastructure in the management of blogs. The enablers for the management, respectively, of the participants in the Social Network, of the points-of-interest (POIs) and of the applications of augmented reality were taken from the Fiware software ecosystem www.fiware.org, which provides thus one of the main backbones for the platform.

The aspect of classification and recommendation of content plays a crucial role in Bread, both for the contents on food, which are instrumental in the bootstrapping of an inter-ethnic community, and for additional related contents, which are exploited to step further into the process of geo-cultural integration. The choice of technology to deploy and manage this kind of extended content access is given by the Probabilistic Topic Models (PTMs) [8]. This choice is justified by a variety of reasons, among which the following are particularly relevant: (i) PTM algorithms have gone through a period of more than 10 years of honing and tuning, that allowed to evaluate and maximize their power, flexibility and robustness in the analysis and classification of large amounts of textual data; (ii) furthermore, they are based on unsupervised learning, which provides for maximal automation in the execution of the analysis and classification tasks, but can also be bent to supervised or semi-supervised modes so as to fit existing classification structures; (iii) there is an excellent open-source software written in Java, and known as Mallet http://mallet.cs.umass.edu/, which makes feasible a quick and cheap transfer of this technology into the application context; (iv) the Bread team has given original contributions in the definition of information retrieval methods based on PTM and applicable to real cases, and has experience in the use for this purpose of Mallet. Therefore Mallet has been chosen as the enabler for this aspect of the architecture. Techniques illustrated in [9] and [10] are used to classify contents into topics, to track "hot topics" and to recommend contents either because they share topics or because they are related through probabilistic transitions. As pointed out in [11], the dichotomy "topic sharing versus probabilistic transitions" among content objects can be thought as an information-theoretic reconstruction of the well-known distinction from social sciences [12] between "strong links" (links within one's inner circle) and "weak links" (links that extend beyond one's inner circle, and thus open up new social perspectives), which fits itself well with Bread's philosophy of initial integration around food, and then of further expansion of such integration through broader themes. Indeed, in this way, items are recommended not only within the initial domain (in this case, food), but also in additional domains that, albeit related, are totally independent, so as to improve and expand the exploration prospects of the user experience. This further feature, which is needed for the specific objectives of geo-cultural integration, provides a significant and original extension of the state of the art in the use of topic models for the purpose of implementation of recommendation systems (for example, with respect to the methodologies illustrated in [13]).

Figure 1 provides a view of the Bread architecture from the standpoint of content flows, while Figs. 2 and 3 depict two cases of content recommendation, the first one within the boundary of food and the second one going beyond such boundary by stepping into the domain of wider interests.

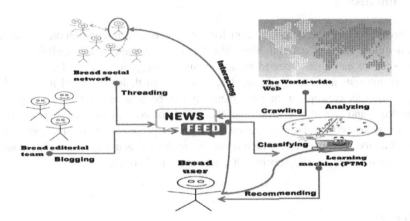

Fig. 1. Content flows in the Bread architecture

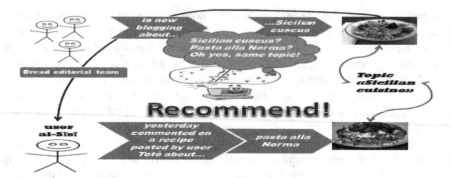

Fig. 2. Recommending about food

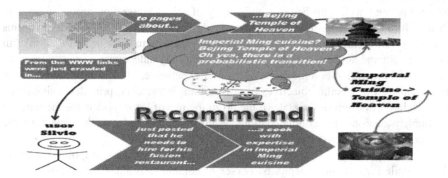

Fig. 3. Recommending about culture

4 Conclusion

We have described the Bread concept for the geo-cultural integration among migrant communities and host communities, which exploits the ancestral conviviality of the experience of eating in order to create an initial integration on the basis of mutual culinary interests and then make the leap towards full-fledged cultural integration. In support of this concept, a specific platform has been developed supporting social networking and dynamic sharing and acquisition of content for the purposes of the Bread way to geo-cultural integration. The prototype phase of this platform has as scope the city of Rome, after which it may be replicated and applied in other contexts with similar, albeit locally specific, characteristics and issues.

References

1. Fondazione Leone Moressa: Rapporto annuale sull'Economia dell'Immigrazione 2014. La forza lavoro degli stranieri, esclusione o integrazione? Il Mulino, Bologna (2014)

2. Predidenza del Consiglio dei Ministri, Dipartimento delle pari opportunità, ISTAT, Dipartimento per le statistiche socilai ed ambientali: I migranti visti dai cittadini (2011)
3. Fox, R.: Food and Eating: an Anthropological Perspective (2003)
4. Mintzl, S., Du Bois, C.: The anthropology of food and eating. Annu. Rev. Anthropol. **31**, 99–119 (2002)
5. Caritas di Roma, Roma Capitale, Provincia di Roma e Regione Lazio: Osservatorio Romano sulle Migrazioni 2014, Roma (2014)
6. Ciurlo, A.: La situazione degli stranieri a Roma. La percezione all'interno delle comunità cattoliche di origine immigrata. In: Le condizioni di vita e di lavoro degli immigrati nell'area romana. Indagine campionaria e approfondimenti tematici. Idos, Roma, pp. 105–116 (2008)
7. Fondazione Leone Moressa: L'influsso della cucina etnica sulle abitudini alimentari degli italiani (2010)
8. Blei, D.: Probabilistic topic models. Commun. ACM **55**(4), 77–84 (2012)
9. Rossetti, M., Pareschi, R., Stella, F., Arcelli, F.: Integrating concepts and knowledge in large content networks. New Gener. Comput. **32**(3–4), 309–330 (2014)
10. Pareschi, R., Rossetti, M., Stella, F.: Tracking hot topics for the monitoring of open-world processes. In: SIMPDA (2014)
11. Pareschi, R., Arcelli Fontana, F.: Information-driven network analysis: evolving the "complex networks" paradigm. Mind Soc. 1–13 (2015). doi:10.1007/s11299-015-0172-1, https://www.researchgate.net/publication/280036227_Information-driven_network_analysis_evolving_the_complex_networks_paradigm?fulltextDi
12. Granovetter, M.: The strength of weakl ties. Am. J. Sociol. **78**(6), 1360–1380 (1973)
13. Wang, C., Blei, D.: Collaborative topic modeling for recommending scientific articles. In : KDD, pp. 448–456 (2011)

IoT to Enhance Understanding of Cultural Heritage: Fedro Authoring Platform, Artworks Telling Their Fables

Fiammetta Marulli[✉]

Department of Electrical Engineering and Information Technologies,
University of Naples Federico II, Naples, Italy
fiammetta.marulli@unina.it

Abstract. Cultural Heritage has got great importance in recent years, in order to preserve countries history and traditions and to support social and economic improvements. Typical IoT smart technologies represent an effective mean to support understanding of Cultural Heritage, by their capability to involve different users and to catch their explicit and implicit preferences, behaviors and contributions. This paper presents FEDRO, an authoring platform, as part of the intelligent infrastructures developed in DATABENC to support a cultural exhibition of "talking" sculptures held in the Southern Italy, in 2015. FEDRO aims to automatically generate textual and users profiled artworks biographies, employed to feed a smart app for guiding visitors during the exhibition. A preliminary experimentation revealed a tangible improvement in the users' experience appreciation during the visit. Quality estimations of generated output were also computed exploiting users' feedbacks, collected through a manual questionnaire, subscribed at the end of their visit.

Keywords: Internet of things · Authoring systems · Text analysis · Semantic web · Domain ontology · Cultural heritage · Natural language generation

1 Introduction and Motivating Example

Internet of Things (IoT) represents an effective mean to support understanding of Cultural Heritage (CH), by enhancing people's awareness about its effective value. Smart cultural sites are a meaningful applications of IoT into CH, aiming to involve visitors with more amazing and personalized experiences in living culture. "Talking" museums exploit a novel approach in the story telling of an art exhibition. More generally, cultural objects and sites (sculptures, drawings, buildings, etc.) are enabled to tell visitors about their stories, when supported by intelligent infrastructures.

In this scenario, a not trivial and not yet deeply investigated issue concerns the selection and organization of knowledge delivered to users. IoT enables objects to communicate each others, but what they should be able to tell and how they could communicate with their human interlocutors should not be taken for granted.

Users, differencing by cultural and social background, by age and sensitivity, have to be approached in different ways, in order to reach an effective engagement with the

V. Atanasovski, L.-G. Alberto (Eds.): Fabulous 2015, LNICST 159, pp. 270–276, 2015.
DOI: 10.1007/978-3-319-27072-2_35

context they are experimenting. A first effort in this direction could be the proposal of the same contents (artworks biographies) in different appearances.

The proposed FEDRO platform (early demo version at http://www.ilbellooilvero.it/FEDRO) is currently tailored to generate two different types of profiled textual artworks biographies, respectively, for generic or "not specialist" users (an occasional tourist, e.g.) and schoolchildren. In the last case, biographies are more amazing; they are shaped as detailed short fables. Platform name comes from Phaedrus, the most famous fables writer from ancient Latin age.

The adopted approach promises to be scalable and flexible enough to support extensions for other types of users. In this perspective, new lexical ontologies have to be built and integrated in the system. For a better characterization of different users, the contribution of folksonomies is remarkable. They consist in taxonomy of terms generated by collecting users' annotations on multimedia cultural objects during their activities in the web. Knowledge discovery and integration services of not structured implicit and explicit contributions (users' comments, descriptions and any digital trace incoming from Social Networks and User Content Generation Communities (e.g., Wiki Systems)) support the authoring platform.

Finally, users profiled textual artworks descriptions are employed to feed a mobile app, as part of an IoT smart infrastructure, supporting users during an actual "talking" sculpture exhibition. Artworks, provided with smart processing board, interact with their human visitors, by telling their own stories according to the specific type of user.

2 Related Works

Most contributions concerning systems and applications supporting CH, mainly focus on technological and infrastructural issues and contents recommendation strategies. The authors of [1] proposed a network based ticket reservation system which is a localization-based smartphone application with augmented reality.

In [2], a Personalized Location-based Recommender System provides personalized tourism information to its users. According to [3] exchanged data can be opportunely exploited by a set of applications in order to make "smart" systems. Social network is a set of Smart Spaces, each needing particular IoT infrastructures and services to transform the physical spaces into useful smart environments. In [4], authors present the design of an IoT based system infrastructure to support a "talking" museum. They focused on the development of a multi-tier system made of a back end server application for multimedia contents storage and a front-end smart App, to deliver recommended contents according to users profiles and location based services. In [5], authors improve the system described in [4], proposing a semantic enrichment of the cultural contents system, by exploiting Social Networks as further knowledge source.

In [6], a perspective on the support of Artificial Intelligence to CH is given, introducing an ontology based approach to improve the effectiveness of recommendation systems. In [7], folksonomies are employed as the base of a strategy to enhance content based filtering techniques of multimedia objects, by the exploitation of semantic annotation (tags) released by users on cultural digital objects during their web navigation. Users profiles generation, based on YAGO ontology is investigated in [8, 9].

In [10, 11] top level information retrieval, text analysis strategies and sense disambiguation strategies are discussed. A survey investigating some of the most relevant approaches in the areas of automatic text summarization is presented in [12].

Natural Language Generation (NLG) Systems, applied in CH domain, are investigated in [13]. They are employed in order to build structured textual descriptions, based on cultural objects ontologies as lexical vocabulary and documents plan to establish the phrasing structures. The authors propose Natural OWL [20], an effective working implementation of a NLG engine, able to automatically generate simpler or more complex textual descriptions in two different languages, English or Greek. System feeds with a lexical ontology, a micro-plan for text structure and users' profile information. Entities vocabularies are fixed for all type of users and the profiling information are used to modify some text features, as length. So, the general appearance of the textual description keeps quite unchanged but such a system represents an example of authoring system in the CH domain.

3   System Processing Flow and Architecture

A general overview of FEDRO platform architecture and processing flow is shown in Fig. 1. Its users are mainly domain experts, enabled to to fill in original complex artworks textual descriptions (documents corpora) by a friendly GUI. They can select the target audience and language (currently, English and Italian) and new profiled descriptions are provided as output. Additional process inputs are users' profiles tables, lexical dictionaries and domain ontologies, user generated terms taxonomies (folksonomies), sentences taxonomies (containing the phrasal structures and language rules needed during the customized text generation step).

At a glance, the processing flow is composed of the following four steps:

1. *Text Analysis*: Typical text analysis and summarization techniques are applied to input documents corpora; terms and sentences are extracted and disambiguated by the support of lexical and domain ontologies The output is represented by lists of relevant terms and sentences.
2. *Semantic Enhancement*: Lists of terms and sentences are semantically enriched and expanded. Terms are annotated by a detailed description and a list of synonymous, each one provided with a label indicating the most appropriate lexical forms for each type of user. Domain ontologies (for specialist terms), Linked Open Resource Archives and sentences taxonomies are employed to select new simplified sentences, according to semantic similarity criteria.
3. *User Profile Based Elements Tailoring*: Annotated terms and sentences are tailored according to users' profiles. When a user's profile is selected, terms and annotations matching the label profile are selected. Prebuilt users folksonomies, when available, are consulted to refine terms and sentences with those ones more familiar to user's class.
4. *Natural Language Text Generation*: The filtered list of terms (user's vocabulary) and sentences (micro-plan text structure) are provided as ontologies to the NLG engine, finally producing the expected textual description, in the selected language.

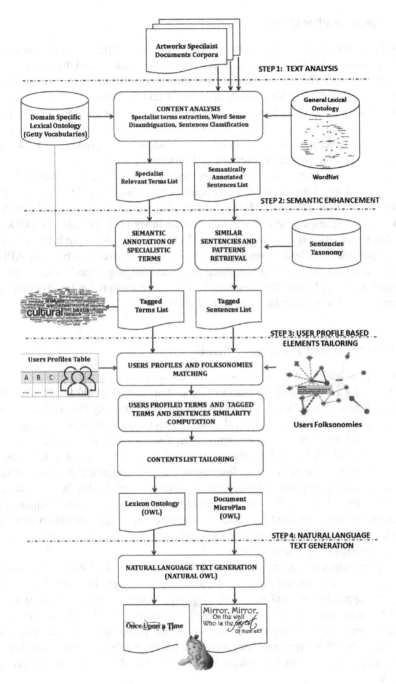

Fig. 1. FEDRO system general architecture and processing flow.

3.1   Implementation Details

FEDRO platform was basically implemented in Java technology, according to a Model View Controller (MVC) architectural pattern. It is characterized by a layered and multi-tier structure. The View Layer is represented by a friendly web user interface for filling in complex descriptions and desired target text features.

The Control layer is a collection of Java servlets, involved in the dispatching and coordination phases of requests among Model modules. The Model layer, is the core of the authoring system consisting in a set of services, responsible for workflow orchestration of data source interactions and processing tasks.

Text analysis is performed by a Python module implemented by the NLTK [14] framework and integrated with Java components by Jython API [15]. As large lexical databases, WordNet [16] and MultiWordNet [17] were employed for English and Italian languages, respectively. The Getty Vocabularies [18], available as LOD, were integrated as specific art domain ontology. Users folksonomies were integrated in the aspect of profiled users lexical ontologies. Ontologies were managed by using API Jena [19]. To generate new textual descriptions in natural language, the Natural OWL [20] framework was employed. This system offers a native support for English and Greek languages. So, it was extended to support Italian language.

3.2   Case Study and Preliminary Results

In Table 1, left and right columns show, respectively, the original complex text, provided by domain expert and the platform generated fable description. Because of the lack of a standard ideal model of output, initially, the similarity between segments of text was measured by applying lexical matching techniques, good for finding semantically identical matches. Basing on experience, a semantic compliance threshold was set to a value of 85 %. A test plan, performed on a 150 generated texts sample, produced a recall value of $\sim$ 70 %. Interesting but less unbiased indications about the effectiveness of the proposed approach, were provided by users' feedback at the end of their visit in the "Il Bello o il Vero" (http://www.ilbellooilvero.it) exhibition.Over than 200 sculptures were exhibited for about 7 months; different schoolchildren visits were scheduled in 15 different days, and each day a different group of 10 artworks fables was proposed by exploiting a mobile app.

An appreciation questionnaire was submitted at the end of the visits, asking to assign a quality score in the range 1– 4 (very much, enough, low, absolutely not) to specify the appreciation level in the visiting experience. Some of measured features were the comprehension and recording level, the clarity and the pleasantness of the proposed narrations. An overall improvement in the comprehension and appreciation level in the exhibition experience was recorded, but more robust and unbiased tests and metrics have to be performed to assess and improve the effectiveness of the proposed approach.

Table 1. A comparison between input text and output simplified textual descriptions.

Input: Technical description (Domain Expert)	Output: Simplified fable description (Schoolchildren)
Carlotta D'Asburgo A Miramare is a model in gypsum and it was realized around 1914 by the sculptor Francesco Jerace. He was born in Polistena in 1853 and he died in Napoli in 1937. It comes from the collezione privata. The plaster model by Francesco Jerace represents The Empress of Mexico Charlotte of Habsburg in Miramare, where the marble was exhibited for the first time in 1999 at the Museo Civico di Castelnuovo. Charlotte is shown seated in front of the castle of Miramare in Trieste, with an eye toward the sea in expectation of the return of melancholy consort Maximilian of Hapsburg. Daughter of Leopold of Belgium, becomes, after the shooting of her husband, the heroine of a nineteenth-century romantic tradition of the last chapter.	Once upon a time, in a country named Italy, there was a man, whose name was Francesco Jerace. This man worked as a sculptor. A sculptor is an artist who is very able in working stones in beautiful shapes. What you are now looking at is named "Carlotta D'Asburgo" Empress of Mexico, portraited when she looked out the balcony of her castle of Miramare, in Trieste, waiting for the return of her husband. This sculpture was made in 1914, in white gypsum and it is stored in another famous Castle, in Naples, in the Southern Italy. This castle is used as a museum. Its name is "Civic Museum of Castelnuovo", built in 1266. Local people call it as Maschio Angioino, from the name of French King Carlo d'Angiò, dominating Southern Italy about in XIII century.

4   Conclusions and Future Work

In this paper an authoring platform supporting IoT smart applications in the CH domain was introduced. Most valuable contribution of this work should be identified in the novel proposed approach, mashing up top level information retrieval and text analysis strategies, with semantic processes, involving lexical and domain ontologies and users generated contents (by UGC systems).

The final aim is to automatically generate customized artworks descriptions for different type of users, feeding smart IoT cultural applications. Approaching people in a right and customized way could significantly enhance people's awareness about the effective value of their territorial richness and the related social and economic opportunities. In this perspective, from current literature, no other contributions are strongly focused on this issue or implement similar approaches for the same aim.

A further novelty aspect is the communication strategy, based on the choice to generate simplified descriptions in the shape of fables, in order to make culture and art environment more charming for children audiences. Current version of the platform is able to generate two different types of profiled textual artworks biographies (general descriptions and short fables). The adopted approach in the platform design promises to be scalable and flexible enough to support extensions for other types of users. New and different lexical ontologies can be built and easily integrated in the system.

As future work, an interesting possibility is the exploitation of different top level text analysis and semantic based strategies and interactive users experiences and evaluations, to improve the quality of generated textual descriptions. Finally, a related open issue, aim of future investigations, is the absence of a standard human or automatic evaluation metrics to establish a text quality baseline.

References

1. Kang, S.K., Kang, H.K., Kim, J.E., Lee, H., Lee, J.B.: A study on the mobile communication network with smart phone for building of location based real time reservation system. IJMUE 7(2), 17–36 (2012)
2. Husain, W., Dih, L.Y.: A framework of a personalized location-based traveler recommendation system in mobile application. Int. J. Multimedia Ubiqui. Eng. 7(3), 11–18 (2012)
3. Amato, F., Chianese, A., Moscato, V., Picariello, A., Sperli, G.: SNOPS: a smart environment for cultural heritage applications. In: Proceedings of the 12th International Workshop on Web Information and Data Management, pp. 49–56 (2012)
4. Chianese, A., Marulli, F., Moscato, V., Piccialli, F.: SmARTweet: A Location-based smart application for Exhibits and Museums. In: Workshop on Cultural Information Systems (CIS2013), collocated with: The 9th International Conference on Signal Image Technology & Internet Based Systems, Kyoto, Japan, 2–5 December 2013
5. Chianese, A., Marulli, F., Piccialli, F., Valente, I.: A novel challenge into multimedia cultural heritage: an integrated approach to support cultural information enrichment. In: Proceedings of 9th International Conference on Signal Image Technology & Internet Based Systems, Kyoto, Japan, 2–5 December 2013
6. Bordoni, L., Ardissono, L., Barceló, J.A., Chella, A., de Gemmis, M., Gena, C., Iaquinta, L., Lops, P., Mele, F., Musto, C., Narducci, F., Semeraro, G., Sorgente, A.: The contribution of AI to enhance understanding of cultural heritage. Intelligenza Artificiale 7(2), 101–112 (2013)
7. Semeraro, G., Lops, P., De Gemmis, M., Musto, C., Narducci, F.: A folksonomy-based recommender system for personalized access to digital artworks. JOCCH 5(3), 11–34 (2012)
8. Pasi, G.: Web Search and Behavior. In: IEEE Intelligent Systems, Trends & Controversies, pp. 14–16 (2014)
9. Calegari, S., Pasi, G.: Personal Ontologies: Generation of user profiles based on the YAGO Ontology. Inf. Process. Manage. 49(3), 640–658 (2013). Elsevier Science
10. Basile, P., de Gemmis, M., Lops, P., Semeraro, G.: A Hybrid strategy for italian word sense disambiguation. In: IRCDL 2009, pp. 108–119 (2009)
11. Gentile, A.L., Basile, P., Semeraro, G.: WibNED wikipedia based named entity disambiguation. In: IRCDL 2009, pp. 51–59 (2009)
12. Nenkova, A., McKeown, K.: A survey of text summarization techniques. In: Aggarwal, C. C., Zhai, C.X. (eds.) Mining Text Data, pp. 43–76. Springer, Heidelberg (2012)
13. Androutsopoulos, I., Lampouras, G., Galanis, D.: Generating natural language descriptions from OWL ontologies: the NaturalOWL system. J. Artif. Intell. Res. 48(1), 671–715 (2013)
14. Natural Language Toolkit. http://www.nltk.org/
15. Jython: Python for the Java Platform. http://www.jython.org/
16. WordNet, a lexical database for English. https://wordnet.princeton.edu/
17. MultiWordNet. http://multiwordnet.fbk.eu/
18. Getty Vocabularies. http://www.getty.edu/research/tools/
19. Apache JENA. https://jena.apache.org/
20. Galanis, D., Karakatsiotis, Androutsopoulos, G.: How to install NaturalOWL (2008)

Estimation of Sparse Time Dispersive SIMO Channels with Common Support in Pilot Aided OFDM Systems Using Atomic Norm

Slavche Pejoski$^{(\boxtimes)}$ and Venceslav Kafedziski

Faculty of Electrical Engineering and Information Technologies,
University Saints Cyril and Methodious Skopje, Skopje, Republic of Macedonia
{slavchep,kafedzi}@feit.ukim.edu.mk

Abstract. We consider the problem of estimation of sparse time dispersive channels in pilot aided OFDM systems on Single Input Multiple Output (SIMO) channels, i.e. with a single transmit and multiple receive antennas. In such systems the channels are inherently continuous-time and sparse, and there is a common support of the channel coefficients of channels associated with different antennas, resulting from the same scatterer. To exploit these properties, we propose a new channel estimation algorithm that combines the atomic norm minimization of the Multiple Measurement Vector (MMV) model, the MUSIC and the least squares (LS) methods. The atomic norm minimization of the MMV model allows to exploit the common support assumption and the continuous-time nature of the channels, MUSIC allows for simple joint estimation of the delays corresponding to the same scatterer, and LS allows for estimation of the path gains. To evaluate the proposed algorithm, we compare its performance with the case when the common support assumption is not used.

Keywords: Channel estimation · Joint atomic norm minimization · SIMO channel · Pilot aided OFDM

1 Introduction

Channel estimation is essential in contemporary communication systems. Many of these systems are OFDM based and use pilot subcarriers for channel estimation. Additionally, most systems are designed to work with multiple antennas at the receive end. Here we consider such systems in a scenario where the channels between the transmit and the receive antennas are time dispersive and sparse in the sense that there are few strong channel paths that are resolvable. With the introduction of compressed sensing (CS), sparse channels have received significant attention [1–4], but CS, in its ordinary form, is not well suited for channel estimation since the delays of different paths can be arbitrary within a certain range (due to the channel continuous-time nature) and CS requires the delays to be on a predefined grid of delays. The recent framework of atomic norm

© Institute for Computer Sciences, Social Informatics and Telecommunications Engineering 2015
V. Atanasovski, L.-G. Alberto (Eds.): Fabulous 2015, LNICST 159, pp. 277–284, 2015.
DOI: 10.1007/978-3-319-27072-2_36

minimization [5,6] allows for estimation of sparse quantities not falling on a pre-defined grid. In [7], we used this framework to propose an algorithm for channel estimation of sparse time dispersive channel in pilot aided OFDM system with single antennas at both the transmit and receive ends. Here we extend the algorithm to the SIMO case. It has been shown in [8,9] that when the signal to noise ratio is not too high, the delays of the paths corresponding to the same scatterer, received on different receive antennas, are not clearly distinguishable and can be treated as being the same. This leads to the common support assumption of the coefficients in the channel impulse responses, which we exploit to jointly estimate the delays corresponding to the same scatterer, by modifying the algorithm from [7]. In fact, we replace the atomic norm minimization from [7] with the atomic norm minimization for the Multiple Measurement Vector (MMV) model [10,11]. The algorithms presented in [8,9] require that the pilot subcarriers are equidistant, and in the proposed algorithm we place them at random positions [7], resulting in the ordinary CS subsampling.

The novelty of this paper comes from introducing the atomic norm minimization in the estimation of sparse time dispersive channels with common support in pilot aided OFDM SIMO systems.

The paper is organized as follows. In Sect. 2 we describe the OFDM channel estimation problem in time dispersive SIMO channels, its connection to the atomic norm minimization of the MMV model and the new algorithm. In Sect. 3 we show simulation results. Section 4 concludes the paper.

2   Problem and Algorithm Description

We investigate an OFDM system with a single transmit antenna and N_r receive antennas. The system uses N subcarriers to transmit pilot or data symbols. The OFDM signal between the transmit antenna and the r-th receive antenna is sent through a time dispersive channel whose baseband channel impulse response, when I specular (point) scatterers are present, during a single frame transmission (assuming a block fading model), is [2,4]:

$$h_r(\tau) = \sum_{i=0}^{I-1} h_{r,i}\delta(\tau - \tau_{r,i}) \qquad (1)$$

where $h_{r,i}$ and $\tau_{r,i}$ are the complex gain and the delay associated with the i-th path. For this channel model, the channel estimation is carried out for each block and the pilots are used in a single OFDM symbol in each block. At the receiver, after processing the signal at antenna r, $r = 1, ..., N_r$ we obtain:

$$Y_{0_r}(n) = H_r(n)X(n) + W_r(n), \quad n = 0, ..., N - 1 \ \ r = 1, ..., N_r \qquad (2)$$

where $X(n)$ is the pilot/data symbol sent on the n-th subcarrier, $W_r(n)$ is the noise sample at the n-th subcarrier and r-th antenna (noise samples are independent in both the frequency and space coordinates and are modeled as zero mean circularly symmetric complex Gaussian variables with variance $\sigma_{n_0}^2$)

$$H_r(n) = \sum_{i=0}^{I-1} h_{r,i} e^{-j2\pi \frac{n}{N} \frac{\tau_{r,i}}{T_s}}, \quad n = 0, ..., N - 1 \quad r = 1, ..., N_r \qquad (3)$$

and T_s is the sampling interval. We introduce a constant L, such that $0 \leq \tau_{r,i} \leq L \leq L_{cp}$ (where L_{cp} is the length of the cyclic prefix), and, assume that L is an integer of the form $L = N/D$ for an integer D. In the rest of the paper, the estimation of $H_r(n)$ for $n = 0, ..., N - 1$ and $r = 1, ..., N_r$ is termed the channel estimation problem. We set $\mathbf{H}_r = [H_r(0), H_r(1), ..., H_r(N - 1)]^T$.

Since the true $\tau_{r,i}$'s are continuous, the estimation of $H_r(n)$ can be formulated as a CS problem based on the atomic norm minimization [5,6,10,11] (such formulation for the SISO channel is proposed in [7] but it does not exploit the common support assumption, and, thus, it can be used only for independent channel estimation for each r). To decrease the complexity of the solution for such formulation, as explained in [7], the pilot subcarriers are allocated at P positions (since the channel is sparse $P < L$) n_p, $p = 0, ..., P - 1$, that create a randomly chosen subset of the set of the equidistant L positions which are at integer multiples of N/L i.e. $n_p \in \{0, \frac{N}{L}, ..., \frac{(L-1)N}{L}\}$. With such a pilot allocation scheme, setting $n_p' = n_p \frac{L}{N}$, $p = 0, ..., P - 1$, using equi-powered (constant amplitude and random phase) pilot symbols and dividing the received samples $Y_{0_r}(n_p)$ with $X(n_p)$ we obtain:

$$Y_r(n_p' \frac{N}{L}) = \sum_{i=0}^{I-1} h_{r,i} e^{-j2\pi \frac{\tau_{r,i}}{LT_s} n_p'} + W_{1_r}(n_p' \frac{N}{L}) \qquad (4)$$

where $W_{1_r}(n_p' \frac{N}{L})$ are zero mean circularly symmetric complex Gaussian variables with variance σ_n^2, independent in both the frequency and space coordinates. Equation (4) represents a model with subsampled measurements of a signal in noise. It should be noted that the subcarriers not carrying pilot symbols can be used to transmit data symbols which increases the system capacity.

For clarity, we first introduce the atomic norm and an algorithm for independent channel estimation (based on [7]) and then extend it to the MMV model. The atomic norm of $\mathbf{x} \in \mathbb{C}^{U \times 1}$ [5] is:

$$||\mathbf{x}||_{\mathcal{A}} = \inf_{\substack{c_i \geq 0 \\ \phi_i \in [0,2\pi) \\ f_i \in [0,1)}} \{\sum_i c_i : \mathbf{x} = \sum_i c_i \mathbf{a}(f_i, \phi_i)\} \qquad (5)$$

where $\mathcal{A} = \{\mathbf{a}(f, \phi) : f \in [0, 1), \phi \in [0, 2\pi)\}$ is the set of atom vectors $\mathbf{a}(f, \phi)$ whose components are $a_u(f, \phi) = e^{-j(2\pi f u + \phi)}$ for $u = 0, ..., U - 1$, and $c_i \in \mathbb{R}$. As explained in [5], the SDP form of $||\mathbf{x}||_{\mathcal{A}}$ is:

$$||\mathbf{x}||_{\mathcal{A}} = \inf_{\mathbf{x}, \mathbf{u}, t} \{\frac{\text{trace}(\text{Toep}(\mathbf{u}))}{2U} + \frac{t}{2} : \begin{bmatrix} \text{Toep}(\mathbf{u}) & \mathbf{x} \\ \mathbf{x}^* & t \end{bmatrix} \succeq 0\} \qquad (6)$$

where $\succeq 0$ stands for a positive semidefinite matrix, $\mathrm{Toep}(\mathbf{u})$ is a Toeplitz matrix created using the elements of $\mathbf{u}$ and $\mathrm{trace}(\cdot)$ is the matrix trace.

In the approach with independent channel estimation for each $r, r = 1, \ldots, N_r$, we estimate each $\mathbf{H}_r$ as in [7]. We use the mapping $f_i = \frac{\tau_{r,i}}{LT_s} \in [0,1)$, $c_i e^{-j\phi_i} = h_{r,i}$, $U = L$, introduce the notation $\mathbf{y}_r = [Y_r(n_0'\frac{N}{L}), \ldots, Y_r(n_{P-1}'\frac{N}{L})]^T$, $\mathbf{H}_{L,r} = [H_r(0), \ldots, H_r(\frac{(L-1)N}{L})]^T$ and $\mathbf{H}_{P,r} = [H_r(n_0'\frac{N}{L}), \ldots, H_r(n_{P-1}'\frac{N}{L})]^T$, and estimate $\mathbf{H}_{L,r}$ for the subsampled signal in noise scenario as [7]:

$$\min_{\mathbf{H}_{L,r}} \mu \|\mathbf{H}_{L,r}\|_{\mathcal{A}} + \frac{1}{2}\|\mathbf{y}_r - \mathbf{H}_{P,r}\|_2^2 \tag{7}$$

where μ is a constant. Using the SDP form of the atomic norm (6) and the reconstruction algorithm in the subsampled noisy case (7), the estimates of $\mathbf{H}_{L,r}$ and $\mathbf{u}_r$ can be obtained as:

$$[\hat{\mathbf{H}}_{L,r}, \hat{\mathbf{u}}_r] = \arg\min_{\mathbf{H}_{L,r}, \mathbf{u}_r, t_r} \mu \left(\frac{\mathrm{trace}(\mathrm{Toep}(\mathbf{u}_r))}{2L} + \frac{t_r}{2} \right)$$

$$+ \frac{1}{2}\|\mathbf{y}_r - \mathbf{H}_{P,r}\|_2^2$$

$$\text{subject to } \begin{bmatrix} \mathrm{Toep}(\mathbf{u}_r) & \mathbf{H}_{L,r} \\ \mathbf{H}_{L,r}^* & t_r \end{bmatrix} \succeq 0 \tag{8}$$

where μ can be estimated as $\frac{\rho}{\rho-1}\sqrt{L(\ln \overline{M} + \ln(\pi\rho) + 1)}\sigma_n$ with $\rho = \lim_{k\to\infty} \rho_k$, $\rho_{k+1} = 2\ln \rho_k + 2\ln(\pi\overline{M}) + 3$ for $\rho_0 > 2$ and $\overline{M} = n_{P-1}' - n_0' + 1$ [6].

As explained in [7], the estimates $\hat{\tau}_{r,i}$ of $\tau_{r,i}$ can be obtained from the Toeplitz matrix $\mathrm{Toep}(\hat{\mathbf{u}}_r)$ using root MUSIC. As in [7] we assume that I is known (otherwise, it can be estimated as explained in [6]). Having obtained $\hat{\tau}_{r,i}$'s, we estimate the $h_{r,i}$'s using the LS method:

$$\hat{\mathbf{h}}_{I,r} = \arg\min_{\mathbf{h}_{I,r}} \|\mathbf{D}_r \mathbf{h}_{I,r} - \mathbf{y}_r\|_2^2 \tag{9}$$

where $\mathbf{D}_r$ is a $P \times I$ matrix with elements $[\mathbf{D}_r]_{p,i} = e^{-j2\pi \frac{\hat{\tau}_{r,i}}{LT_s} n_p'}$, $i = 0, \ldots, I-1$, $p = 0, \ldots, P-1$ and $\mathbf{h}_{I,r}$ is an $I \times 1$ vector that contains the $h_{r,i}$'s. The estimated $\hat{\tau}_{r,i}$'s and $\hat{h}_{r,i}$'s are used in (3) instead of the $\tau_{r,i}$'s and the $h_{r,i}$'s to estimate $\mathbf{H}_r$. To obtain the estimates of $\mathbf{H}_r$ of all N_r channels the procedure is repeated N_r times ($r = 1, \ldots, N_r$). It should be noted that if the correlations among the channels are available at the receiver, $\hat{\mathbf{h}}_{I,r}$ can be obtained as an MMSE estimate instead of using the LS method, which may improve the method performance, but the evaluation of such improvement is left for future work.

If the signal to noise ratio is not high, then it can be assumed that [8,9]:

$$\tau_{1,i} \approx \tau_{2,i} \approx \ldots \approx \tau_{N_r,i} \text{ for } i = 1, \ldots, I \tag{10}$$

$$h_{1,i} \neq h_{2,i} \neq \ldots \neq h_{N_r,i} \text{ for } i = 1, \ldots, I \tag{11}$$

which means that the different channels have common support. It should be noted that the correlation between $h_{r,i}$ for different r and given i depends on the system parameters (carrier frequency and distance between receive antennas). The expressions for calculating its value can be found in [9], and, for current communication systems its value is below 0.5 [8].

Based on (10) and (11) we reformulate the channel estimation problem as an atomic norm minimization of the MMV model. Namely, the definition of the atomic norm of matrix $\mathbf{X}$ of dimensions $U \times N_r$ is [10,11]:

$$\|\mathbf{X}\|_{\mathcal{A}} = \inf_{\substack{b_i \geq 0, b_i \in \mathbb{R} \\ \psi_i \in \mathbb{C}^{1 \times N_r}, \|\psi_i\|_2 = 1 \\ f_i \in [0,1)}} \left\{ \sum_i b_i : \mathbf{X} = \sum_i b_i \mathbf{a}(f_i, 0)\psi_i \right\} \tag{12}$$

When $b_i \neq 0$ in (12), $\mathbf{a}(f_i, 0)$ can be included in the creation of each column of $\mathbf{X}$ with arbitrary phase and gain that are included in the value of the corresponding element of ψ_i (the influence of the gains is partially contained in ψ_i and in b_i). So, each column of $\mathbf{X}$ is constructed of the same atoms $\mathbf{a}(f_i, 0)$ but mixed with different complex gains which means that each column of $\mathbf{X}$ can be considered as a different measurement vector. By constructing $\mathbf{H}_L = [\mathbf{H}_{L,1}, \mathbf{H}_{L,2}, ..., \mathbf{H}_{L,N_r}]$, $\mathbf{H}_P = [\mathbf{H}_{P,1}, \mathbf{H}_{P,2}, ..., \mathbf{H}_{P,N_r}]$ and $\mathbf{Y} = [\mathbf{y}_1, \mathbf{y}_2, ..., \mathbf{y}_{N_r}]$ the joint estimation of the channel delays can be carried out using an SDP program for the atomic norm minimization of the MMV model [11]:

$$[\hat{\mathbf{H}}_L, \hat{\mathbf{u}}] = \arg \min_{\mathbf{H}_L, \mathbf{u}, \mathbf{W}} \mu_X \left(\frac{\text{trace}(\text{Toep}(\mathbf{u}))}{2} + \frac{\text{trace}(\mathbf{W})}{2} \right)$$

$$+ \frac{1}{2}\|\mathbf{Y} - \mathbf{H}_P\|_2^2$$

$$\text{subject to } \begin{bmatrix} \text{Toep}(\mathbf{u}) & \mathbf{H}_L \\ \mathbf{H}_L^* & \mathbf{W} \end{bmatrix} \succeq 0 \tag{13}$$

where $\text{Toep}(\mathbf{u})$ is of the form $\text{Toep}(\mathbf{u}) = \mathbf{A}\mathbf{K}\mathbf{A}^H$ for $\mathbf{A} = [\mathbf{a}(f_0, 0) \, ... \, \mathbf{a}(f_{I-1}, 0)]$, $\mathbf{K} = \text{diag}([k_0 \, ... \, k_{I-1}])$ $(k_i, i = 0, ..., I-1$ are positive real numbers). Using $\text{Toep}(\hat{\mathbf{u}})$ from (13), the estimation of $\tau_{r,i}$ is jointly carried out for all $r = 1, ..., N_r$ using root MUSIC [7]. Having obtained $\hat{\tau}_{r,i}$, the $h_{r,i}$'s are estimated using (9). In (13), μ_X can be estimated as $\sigma_n \sqrt{1 + \frac{1}{L}} \sqrt{N_r + \ln \alpha N_r + \sqrt{2N_r \ln \alpha N_r} + \sqrt{\frac{\pi N_r}{2}} + 1}$ for $\alpha = 4\pi \overline{M} \ln L$, which is obtained by combining the results from [6] and [11].

3   Numerical Results

To evaluate the performance of the proposed algorithm we carried out Matlab simulations. We assumed $N = 512$ and $L = 64$ in the OFDM system and used CVX [12] for solving the SDP programs. In each simulation run we used different realizations of the channel impulse responses. To generate the $\tau_{r,i}$'s we first generated I values τ_i from a uniform distribution on $[2T_s, (L-2)T_s)$ such that $|\tau_i - \tau_j| \geq 1.5T_s$ for $i \neq j$ (see [5–7]), then generated $\Delta\tau_{r,i}$'s for $r = 1, ..., N_r$ and $i = 1, ..., I$ to have a uniform distribution on $[-\frac{T_s}{50}, \frac{T_s}{50}]$, and obtained the $\tau_{r,i}$'s as $\tau_{r,i} = \tau_i + \Delta\tau_{r,i}$. We generated the channel gains $h_{r,i}$ as zero mean and unit variance circularly symmetric complex Gaussian variables, independent in both the frequency and space variable. We chose the P pilot positions from the L available using equal probability for each position. We called the algorithm that uses (13) 'JAtomSR' and we called the algorithm that uses (8) 'AtomSR'. Additionally, when appropriate, we showed the MSE of the LS estimates obtained if all N subcarriers were used as pilot subcarriers transmitting equi-powered symbols and the estimation was carried out as $H_r(n) = Y_{0_r}(n)/X(n), n = 0, \ldots, N-1, r = 1, \ldots, N_r$ (termed 'Full LS'). In (8) we used μ obtained by scaling the value below (8) by $1/1.4$ and in (13) for μ_X we used the value below (13) scaled by $1/1.7$. To obtain each point in each plot we averaged the results from 500 simulation runs. As a performance criterion we used the average per sample and per antenna mean squared error defined as:

$$MSE = \mathbb{E}\left[\frac{1}{NN_r}\sum_{r=0}^{N_r}\sum_{n=0}^{N-1}|\hat{H}_r(n) - H_r(n)|^2\right] \quad (14)$$

A performance comparison in terms of P and I is shown in Fig. 1. The lower bound, assuming perfect knowledge of $\tau_{r,i}$'s prior to the LS step (termed 'Known delays') is also shown. JAtomSR shows significant performance gain over AtomSR due to the utilization of the common support assumption, and its performance is very close to the lower bound. The improvement is highest in regions where P is small and/or I is high, and as P increases or I decreases the improvement decreases. By comparing Full LS and JAtomSR in Fig. 1(b) we conclude that exploiting the channel sparsity leads to reduced MSE even when low number of pilot subcarriers are used. It should be noted that the Full LS algorithm has low complexity, negligible compared to JAtomSR.

Performance comparison in terms of N_r and the inverse noise power $10\log_{10}\frac{1}{\sigma_n^2}$ is shown in Fig. 2. The improvement of JAtomSR over AtomSR, shown in Fig. 2(a), increases as N_r increases, but the improvement slope is highest for $N_r = 2$ and

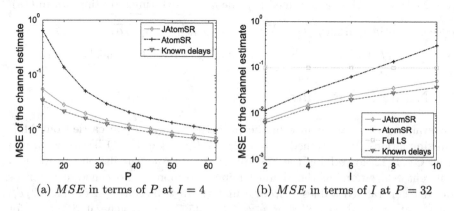

(a) MSE in terms of P at $I = 4$ (b) MSE in terms of I at $P = 32$

Fig. 1. The MSE in terms of P and I at $10\log_{10}\frac{1}{\sigma_n^2} = 10dB$, $N_r = 5$

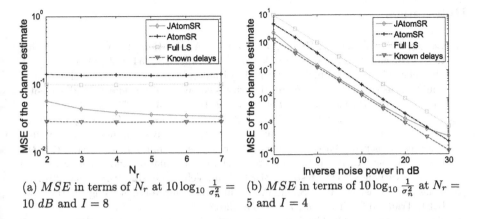

(a) MSE in terms of N_r at $10\log_{10}\frac{1}{\sigma_n^2} = 10\,dB$ and $I = 8$

(b) MSE in terms of $10\log_{10}\frac{1}{\sigma_n^2}$ at $N_r = 5$ and $I = 4$

Fig. 2. The MSE in terms of N_r and the inverse noise power at $P = 32$

decreases with the increase of N_r. Figure 2(b) shows that the improvement of JAtomSR compared to AtomSR is almost constant for broad range of inverse noise powers. However, in the high inverse noise power region the performance of AtomSR becomes comparable to and even better than the performance of JAtomSR. In this region, using the common support assumption does not help anymore. Namely, here the noise power is very low and AtomSR is capable of estimating the $\tau_{r,i}$ with such a precision that the evaluated different delays at different antennas, associated with the same scatterer, significantly decrease the MSE. The complexity analysis of JAtomSR is left for future work.

4 Conclusion

We proposed the use of atomic norm in the estimation of sparse time dispersive SIMO channels with common support in pilot aided OFDM systems. The proposed algorithm uses specific subsampled subcarrier pilot allocation scheme and is based on the atomic norm minimization of the Multiple Measurement Vector model to jointly estimate the delays of the paths at different antennas, corresponding to the same scatterer. The simulation results show that the performance improvement compared to the algorithm that does not use the common support assumption, increases with the increase of the number of receive antennas and is significant in the low to medium SNR region. At high SNR the common support assumption does not hold and the performance of the proposed algorithm degrades. The proposed algorithm can be also used in a MIMO OFDM system, where specific orthogonal pilot patterns are used in the different OFDM symbols of the training sequence, which allows the estimation of the channels between any transmit and each receive antenna.

References

1. Berger, C.R., Wang, Z., Huang, J., Zhou, S.: Application of compressive sensing to sparse channel estimation. IEEE Commun. Mag. **48**, 164–174 (2010)
2. Taubock, G., Hlawatsch, F., Eiwen, D., Rauhut, H.: Compressive estimation of doubly selective channels in multicarrier systems: leakage effects and sparsity-enhancing processing. IEEE J. Sel. Top. Sig. Process. **4**(2), 255–271 (2010)
3. Cheng, P., Chen, Z., Rui, Y., Guo, Y.J., Gui, L., Tao, M., Zhang, Q.T.: Channel estimation for OFDM systems over doubly selective channels: a distributed compressive sensing based approach. IEEE Trans. Comm. **61**, 4173–4185 (2013)
4. Hu, D., Wang, X., He, L.: A new sparse channel estimation and tracking method for time-varying OFDM systems. IEEE Tran. Veh. Tech. **62**, 4848–4653 (2013)
5. Tang, G., Bhaskar, B.N., Shah, P., Recht, B.: Compressed sensing off the grid. IEEE Trans. Inf. Theor. **59**, 7465–7490 (2013)
6. Yang, Z., Xie, L.: On Gridless sparse methods for line spectral estimation from complete and incomplete data. IEEE Trans. Sig. Process. **63**, 3139–3153 (2015)
7. Pejoski, S., Kafedziski, V.: Estimation of sparse time dispersive channels in pilot aided OFDM using atomic norm. IEEE Wirel. Commun. Lett. **4**, 397–400 (2015)
8. Barbotin, Y., Hormati, A., Rangan, S., Vetterli, M.: Estimation of sparse MIMO channels with common support. IEEE Trans. Comm. **60**, 3705–3716 (2012)
9. Barbotin, Y., Vetterli, M.: Fast and robust parametric estimation of jointly sparse channels. IEEE J. Emerg. Sel. Top. Circ. Syst. **2**, 402–412 (2012)
10. Yang, Z., Xie, L.: Exact Joint Sparse Frequency Recovery via Optimization Methods (2014). arXiv:1405.6585
11. Li, Y., Chi, Y.: Off-the-Grid Line Spectrum Denoising and Estimation with Multiple Measurement Vectors (2014). arXiv:1408.2242
12. Grant, M., Boyd, S.: CVX: Matlab Software for Disciplined Convex Programming, version 2.0 beta (2013). http://cvxr.com/cvx

Outage Probability of Dual-Hop MIMO Relay Systems with Direct Links

Jovan Stosic[1]([✉]) and Zoran Hadzi-Velkov[2]

[1] Tenders and Sales Support Department, Makedonski Telekom AD,
Kej 13 Noemvri 6, 1000 Skopje, Macedonia
jstosic@t-home.mk
[2] Faculty of Electrical Engineering and Information Technology,
Saints Cyril and Methodius University, Rugjer Boskovic Bb, 1000 Skopje, Macedonia
zoranhv@feit.ukim.edu.mk

Abstract. In this paper we present approximations of the outage probability for an amplify-and-forward MIMO relaying system with three nodes, which employs multiple antennas at the nodes and orthogonal space-time block coding (OSTBC) transmission over a flat Rayleigh fading. In the amplify-and-forward relay, the incoming signal is decoupled, amplified and forwarded to the destination. Under assumption of availability of full channel state information at the relay and destination and availability of direct link between the source and destination we derived expression for approximation of the outage probability which is sufficiently accurate in the entire SNR range of practical interest. The results obtained by this approximation are compared with the approximations for outage probability of the system without direct link to the destination.

Keywords: Outage probability · Amplify-and-forward · MIMO relay system · Direct link

1 Introduction

Multiple-input multiple-output (MIMO) technology is becoming commonplace in the contemporary communication systems since it offers significant performance improvements in terms of their capacity and reliability, achieved through exploiting the multipath propagation in the wireless medium. Wireless systems with multiple antennas are currently used in local area networks (802.11n, 802.11ac) and in cellular systems such as LTE and LTE advanced. Partly motivated by the MIMO concept, a user cooperation has emerged as an additional breakthrough concept in wireless communications, called cooperative diversity, which has the potential to revolutionize the next generation communication systems by offering additional capacity and reliability improvements with small additional signal processing and cost [1].

In the literature (e.g. [2–7]) for the implementation of the MIMO AF relaying system a specific *amplify and forward* (AF) relaying scheme called Decouple-and-Forward (DCF) relaying is used that has been proposed by Lee et al. in [2].

© Institute for Computer Sciences, Social Informatics and Telecommunications Engineering 2015
V. Atanasovski, L.-G. Alberto (Eds.): Fabulous 2015, LNICST 159, pp. 285–291, 2015.
DOI: 10.1007/978-3-319-27072-2_37

DCF is linear processing technique by which the relay converts multiple spatial streams of the received OSTBC signal into a single spatial stream signal without symbol decoding.

In this paper we derived simple universal approximations for the outage probability of the amplify-and-forward MIMO relay system with direct link, consisted of a source, a decouple-and-forward half-duplex relay and a destination, each equipped with multiple antennas and utilizing an OSTBC transmission technique in a Rayleigh fading environment. The results are compared with the approximations of the outage probability of a dual hop decouple-and-forward relaying system that already exist in literature [4].

In [3–7] we analyzed the performance of the amplify-and-forward MIMO relay systems without direct link from the source to the destination. This analysis is applicable when the sent signal from the source to the destination is very weak or it does not exist at the destination. In such case the destination is reconstructing the sent signal by processing the signal sent by the relay. Hence we call such system a cascade amplify-and-forward MIMO relay system.

In [10] it is shown that the use of the relay which is helping the communication between the source and the destination might increase the capacity of the system. According [11] the total end-to-end instantaneous SNR of an amplify-and-forward relay system is a sum of two random variables: the SNR of the direct component from the source to the destination (γ_1) and the end-to-end SNR - γ_2 of the component that passes via the relay (Fig. 1). We study the outage probability of this relay system under the assumption that γ_1 of the direct transmission branch is statistically independent from γ_2 of the relay transmission branch.

The remainder of this paper is organized as follows. Next section presents the system model. In Sect. 3 we derive the simple expressions for the probability density function (PDF) of the amplify-and-forward MIMO relay system with and without direct link to the destination and then derive the closed form expression for approximation of the outage probability of the amplify-and-forward MIMO relay system with direct link to the destination. Numerical results are presented in Sects. 4 and 5 concludes the article.

2   System Model

The system model is presented in Fig. 1 where the upper branch of the system represents the cascade amplify-and-forward MIMO relay system, and the lower branch of the system represents the direct transmission link from the source to the destination. It consists of a source, an amplify-and-forward MIMO relay and a destination. Each of the three nodes are equipped with N antennas and utilize OSTBC transmission. The relay employs a decouple-and-forward transmission scheme in which if the additive channel noise is neglected, the estimate of the transmitted symbol at the relay can be mathematically expressed as product of the transmitted symbol and the sum of the squared modulus of the MIMO channel coefficients. After the relay decouples the OSTBC signal it re-encodes the decoupled symbols by usage of OSTBC, amplifies each of them separately and transmits them over the relay-destination hop.

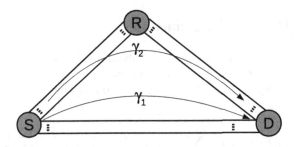

Fig. 1. Dual-hop amplify-and-forward MIMO relay system with direct link to the destination

We consider $NxNxN$ relay configuration, where the source, the relay and the destination are each equipped with N antennas. We assume that there is no spatial correlation between the signals transmitted or received in different antennas. The amplify-and-forward relay applies variable-gain amplification of its input signal, which requires the instantaneous channel state information of the source-relay hop being available to the relay [12]. The destination is also assumed to have a full channel state information of the relay-destination and source-destination hops for coherent demodulation. The source-relay, relay-destination and source-destination hops are modeled as the independent MIMO Rayleigh channels with channel coefficients between the i-th transmit antenna and j-th receive antenna, considered as independent circularly-symmetric complex Gaussian random processes with zero mean and unit variance. Therefore, the squared envelope of signal transmitted over channel follows the exponentially decaying PDF [13] with unit mean squared values. The source transmits with power P. The utilized OSTBC codes are designated as three digit codes, NKL, where N is the number of antennas, K is the number of code symbols transmitted in a code block, and L is the number of required time slots for single codeword [8].

We assume that the relay branch of the system operates in half-duplex mode, divided in two phases (phase 1 and phase 2). The source transmits towards relay during phase 1, then relay transmits towards destination during phase 2. Since we assume that the source employs the OSTB encoding in the phase 1, group of K information symbols are transmitted over the N transmit antennas in L successive time slots. During the phase 2 the $NxNxN$ system's relay decouples, amplifies, OSTB encodes and transmits the K received symbols to the destination.

We have focused on several practical OSTBC schemes, such as 222, 334 and 434, and established their respective approximate outage probabilities when applied in the considered system depicted on Fig. 1 with codeword matrices picked according [8,9] and given with [3, Eq. (32)], [4, Eq. (15)] and [7, Eq. (20)]

with average power per symbol $E = P \cdot c$, $c = L/(KN)$. The received symbols in a single relay antenna for 222, 334 and 434 OSTB codes are decoupled according to [3, Eq. (34)] i.e. [7, Eq. (22)].

3   Outage Probability Analysis

The outage probability is defined as the probability that the instantaneous SNR falls below a predetermined threshold ratio γ_{th}. For the cascade amplify-and-forward MIMO relay channel the approximation of the outage probability is [4]:

$$P_{\text{out}} = F_\Gamma(\gamma)|_{\gamma=\gamma_{th}} \approx 1 - \sum_{n=0}^{m-1} \frac{(b+1)^n}{n!} \left(\frac{\gamma_{th}}{\overline{\gamma}}\right)^n \exp\left(-\frac{(b+1)\gamma_{th}}{\overline{\gamma}}\right), \qquad (1)$$

where and $F(\ldots)$ designates the Cumulative Distribution Function (CDF) approximation of the instantaneous end-to-end SNR which is obtained by taking the terms with $k = 0$ in [3, Eq. (22)] i.e. [4, Eq. (12)] and $\overline{\gamma}$ is the average SNR per symbol. This expression can be used for calculation of the outage probability for the $Nx1xN$ system ($m = N$ and $b = c = L/(KN)$) and for the $NxNxN$ system ($m = N^2$ and $b = 1$) where b is the power normalization factor. In this paper we focus on $NxNxN$ system for which we select $b = 1$. The tight approximation of the PDF is given with [3, Eq. (24)] and its accuracy is presented in the discussion of [3, Sect. (5)] and depicted on [3, Figs. (2)–(7)]. The simplification of [3, Eq. (24)] is necessary in order to simplify the mathematical analysis of the amplify-and-forward MIMO relay system with direct link to the destination. The accuracy of this approach of simplification is checked for the cascade amplify-and-forward MIMO relay system through the analysis of the approximation of error probability [7, Eq. (19)] given in [7, Sect. (5)] and the approximation of outage probability in [4, Eq. (14)] presented in [4, Sect. (5)].

For the derivation of the simplified PDF of cascade amplify-and-forward MIMO relay channel the second term in (1) may be express through Gamma and incomplete upper Gamma function [14, Eq. (8.350.2)] by using of [14, Eq. (8.352.2)]. If we use [15, Eq. (6.5.3)] we obtain the following expression for the CDF of the cascade amplify-and-forward MIMO relay system:

$$F_\Gamma(\gamma) \approx 1 - \frac{\Gamma\left(m, \frac{(b+1)\gamma}{\overline{\gamma}}\right)}{\Gamma(m)} = \frac{\gamma\left(m, \frac{(b+1)\gamma}{\overline{\gamma}}\right)}{\Gamma(m)}, \qquad (2)$$

where $\gamma(\ldots)$ is lower incomplete Gamma function [14, Eq. (8.350.1)]. CDF function given in (2) is CDF of the random variable that is following the gamma PDF with shape parameter m and scale parameter $\theta = \overline{\gamma}/(b+1)$, hence the instantaneous end-to-end SNR [3, Eq. (8)] for cascade amplify-and-forward MIMO relay channel might be approximated by random variable which follows Gamma PDF:

$$f(\gamma) = \frac{1}{\theta^m \cdot \Gamma(m)} \gamma^{m-1} e^{-\frac{\gamma}{\theta}} = \frac{(b+1)^m}{\overline{\gamma}^m \cdot \Gamma(m)} \gamma^{m-1} e^{-\frac{(b+1)\gamma}{\overline{\gamma}}}, \quad \theta = \frac{\overline{\gamma}}{b+1}. \qquad (3)$$

We assume that direct transmission branch is under the influence of Rayleigh fading, hence its instantaneous SNR follows Gama PDF, and the instantaneous SNR in the relay transmission branch is distributed by (3) in which we select $b = 1$ since we consider the NxNxN system configuration:

$$f_{\Gamma_1} := \frac{1}{\overline{\gamma}^m \cdot \Gamma(m)} \gamma^{m-1} e^{-\frac{\gamma}{\overline{\gamma}}}, \quad f_{\Gamma_2} := \frac{2^m}{\overline{\gamma}^m \cdot \Gamma(m)} \gamma^{m-1} e^{-\frac{2 \cdot \gamma}{\overline{\gamma}}}. \tag{4}$$

The resulting random variable is sum of two random variables each following Gamma PDF with different scale parameter: $\Gamma = \Gamma_1 + \Gamma_2$. In arbitrary case the sum of n random variables which follow gamma PDFs with different shape and scale parameters is:

$$Y = X_1 + X_2 + \ldots + X_n, \quad f_i(x_i) = \frac{x_i^{\alpha_i}}{\theta_i^{\alpha_i} \cdot \Gamma(\alpha_i)} e^{-\frac{x_i}{\theta_i}}. \tag{5}$$

The random variable Y is distributed by following PDF [16]:

$$g(y) = C \cdot \sum_{k=0}^{\infty} \frac{\delta_k \cdot y^{\rho+k-1}}{\Gamma(\rho+k) \cdot \theta_l^{\rho+k}} e^{-\frac{y}{\theta_l}}, \quad \theta_l = \min_i(\theta_i), \quad \rho = \sum_{i=1}^{n} \alpha_i,$$

$$C = \prod_{i=1}^{n} \left(\frac{\theta_l}{\theta_i}\right)^{\alpha_i}, \quad \delta_{k+1} = \frac{1}{k+1} \cdot \sum_{i=1}^{k+1} i \cdot \gamma_i \cdot \delta_{k+1-i}, \quad k = 0, 1, 2, \, \delta_0 = 1,$$

$$\gamma_k = \frac{1}{k} \sum_{i=1}^{n} \alpha_i \left(1 - \frac{\theta_l}{\theta_i}\right)^k, \quad k = 1, 2, \ldots \tag{6}$$

We simplify the parameters given in (6) for the case of two random variables:

$$\theta_l = \frac{\overline{\gamma}}{b+1}, \quad \rho = 2 \cdot m, \quad C = (b+1)^{-m}, \quad \delta_i = \frac{(m)_i}{i!} \cdot \left(\frac{b}{b+1}\right)^i, \tag{7}$$

where $(\ldots)_{\ldots}$ represents pochhammer symbol. In case of NxNxN system ($b = 1$) parameters in (7) are:

$$\theta_l = \frac{\overline{\gamma}}{2}, \quad \rho = 2 \cdot m, \quad C = 2^{-m}, \quad \delta_i = \frac{(m)_i}{i!} \cdot \left(\frac{1}{2}\right)^i. \tag{8}$$

If parameters from (8) are introduced in expression for $g(y)$ in (6) we obtain the PDF of the random variable Γ representing the instantaneous SNR in the destination of amplify-and-forward MIMO relay system with direct link:

$$f_\Gamma(\gamma) = \sum_{k=0}^{\infty} \frac{(m)_k}{k!} \cdot \frac{\gamma^{2m+k-1} 2^m}{\Gamma(2m+k) \cdot \overline{\gamma}^{2m+k}} \cdot e^{-\frac{2 \cdot \gamma}{\overline{\gamma}}}. \tag{9}$$

If (9) is introduced in $P_{\text{out}} = F_\Gamma(\gamma)|_{\gamma=\gamma_{th}}$ we obtain the outage probability of amplify-and-forward MIMO relay system with direct link to the destination:

$$P_{out} = 1 - \sum_{k=0}^{\infty} \frac{(m)_k}{k! \cdot 2^{m+k}} \cdot \frac{\Gamma\left(2m+k, \frac{2 \cdot \gamma_{th}}{\overline{\gamma}}\right)}{\Gamma(2m+k)}. \tag{10}$$

4 Numerical Results

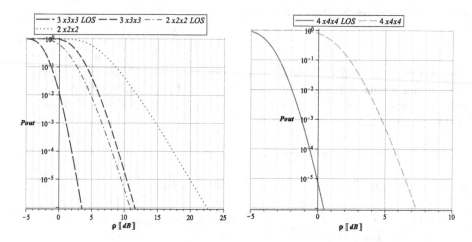

Fig. 2. Outage probability for $N \times N \times N$ 222/334/434 OSTBC system with and without direct link to the destination for $\gamma_{th} = 5\,dB$

On Fig. 2 we present the comparison of the outage probability for amplify-and-forward MIMO relay system with and without direct link to the destination for $\gamma_{th} = 5\,dB$. The curves on these figures are obtained by usage of the expressions (1) and (10) which are based on the approximation of the PDF of the cascade MIMO relay channel given with (3). From Fig. 2 we conclude that the systems with direct link has much lower outage probability in comparison to the systems without direct link, as it could be expected from the information theoretic analysis given in [10]. For example, for the $2 \times 2 \times 2$ system for $\rho = 10\,dB$ (where ρ is the average SNR per symbol per node) the outage probability of the system without direct link is $4 \cdot 10^{-2}$, and the outage probability of the same system with direct link is $4 \cdot 10^{-6}$ resulting in four order of magnitude improvement. Moreover, from Fig. 2 it is obvious that the systems with direct link has greater diversity gain compared to the cascade systems. The difference in diversity gain is reduced by increase of the number of antennas.

5 Conclusion

In this paper we have analyzed the dual-hop relay system with multiple antennas at the source, the relay and the destination that utilize OSTBC and amplify-and-forward relaying schemes. We analyzed the outage probability of this system in case when direct link to the destination is available. For such relay system we have derived generalized closed form expressions for approximation of the outage probability (10). We compared the results obtained with this approximation with results from the literature for amplify-and-forward MIMO relay systems without direct link to the destination. The amplify-and-forward MIMO relay system with direct link to the destination shows significant outage probability improvement yielding to significant diversity gain.

References

1. Sendonaris, A., Erkip, E., Aazhang, B.: User cooperation diversity Part I and Part II. IEEE Trans. Commun. **51**(11), 1927–1948 (2003)
2. Lee, I.-H., Kim, D.: Decouple-and-forward relaying for dual-hop alamouti transmissions. IEEE Commun. Lett. **12**(2), 97–99 (2008)
3. Stosic, J., Hadzi-Velkov, Z.: Simple tight approximations of the error performance for dual-hop MIMO relay systems in Rayleigh fading. AEU Int. J. Electr. Commun. **67**(10), 854–960 (2013)
4. Stosic, J., Hadzi-Velkov, Z.: Outage probability approximations for dual-hop amplify-and-forward MIMO relay systems in Rayleigh fading. In: Proceedings of 11th International Conference on Telecommunication in Modern Satellite, Cable and Broadcasting Services (TELSIKS 2013), Nis, Serbia (2013)
5. Stosic, J., Hadzi-Velkov, Z.: Performance analysis of dual-hop MIMO systems. In: Proceedings of 2nd Conference on Information and Communication Technologies' Innovations (ICT Innovations 2010), Ohrid, Macedonia (2010)
6. Stosic, J., Hadzi-Velkov, Z.: Performance analysis of dual-hop dual-antennas MIMO systems in Rayleigh fading. In: Proceedings of 2nd International Congress on Ultra Modern Telecommunications and Control Systems (ICUMT 2010), Moscow, Russia (2010)
7. Stosic, J., Hadzi-Velkov, Z.: Approximate performance analysis of dual-hop decouple-and-forward MIMO relaying. In: Proceedings of 11th International Conference on Electronics, Telecommunications, Automation and Informatics, Macedonia (2013)
8. Jafarkhani, H.: Space Time Coding Theory and Practice. Cambridge University Press, Cambridge (2005)
9. Tarokh, V., Jafarkhani, H., Calderbank, A.R.: Space-time block codes from orthogonal designs. IEEE Trans. Inf. Theor. **45**(5), 1456–1467 (1999)
10. Cover, T.M., Gamal, A.E.: Capacity theorem for the relay channels. IEEE Trans. Inf. Theor. **25**(5), 527–584 (1979)
11. Gamal, A.E., Kim, Y.-H.: Network Information Theory. Cambridge University Press, Cambridge (2011)
12. Hasna, M.O., Alouini, M.S.: A performance study of dual-hop transmissions with fixed gain relays. IEEE Trans. Wirel. Commun. **3**(6), 1963–1968 (2004)
13. Simon, M.K., Alouini, M.S.: Digital Communication Over Fading Channels, 2nd edn. Wiley, New York (2005)
14. Gradshteyn, I.S., Ryzhik, I.M.: Table of Integrals, Series, and Products, 6th edn. Academic Press, Burlington (2000)
15. Abramowitz, M., Stegun, I.A.: Handbook of Mathematical Functions with Formulas, Graphs, and Mathematical Tables, 9th edn. Dover, New York (1970)
16. Moschopoulos, P.G.: The distribution of the sum of independent gamma random variables. Ann. Inst. Statist. Math. **37**(1), 541–544 (1985)

Resource Allocation in Energy Harvesting Communication Systems

Ivana Nikoloska$^{(\boxtimes)}$, Zoran Hadzi-Velkov, and Hristina Cingoska

Faculty of Electrical Engineering and Information Technologies,
Saints Cyril and Methodius University, Skopje, Macedonia
{ivanan,zoranhv,cingoska}@feit.ukim.edu.mk

Abstract. We consider a point-to-point wireless communication link, with a perpetual energy source, since a base station, sends energy to energy harvesting nodes. These nodes employ a so called "harvest than transmit" protocol, hence they use the harvested energy to send information in the uplink. We present 3 ways of maximizing the achievable throughput, one via optimizing the base station output power, the second via optimizing the duration of the Energy Harvesting phase and a novel transmission scheme that jointly optimizes both the Base Station output power as well as the Energy Harvesting phase duration. This third scheme, is the main contribution of this paper.

Keywords: Energy harvesting · Wireless power transfer · Resource allocation

1 Introduction

Energy is a major constraint for wireless networks. Perpetual operation of Wireless Sensor Networks (WSNs) can be enabled be energy harvesting, because of its capability to provide endless system operation [1,2]. Since the arrival of energy packets may be insufficient, which puts in question the reliability of communication, dedicated far-field radio frequency (RF) radiation may be used as energy supply for EH transmitters, an approach known as wireless power transfer (WPT) [5,6]. The WPT can be realized as a simultaneous wireless information and power transfer (SWIPT) [7], or, alternatively, over a dedicated (either time or frequency) channel for energy transfer. The latter option makes wireless powered communications networks (WPCNs) possible. These WPCNs typically share a common channel, based upon time-division multiple access (TDMA).

In [8], the authors determine the optimal TDMA scheme among the half-duplex nodes (either BS or EHNs), depending on the channel fading states. Separated frequency channels for energy broadcast and information transmissions (IT) were studied in [9] and an optimal time-sharing scheme for WPCNs was derived. Furthermore, [10] studies the WPCN with full-duplex nodes, where the BS is equipped with two antennas. The authors in [12], consider WPCNs, where the nodes choose between two power levels, a constant desired power, or a lower power when its EH battery has stored insufficient energy. Finally, in [13],

© Institute for Computer Sciences, Social Informatics and Telecommunications Engineering 2015
V. Atanasovski, L.-G. Alberto (Eds.): Fabulous 2015, LNICST 159, pp. 292–298, 2015.
DOI: 10.1007/978-3-319-27072-2_38

a three-node relaying system, was considered, where both source and relay harvest energy from the BS, by using WPT.

The above-referenced works propose optimal (either time or power) allocation schemes (except for [12]). In this paper, we employ these approaches for our system model and we propose a novel optimal scheme, that jointly allocates the BS broadcasting power and the TDMA slots.

The rest of this paper is organized as follows. Section 2 presents the system and channel model. Optimal power allocation is presented in Sect. 3 and optimal EH phase duration is presented in Sect. 4. Section 5 presents the novel joint optimization scheme and Sect. 6 presents numerical results. Finally, Sect. 7 concludes the paper and proof of the optimal solution of the novel scheme is presented in the Appendix.

2   System and Channel Model

We consider a point-to-point link consisting of a half-duplex BS and a half-duplex EHN, which operate in fading environment. The BS broadcasts RF energy to the EHN, whereas the EHN transmits information back to the BS. The EHN is equipped with rechargeable EH batteries that harvest the RF energy broadcasted from the BS. The IT from EHN to BS (IT phase), and the WPT from BS to EHN (EH phase) are realized as successive signal transmissions using TDMA over a common channel, where each TDMA frame/epoch is of duration T. Each (TDMA) epoch consists of an EH phase and an IT phase. The channel between the BS and the EHN is a quasi-static block fading channel, which is constant during a single block but changes independently from one block to the next. The duration of one fading block is assumed equal to T, and one block coincides with a single epoch. In epoch i, the fading power gains of the BS-EHN channel is denoted by x'_i. For convenience, these gains are normalized by the additive white gaussian noise (AWGN) power, yielding $x_i = x'_i/N_0$ with an average value of $\Omega = E[x'_i]/N_0$, where $E[\cdot]$ denotes expectation. The channels are assume to be reciprocal, i.e., in epoch i, the gains of BS-EHN and EHN-BS channels are the same.

3   Throughput Maximization with Optimal Output Power

Let us consider $M \to \infty$ epochs. In epoch i, the BS transmits power, denoted by p_i. In the same epoch, the duration of the EH phase is, $\tau_0 T$. Note, that τ_0 is not included in the optimization.

During the EH phase of epoch i, the amount of harvested power by the EHN is $E_i = N_0 p_i x_i \tau_0 T$. Moreover, during the IT phase, this EHN spends its total amount of harvested energy, E_i, for transmitting a complex-valued Gaussian codeword of duration $(1 - \tau_0) T$, comprised of $n \to \infty$ symbols, with an output transmit power $P(i) = \frac{E_i}{(1-\tau_0) T} = \frac{N_0 p_i x_i \tau_0}{1-\tau_0}$, and an information rate, $R(i) = (1 - \tau_0) \log (1 + P(i) x_i) = (1 - \tau_{0i}) \log \left(1 + \frac{a_i p_i \tau_0}{1-\tau_0}\right)$, where $a_i = N_0 x_i^2$.

During the $M \to \infty$ epochs, the average throughout, we maximize overall according to

$$\max_{p_i, \forall i} \frac{1}{M} \sum_{i=1}^{M} (1 - \tau_0) \log \left(1 + a_i p_i \frac{\tau_0}{1 - \tau_0} \right)$$

$$C1 : \frac{1}{M} \sum_{i=1}^{M} p_i \tau_0 \leq P_{avg}$$

$$C2 : p_i \geq 0, \forall i \tag{1}$$

Equation 1 is a convex optimization problem. It's optimal power allocation is as follows:

Theorem 1. *The optimal BS transmit power is given by*

$$p_i^* = \frac{1 - \tau_0}{\tau_0} \left(\frac{1}{\lambda} - \frac{1}{a_i} \right) \tag{2}$$

The constant λ is found such that the constraint $C1$ in (1) holds with equality.

4   Throughput Maximization with Optimal EH Phase Duration

Another way to maximize the achievable throughput is by optimizing the duration of the energy harvesting phase, i.e. τ_{0i}. Here, p is not included in the optimization, hence p has a pre-determined fixed value. We solve the following convex optimization problem:

$$\max_{\tau_{0i}, \forall i} \frac{1}{M} \sum_{i=1}^{M} (1 - \tau_{0i}) \log \left(1 + a_i \, p \, \frac{\tau_{0i}}{1 - \tau_{0i}} \right)$$

$$C1 : \frac{1}{M} \sum_{i=1}^{M} p \tau_{0i} \leq P_{avg}$$

$$C2 : 0 < \tau_{0i} < 1, \forall i \tag{3}$$

The following theorem presents the optimal solution of 3:

Theorem 2. *The optimal τ_{0i} is the solution of the following transcendental equation:*

$$- \log \left(1 + \frac{a_i p \tau_{0i}}{1 - \tau_{0i}} \right) + \frac{a_i p}{1 - \tau_{0i} + a_i p \tau_{0i}} = \lambda p \tag{4}$$

The constant λ is found such that the constraint $C1$ in (3) holds with equality.

5   Throughput Maximization via Joint Optimization

We present a novel transmission scheme by jointly optimizing both the BS transmission power, p_i and the duration of the energy harvesting phase τ_{0i}. To this end we solve:

$$\max_{p_i,\tau_{0i},\forall i} \frac{1}{M} \sum_{i=1}^{M} (1 - \tau_{0i}) \log \left(1 + a_i\, p_i \frac{\tau_{0i}}{1 - \tau_{0i}} \right)$$

$$C1 : \frac{1}{M} \sum_{i=1}^{M} p_i \tau_{0i} \leq P_{avg}$$
$$C2 : 0 \leq p_i \leq P_{max}, \forall i$$
$$C3 : \tau_{0i} > 0, \forall i. \tag{5}$$

The optimization problem in (5) is non-convex because of the products and ratios of the optimization variables p_i and τ_{0i}. However, if we introduce the new variable, $e_i = p_i\,\tau_{0i}$, (5) is transformed into a convex optimization problem, as:

$$\max_{e_i,\tau_{0i},\forall i} \frac{1}{M} \sum_{i=1}^{M} (1 - \tau_{0i}) \log \left(1 + a_i \frac{e_i}{1 - \tau_{0i}} \right)$$

$$\bar{C}1 : \frac{1}{M} \sum_{i=1}^{M} e_i \leq \bar{P}$$
$$\bar{C}2 : 0 \leq e_i \leq P_{max}\,\tau_{0i}, \forall i$$
$$C3 : \tau_{0i} > 0, \forall i. \tag{6}$$

Concavity of $(1 - \tau_{0i}) \log \left(1 + a_i \frac{e_i}{1-\tau_{0i}} \right)$ can be argued from the fact that the function $(1 - \tau_{0i}) \log \left(1 + a_i \frac{e_i}{1-\tau_{0i}} \right)$ is the perspective of the strictly concave function $\log (1 + a_i e_i)$. Since this operation preserves concavity, $(1 - \tau_{0i}) \log \left(1 + a_i \frac{e_i}{1-\tau_{0i}} \right)$ is also concave [14]. Linear constraints in (6) form a convex feasible set, therefore, (6) is a convex optimization problem.

Theorem 3. *The optimal BS transmit power is given by*

$$p_i^* = \begin{cases} P_{max}, & a_i > \lambda \\ 0, & otherwise. \end{cases}$$

The optimal duration of the EH phase, τ_{0i}^*, is the root of the following transcendental equation,

$$\lambda P_{max} + \log \left(1 + \frac{a_i P_{max} \tau_{0i}}{1 - \tau_{0i}} \right) = \frac{a_i P_{max}}{1 - \tau_{0i} + a_i P_{max} \tau_{0i}}, \tag{7}$$

The constant λ is found such that the constraint C1 in (1) holds with equality.

Proof. Please refer to the Appendix.

Theorem 3 shows that an optimal policy requires binary power allocation and time allocation as shown in (7).

6   Numerical Results

We illustrate our results for a point-to-point EH system in Rayleigh fading environment. The AWGN power is set to $N_0 = 10^{-12}$ W, and the deterministic path loss (PL) of the BS-EHN channel is $PL = 60$ dB. Thus, $E[x'_{1i}] = 1/PL$ and $\Omega_1 = 1/(N_0\,PL) = 10^6$.

Figure 1, compares (1) achieved throughput for optimal BS output power (and fixed duration on 0.5 and 0.7), (2) achieved throughput with optimal duration (and output power equal to P_{avg}) and (3) achieved throughput with joint optimization. It is clearly shown that the novel scheme outperforms the previously mentioned.

As shown on Fig. 1, the power allocation scheme when τ_{0i} is relatively large (0.7), gives worst performance. In this case $1 - \tau_{0i}$ i.e. the duration of the information transmission, is small, thus a smaller throughput is achieved. As the value of τ_{0i} decreases (to 0.5 in this scenario), the throughput becomes larger. The time allocation scheme, only outperforms power allocation when the duration of the IT phase is small. In any case, joint allocation always performs best.

7   Conclusions

We reviewed transmission schemes that optimize the BS output power and duration of the EH phase respectively. Also, a transmission scheme was proposed for the jointly optimal power allocation of the BS, and TDMA time sharing, for wireless powered communication links. The proposed scheme clearly outperforms any knows solution so far.

Joint optimization of time and power can be efficiently used in practical scenarios when a single transmitter is concerned. In the future, we will develop similar practical schemes for arbitrary number of transmitters.

A Proof of theorem 3

We obtained a convex optimization problem, whose Lagrangian is given by

$$L'(e_i, \tau_{0i}, \lambda) = \frac{1}{M} \sum_{i=1}^{M} (1 - \tau_{0i}) \log\left(1 + a_i \frac{e_i}{1 - \tau_{0i}}\right)$$

$$-\lambda \frac{1}{M} \sum_{i=1}^{M} (e_i - \bar{P}) + q_i e_i - \mu_i(e_i - P_{max}\tau_{0i}). \qquad (8)$$

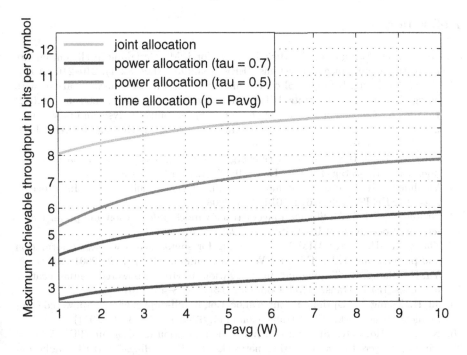

Fig. 1. Maximum achievable throughput vs. relay average output power

where the Lagrange multiplier λ is associated with the constraint $\bar{C}1$, whereas q_i and μ_i correspond to the left-hand side and the right-hand side of $\bar{C}2$, respectively.

According to the Karush-Juhn-Tucker (KKT) conditions, complementary slackness should be satisfied, $\forall i$: $q_i e_i = \mu_i(e_i - P_{max}\tau_{0i}) = 0$, where $q_i \geq 0$ and $\mu_i \geq 0$. Related to the complementary slackness, we consider the following 3 cases:

<u>Case 1</u>: When $\alpha_i = 0$, from the definition of α_i, θ_i is also 0. Naturally, no power is allocated in epoch i, i.e. $p_i = 0$ [11].

<u>Case 2</u>: When $0 < e_i < P_{max}\tau_i$, the slackness conditions require $\mu_i = 0$ and $q_i = 0$. In this case, according to the derivative with respect to e_i, the optimal e_i is given by $e_i = (1 - \tau_{0i})\left(\frac{1}{\lambda} - \frac{1}{a_i}\right)$. However, if we introduce the previous into the derivative with respect to τ_{0i}, we obtain $1 - \lambda/a_i = \log(a_i/\lambda)$, which is satisfied iff $a_i = \lambda$. However, $a_i = \lambda$, $\forall i$, is unlikely event, and therefore, the optimal e_i does not belong to the interval $0 < e_i < P_{max}\tau_{0i}$.

<u>Case 3</u>: When $e_i = P_{max}\tau_{0i}$, the slackness conditions require $q_i = 0$ and $\mu_i > 0$. In this case, $\mu_i = \frac{a_i}{1 + \frac{a_i P_{max}\tau_{0i}}{1 - \tau_{0i}}} - \lambda > 0$, or equivalently $\frac{1 - \tau_{0i}}{\tau_{0i}}\left(\frac{1}{\lambda} - \frac{1}{a_i}\right) > P_{max}$, which yields the condition $a_i > \lambda$. Introducing μ_i and $e_i = P_{max}\tau_{0i}$ into the derivative with respect to τ_{0i}, we finally obtain (7).

References

1. Gunduz, D., Stamatiou, K., Michelusi, N., Zorzi, M.: Designing intelligent energy harvesting communication systems. IEEE Commun. Mag. **52**(1), 210–216 (2014)
2. Ho, C.K., Zhang, R.: Optimal energy allocation for wireless communications with energy harvesting constraints. IEEE Trans. Sig. Proccess. **60**(9), 4808–4818 (2012)
3. Krikidis, I., Charalambous, T., Thompson, J.S.: Stability analysis and power optimization for energy harvesting cooperative networks. IEEE Sig. Process. Lett. **19**(1), 20–23 (2011)
4. Ding, Z., Poor, H.V.: Cooperative energy harvesting networks with spatially random users. IEEE Sig. Process. Lett. **20**(12), 1211–1214 (2013)
5. Varshney, L.R.: Transporting information and energy simultaneously. In: Proceedings of IEEE ISIT, pp. 1612–1616, July 2008
6. Grover, P., Sahai, A.: Shannon meets Tesla: wireless information and power transfer. In: Proceedings of IEEE ISIT, pp. 2363–2367, June 2010
7. Zhang, R., Ho, C.K.: MIMO broadcasting for simultaneous wireless information and power transfer. IEEE Trans. Wireless Commun. **12**(5), 1989–2001 (2013)
8. Yu, H., Zhang, R.: Throughput maximization in wireless powered communication networks. IEEE Trans. Wirel. Commun. **13**(1), 418–428 (2014)
9. Ju, H., Zhang, R.: Optimal resource allocation in full-duplex wireless-powered communication network. IEEE Trans. Commun. **62**(10), 3528–3540 (2014)
10. Kang, X., Ho, C.K., Sun, S.: Optimal time allocation for dynamic-TDMA-based wireless powered communication networks. In: Proceedings of IEEE Globecom 2014, Signal Processing for Communications Symposium, December 2014
11. Orhan, O., Gunduz, D., Erkip, E.: Throughput maximization for an energy harvesting communication system with processing cost. In: Information Theory Workshop (ITW), pp. 84–88, 03 September 2012
12. Morsi, R., Michalopoulos, D.S., Schober, R.: Performance analysis of wireless powered communication with finite/infinite energy storage, October 2014. arXiv:1410.1805v2
13. Chen, H., et al.: Harvest-then-cooperate: wireless-powered cooperative communications, March 2015. arXiv:1404.4120v2
14. Boyd, S., Vandenberghe, L.: Convex Optimization. Cambridge University Press, Cambridge (2004)

Advanced QoS-Based User-Centric Aggregation (AQUA) for 5G Mobile Terminals in Heterogeneous Wireless and Mobile Networks

Tomislav Shuminoski[✉] and Toni Janevski

Faculty of Electrical Engineering and Information Technologies,
Saints Cyril and Methodius University, Skopje, Republic of Macedonia
{tomish, tonij}@feit.ukim.edu.mk

Abstract. The paper is presenting an advanced QoS provisioning module with vertical multi-homing framework for future 5G mobile terminals (5GMT) with radio network aggregation capability and traffic load sharing in heterogeneous mobile and wireless environments. The proposed 5GMT framework is leading to high performance utility networks with high QoS provisioning for any given multimedia service and multi-RAT capabilities. It is using vertical multi-homing and virtual QoS routing algorithms within the mobile terminal, that is able to handle simultaneously multiple radio network connections via multiple wireless and mobile network interfaces. The performance of our proposed 5GMT is evaluated using simulations with multimedia traffic in heterogeneous wireless and mobile networks under different network conditions.

Keywords: 5G · Quality of service · User-centric · Vertical multi-homing

1 Introduction

The novel scientific research and development directions are undoubtedly leading to profound changes in the design of 5G mobile equipments, networks and services. This paper provides advanced mobile technology framework that could lead to high performance utility networks with high QoS provisioning for any given multimedia service. Looking beyond network implementations and improvements, the 5G networks will require smarter devices capable to provide a broad range of multimedia services (voice, data and video) to mobile users, with ubiquitous mobility, mobile broadband connections, enormous processing power of the mobile equipment, machine-to-machine communications, massive MIMO, better network utilization and load balancing, advanced QoS support, as well as bigger memory space and longer battery life of mobile terminals, which will provide enough storage capability for control information and enormous spectrum for advanced capabilities [1–8]. The 5G networks are expected to be deployed beyond 2020, but currently we have operator-centric approach implemented in 3G mobile networks and service-centric approach in 4G mobile networks [9]. In the future generation mobile networks, the 5G is moving towards the user-centric (or device-centric) concept [1–7].

© Institute for Computer Sciences, Social Informatics and Telecommunications Engineering 2015
V. Atanasovski, L.-G. Alberto (Eds.): Fabulous 2015, LNICST 159, pp. 299–306, 2015.
DOI: 10.1007/978-3-319-27072-2_39

2   Related Works

The main motivation for our QoS provisioning framework could be found in [5–8] and [10, 11]. Device-centric multi-RAT architectures, native support of machine-to-machine communications and smarter devices are part of the main trend for 5G [1]. Our framework and design of a novel mobile terminal is a next step from our previous work on adaptive QoS provisioning in heterogeneous wireless and mobile IP networks [13–15]. Those papers were introducing a novel adaptive QoS provisioning module that provides the best QoS and lower cost for a given multimedia service by using one or more wireless technologies at a given time. The performance of our adaptive QoS algorithm, in the above mentioned papers, was evaluated using simulation with dual-RAT UMTS/WLAN mobile equipments. However, the drawback of such adaptive QoS framework lies in its applicability to single RAT at a given time, even in the cases when it is probably the best connection for a given service traffic. In that way, one step forward is made by using simultaneously all available RATs at a same time by combining different traffic flows from different RATs using vertical multi-homing. Another paper [16] is dealing with a network selection algorithm based on Fuzzy Multiple Attribute Decision Making. That algorithm considers the factors of Received Signal Strength, monetary cost, bandwidth, velocity and user preference. It defines a network selection function that measures the efficiency in the utilization of radio resources in given networks. Again, there is a selection of only one network. The main base for developing our novel QoS routing algorithm for our 5GMT can be found in [17] and for the vertical multi-homing features in [10, 11]. The proposed general scheme is trying to solve the access network selection problem in the heterogeneous wireless and mobile network scenario and has been used to present and design a general multicriteria software assistant that can consider the user, operator, and/or the QoS view points. Combined fuzzy logic (FL) and genetic algorithms (GAs) have been used to give the proposed scheme the required scalability, flexibility, and simplicity. On the other side, [18] presents a joint radio resource management strategy based on reinforcement learning mechanisms that control a fuzzy-neural algorithm to ensure certain QoS constraints. The fuzzy logic allows for a very simple handling of the joint radio resource manager simply by activating a set of rules. In comparison with all related works, we must to emphasize that our framework is implemented on IP level, is able to combine different traffic flows from different multimedia services and in the same time is able to use several RATs, achieving superior results and high QoS provisioning.

3   System Model and AQUA Algorithm

The proposed novel 5GMT is multi-RAT node, with several (n) interfaces, each for different RAT (overall n RATs). According to [5, 6] physical and OWA (Open Wireless Architecture) define the wireless technology: Medium Access Layer (MAC) and Physical layer. One may emphasize that on OWA layer can be added any present or future RAT with their defined MAC and Physical layers.

However, the main focus of the work in this paper is on IP layer and above, by using different RATs below. With all-IP concept adopted in all IEEE networks, and the

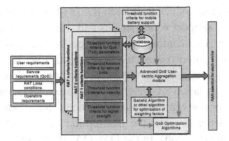

Fig. 1. Advanced QoS routing and RAT selection mobile.

same concept is adopted in 3GPP 4G mobile networks and beyond (5G), the network layer everywhere will be IP. However, separation of this layer into two sublayers will be necessary. The Upper IP Network Layer (UIPNL) has one unified IPv6 address within, and is nominated for routing as well as for creation of sockets to the upper open transport layer (OTL) and to the application layer. Moreover, 5GMT will be suitable to have Open Transport Protocol (OTP) that is possible to be downloaded and installed. Such MTs shall have the possibility to download (e.g., modifications and adaptation of TCP for the mobile and wireless networks, RTP, Stream Control Transmission Protocol (SCTP) [19], Datagram Congestion Control Protocol (DCCP) [20], some future transport protocol, etc.) version which is targeted to a specific wireless and mobile technology installed at the base stations, with multi-homing support [10, 11]. More detail description for the OSI layers in future 5GMT designs is given in [5, 7, 12]. The core of our work is development of novel adaptive QoS Module with advanced QoS user-centric aggregation algorithm and with vertical multi-homing features. We will refer to it as Advanced QoS-based User-centric Aggregation (AQUA) algorithm, which is defined independently from different wireless and mobile technologies, uses Multi-RAT interfaces. It is implemented between UIPNL and LIPNL, which will be able to provide intelligent QoS management and routing over variety of RATs at the same time. The building components of AQUA for radio networks selection with vertical multi-homing and routing in heterogeneous RAT environment are shown in Fig. 1. The data measurements for different selection criteria, including user require-ments, QoS requirements, operator requirements, as well as radio link conditions in different RATs present in the user's moving area are inputs for the n sets of parallel criteria functions (CFs), one set per each RAT. One RAT CF is shaping and filtering the outputs from the previous four components into four interior threshold functions: the first is shaping the QoS parameters, the second is shaping the service price if the service stream is going over that RAT, the third is shaping velocity support and the last is shaping the signal strength detected in mobile terminal from RAT base station(s). Any of those four threshold criteria functions is giving on its output only one value (as a real number within the limits of [0, 1]). However, our solution is allowing person-alization. The central component is AQUA module with capability to select one optimization algorithm (OA), which as inputs uses: the outputs of the n sets of parallel criteria functions (CFs), four values from each RATs (4*n in total) and the output of the threshold CF for battery support which shapes and filtrates the outputs from the user's mobile battery life-time. This central component of AQUA algorithm is in continuous communication and interaction (connected permanently) with: the Generic Algorithm (GA) module, QoS OAs database. The GA [17] (or other OA, like Linear Programming (LP)) is doing the optimization of weighting coefficients (factors) of different input criteria for each RAT for a given multimedia service. That is, each criterion may have different weight that depends upon the assumption of its impact on the best RAT selection process (i.e. the decision). In the QoS OAs database is stored information for QoS parameters for all services, together with the measured data and OAs which can be used for solving the optimization problem. Finally, the AQUA module is targeted for the selection of wireless and mobile networks in heterogeneous environment, so the decision as an outcome should select the best RATs (among all present RATs) and will rank them in certain order. The ranking order accrues from the ranking value that has each of the RAT ranking functions (RFs). If we calculate the inputs from the threshold CFs as a real numbers within the limits of [0, 1], then the i-th RAT RF can be yield as follows:

$$RF_{RAT\_i} = \frac{QoSt_i * W_{QoS} + Ct_i * W_C + Vt_i * W_V + SSt_i * W_{SS} + Bt_i * W_B}{W_{QoS} + W_C + W_V + W_{SS} + W_B} \quad (1)$$

$$\text{where } 1 \leq i \leq n \text{ and } W_{QoS} + W_C + W_V + W_{SS} + W_B = 1 \quad (2)$$

where W_{QoS}, W_C, W_V, W_{SS}, W_B are assigned weight factors for the criteria functions of: QoS parameter, service price, velocity of the mobile terminal, signal strength and mobile terminal battery support, respectively. Those values of weight factors are assigned using a particular method of optimization, i.e. GAs, where their value is obtained through the process of moving the GA OA to the pre-specified goal. On the other hand, after passing the four interior threshold functions for i-th RAT CF (see Fig. 1), the outputs (shaped values) from QoS parameters are $QoSt_i$, from service price are Ct_i, from velocity support are Vt_i, and from detected signals strength are SSt_i. The shaped output value of the threshold CF for battery support is Bt_i. So, the final step is selection of the best RAT, by choosing the RAT (from all available RATs) which has the highest value for his RF (1), for a given service:

$$\max_{service\_j} \{Optimal(RF_{RAT\_i})\} \quad (3)$$

subject to $W_{QoS} \leq 1$, $W_C \leq 1$, $W_V \leq 1$, $W_{SS} \leq 1$, $W_B \leq 1$ and (2) where $1 \leq j \leq 3$.

$$(4)$$

Above we have defined the optimization problem. Where $service\_j$ is the given service (i.e. $j = 1$, video, $j = 2$, audio and $j = 3$ data), and $Optimal(RF_{RAT\_i})$ is the optimal function value for the i-th RAT RF, calculated by OA. To summarize, we choose that RAT_i technology with maximal value for it's optimal RAT RF ($Optimal(RF_{RAT\_i})$).

4   Simulation Results and Analysis

The simulation scenario consists of three RATs. Each RAT is represented with single base station with different radius of network coverage. All base stations (from all RATs) are positioned in the center of the simulation area, with coordinates (0, 0). RAT1, RAT2 and RAT3 have cell radiuses of 5 km, 2.5 km and 250 m, adequately. Network capacity for the given three RATs is set to: RAT1_C = 307200 kbit/s, RAT2_C = 1048576 kbit/s, and RAT3 = 614400 kbit/s. The values are carefully chosen in order to correspond with the certain standardized capacities of the following RATs: LTE, Mobile WiMAX 2.0 (IEEE 802.16 m) and IEEE 802.11n, and with aim to obtain generally more realistic conclusions from the proposed solution. At the beginning of the simulation, the MTs are randomly scattered within the area of 5×5 km^2. For MTs physical mobility, we adopted 2-dimensional implementation of the Gauss-Markov Mobility model [21] considering average speeds in the range of 30-180 km/h, and providing high level of randomness for user mobility. Moreover, this simulation scenario provides total network coverage for all MTs (RAT1, RAT2 and RAT3 coverage, or minimum RAT1 coverage). The multimedia service flow model in the proposed form predicts the existence of three types of services that are defined by its required bit rate (bandwidths) and its starting time and duration. The first service type is video conference, defined by a low bit rate (128 kbit/s) and small propagation time. The second service type, the video-streaming, is defined by medium bit rate (256 kbit/s) and low propagation time. The third service type is data service with high bit rate (512 kbit/s) and can handle higher delays, but requiring no packet delivery error. During the simulation for a given number of ordinary active mobile users N, each user is randomly assigned to one of the three types of services defined above. On the other side, when the users have 5GMT with AQUA module within, for each user are randomly assigned all three (or minimum two) types of multimedia services. There are five cases for this scenario: in the first case all MTs are enhanced with AQUA module with GA optimizations in our three-RAT MT with three interfaces and with AQUA module. In the second case all MTs are enhanced with LP optimization of weighting coefficients of different input criteria for each RAT for a given multimedia service (for the optimization problem of each i-th RAT RF), instead of having GA module. We refer to this kind of MT as MT with LP module (LP_MT). In the last three cases, we are using MT without AQUA module and without multi-RAT interfaces, but only with one RAT interface. So, in the third scenario we have MTs which are using only RAT1 technology (i.e. only LTE interface). In the forth and fifth scenarios there are MTs which are using only RAT2 and RAT3, respectively. Furthermore, a comparative simulation analysis regarding the achievable bit rates are shown in Fig. 2, which provides results on the average throughput versus number of MTs for all five cases. The average velocity of the MTs is set on 40 km/h and the total simulation time is 60 s. As can be noticed, the throughput for our 5GMT (R_5GMT), with included AQUA module, for any number of used MTs, is much higher than the average throughput values in the case when we used only MTs that can access only RAT1 (R_RAT1_MT), or in the case when we use only MTs that access RAT2 (R_RAT2_MT) or RAT3 (R_RAT3_MT). Comparing the throughput for the 5GMT (R_5GMT) and the throughput in the case when LP is used as OA within the AQUA module of MT (R_LP_MT), the 5GMT with GA is achieving the highest throughput for any number of MT up to 1100, then is almost equal for very high number of MTs (between 1100 and 1200) with the average throughput values for the LP_MT case, and for higher number of MTs (more then 1200) is getting lower and LP_MT shows superior results. This indicates that 5GMT with GA can be used for low to middle traffic congestion scenarios (up to 1250 TMs), and LP OA can be triggered within AQUA for very high traffic concentration (high number of MTs, i.e. more then 1300).

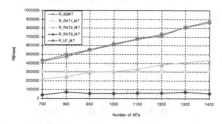
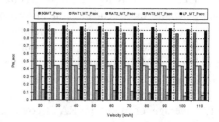

Fig. 2. Throughput vs number of MTs.   **Fig. 3.** Pm_acc vs velocity of MTs.

So, if we have 5GMT with two options for choosing LP or GA OAs, more often we will use 5GMT with GA, and less with LP. Undoubtedly, vertical multi-homing and multi-RAT MTs are achieving superior results regarding the aggregated average throughput per service and optimal RAT decisions. Consequently other MTs three cases which are using only one service per user, and only one RAT, are limited with the capacity and performances provided by that RAT. Furthermore, in Fig. 3 are presented the average access probability ratio (Pm_acc) values for different average speed with 450 MTs and simulation time of 60 s. The multimedia access probability ratio is calculated as ratio of the total number of all successfully multimedia service access attempts from the users and the total number of all multimedia service access attempts (as sum of not successful and successful access attempts). For the first case when we use 5GMTs with AQUA modules with GA algorithm within, the average access probability ratio values are following the MTs with AQUA modules with LP algorithm within for any velocity values. The difference between those two cases is in 0.1 or less in the average access probability ratios. As can be seen, the case with AQUA module with LP algorithm within the MTs is better and shows higher average access probability ratio. In case of congested networks, we can used the LP OA if this QoS parameter (Pm_acc) is crucial for the applications, if not we can still use GA OA, because the difference is not so high, and in return (see Fig. 2) we get more available throughput. Above all the MTs with AQUA module and vertical multi-homing features are showing, undoubtedly, superior results compared with the other three cases when there are MTs without those advantages, just with one RAT interface. If we see the values of case five, with RAT3 MTs, because of the small area coverage and nomadic mobility support, we get the worst average access probability values, and as the average velocities of the MTs are rising – the Pm_acc values are getting smaller.

5 Conclusion

In this paper we have proposed a our 5GMT design targeted to exploit future multi-RAT by using advanced QoS provisioning and with vertical multi-homing features, here-called AQUA module. The proposal is evaluated via simulation results for the key QoS parameters in the analysis, which are throughput and multimedia service access probability ratio. According to the simulation results and analysis, our proposed 5GMT with AQUA and vertical multi-homing performs fairly well under a variety of network conditions.

References

1. Boccardi, F., et al.: Five disruptive technology directions for 5G. IEEE Commun. Mag. **52** (2), 74–80 (2014)
2. Bhushan, N., et al.: Network densification: the dominant theme for wireless evolution into 5G. IEEE Commun. Mag. **52**(2), 82–89 (2014)
3. Bangerter, B., Talwar, S., Arefi, R., Stewart, K.: Networks and devices for the 5G era. IEEE Commun. Mag. **52**(2), 90–96 (2014)
4. Wang, C.X., et al.: Cellular architecture and key technologies for 5G wireless communication networks. IEEE Commun. Mag. **52**(2), 122–130 (2014)
5. Janevski, T.: 5G Mobile phone concept. In: IEEE Consumer Communications and Networking Conference (CCNC), Las Vegas, USA (2009)
6. Lu, W.W.: An open baseband processing architecture for future mobile terminals design. IEEE Wirel. Commun. **15**(2), 110–119 (2008)
7. Tudzarov, A., Janevski, T.: Design for 5G mobile network architecture. Int. J. Commun. Netw. Inf. Secur. (IJCNIS) **3**(2), 112–123 (2011)
8. Noll, J., Chowdhury, M.M.R.: 5G – Service continuity in heterogeneous environments. Wireless Pers. Commun. **57**(3), 413–429 (2010). doi:10.1007/s11277-010-0077-6
9. Rahman, M., Mir, F.: Fourth generation (4G) mobile networks - features, technologies and issues. In: 6th IEE International Conference on 3G Mobile Communication Technologies (3G 2005), London, UK, pp. 1–5, November 2005
10. Rec. ITU-T Y. 2052 (02/2008): Framework of multi-homing in IPv6-based NGN
11. Recommendation ITU-T Y.2056 (08/2011): Framework of vertical multihoming in IPv6-based Next Generation Networks
12. Tudzarov, A., Janevski, T.: Protocols and algorithms for the next generation 5G mobile systems. Netw. Protoc. Algorithms **3**(1), 94–114 (2011). ISSN 1943-3581
13. Janevski, T.: Traffic Analysis and Design of Wireless IP Networks. Artech House, Norwood (2003)
14. Shuminoski, T., Janevski, T.: Novel adaptive QoS provisioning in heterogeneous wireless environment. Int. J. Commun. Netw. Inf. Secur. (IJCNIS) **3**(1), 1–7 (2011). ISSN: 2076-0930
15. Shuminoski, T., Janevski, T.: Novel adaptive QoS framework for integrated UMTS/WLAN environment. Telfor J. **5**(1), 14–19 (2013)
16. Radhika, K., Reddy, A.V.: Network selection in heterogeneous wireless networks based on fuzzy multiple criteria decision making. International Journal of Computer Applications (0975– 8887), Volume 22– No.1, (2011)

17. Alkhawlani, M., Ayesh, A.: Access network selection based on fuzzy logic and genetic algorithms. Adv. Artif. Intell. **8**(1), 1–12 (2008)
18. Giupponi, L., et al.: A novel joint radio resource management approach with reinforcement learning mechanisms. In: Proceedings of the 24th IEEE International Performance, Computing, and Communications Conference (IPCCC 2005), USA, pp. 621–626, (2005)
19. Fu, S., Atiquzzaman, M.: SCTP: state of the art in research, products, and technical challenges. IEEE Commun. Mag. **42**(4), 64–76 (2004)
20. Kohler, E., Handley, M., Floyd, S.: RFC: 4340 Datagram Congestion Control Protocol (DCCP). http://tools.ietf.org/html/rfc4340 (2006). Accessed: 15 May 2015
21. Broyler, D., et al.: Design and analysis of a 3-D gauss-markov mobility model for highly dynamic airborne networks. In: International Telemetering Conference (ITC 2010) (2010)

Design and Implementation of a System for Automatic Sign Language Translation

Vasilkovski Martin[✉]

Faculty of Electrical Engineering and Information Technologies,
Saints Cyril and Methodius University, Karpos 2 BB, 1000 Skopje,
Republic of Macedonia
martin.vasilkovski@gmail.com

Abstract. The communication between hearing and speech impaired people, and the rest of the world is generally done through sign language. However, only less than 1 % of the world's population can communicate using this language and thus setting a barrier in everyday situations. This paper tackles the previous problem by offering a solution based on the concept of smart gloves. A smart glove is a glove equipped with sensing gear, computational power and intelligence that can easily track every movement of a hand and as such, is able to also recognize characteristic positions allowing sign language to text conversion, as well as audio presentation of the letter shown. In addition, the detailed realization process of this kind of glove follows a budget-friendly concept in order to enable financial ease in rebuilding and further development.

Keywords: Smart glove · Sign language · Real time signal processing · Robotics · Hand · Biomedical · Design · Hand-motion capture · Multifinger sensing

1 Introduction

Taking into account that more than 70 million people worldwide use sign language as their primary language, a device which will translate those hand gestures to text or sound may not only be used for that particular everyday use, but also in the fields of education, computer-human interaction and even entertainment. The main idea of this paper is to present the idea of a device that can analyze all hand gestures, interpret them to text and audio, and most importantly that is feasible and economical.

By definition, sign language is a system of communication using visual gestures and signs, as used by deaf people. The sign language manual alphabet does not use the previously mentioned gestures and impressions, on the contrary, it only needs one hand. This leads to the conclusion that making a glove that can translate the manual alphabet with a single handed glove is a more comfortable solution [1]. The idea of a device containing solely sign language translation capabilities is something that can be considered popular at present times [2], but the initial difference and main idea of this paper is to present the idea of a device that can analyze all hand gestures, interpret them to text and audio, and most importantly that is vastly more feasible and economical [3]. For this purpose the author after extensive research and development, created hardware

© Institute for Computer Sciences, Social Informatics and Telecommunications Engineering 2015
V. Atanasovski, L.-G. Alberto (Eds.): Fabulous 2015, LNICST 159, pp. 307–313, 2015.
DOI: 10.1007/978-3-319-27072-2_40

and software that is optimized for the purpose of this system. One algorithm for effective and high precision recognition of letter, visualization, processing of the sensors' signals to achieve stability and precision of expensive and complex industrial bend sensors, and an additional algorithm for optimized stand alone functioning of the system with no processing on a an extra computer needed.

2 Kinematic Model of the Human Hand

The use of all joints on the fingers can be stripped down to four basic movements:

- Flexion and extension;
- Adduction and abduction.

Since all of the movements that are being analyzed are the positions from a completely flattened hand (complete extension) to a hand set as a fist (complete flexion), it is only needed to observe the flexion and extension of each finger.

In order to gain more advanced knowledge of the positions of a particular finger a kinematic model of a hand and finger is needed. However, a complete picture of the position of each join of each finger is not needed for the primary purpose of this project. To simplify the procedure, only one joint of each finger is being observed, and that is the middle (proximal intrephalangeal) joint. For the basic movements used in the manual alphabet, it is postulated that the adjacent joints at each point of time are flexed at approximately half of the angle of the middle joint.

3 Hardware Implementation

What was previously described gives an insight on what the manual alphabet is, how it is used and what is required for it to be used. In order to make use of the ability to measure the movement of the fingers and hand we need a device which will be built by hand. Aside from the choice of computational power, gyroscopic equipment, the most important part of the glove are the flex sensors.

The leading component is the microcontroller, with which the signals are read, gathered and processed. The choice was set on Arduino Mega 260 R3. For the purpose of measuring the movement of the hand, as well as the tilting of it, a 3-axis gyroscope is needed. In this project, a GY-521 gyroscope (with included accelerometer) is used. It has an integrated chip MPU-6050 which gives 16-bit data for each of the axis for both the gyroscope and the accelerometer. The vast majority of letters do not require use of abduction or adduction, but still two of them do. The easiest solution for this was to add normally open (N.O.) contacts, from coiled copper wire.

Choosing the right sensors for the joints of the fingers is the crucial part. Many types can be used, such as: Flex sensors, stretch sensors and optical linear encoders [4], but what proved to be the best choice were piezoresistive flex sensors. These have to be handmade, and they use the effect of piezoresistivity that can be induced by black conductive ESD bags or Velostat material. Piezoresistivity is the ability of certain materials to change their resistance, and with that conductivity, by applying pressure. In this case, using black conductive ESD bags, when pressure is applied the resistance decreases nearly proportionally. Velostat is a packaging material made of a polymeric foil enriched with carbon black to make it electrically conductive. It is used for the protection of items or devices that are susceptible to damage from electrostatic discharge.

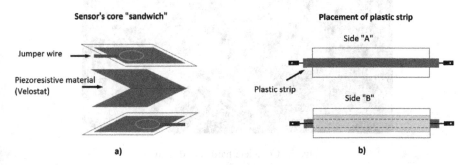

Fig. 1. Constructing the sensor is characterized by two main parts: (a) Core of the sensor; (b) Shell of the sensor

The core of the sensor is the most important part of it, as it is the region which reacts to changes. In order to make it sensitive to external pressure when applied, a sandwich with a couple of layers of piezoresistive material and curled copper wire, as shown in Fig. 1(a) This way, instead of the wires directly touching and conducting electricity with no resistance between them, a thick layer of material that changes resistivity when pressed makes the contact area act as a resistor with variable resistance. Thus when the joint is flexed, the resistance decreases and the current flow increases. A plastic strip is added in order to give the sensor flexibility and to make sure that the pressure applied by the flexing is dispersed equally along the sensing core. The former is illustrated in Fig. 1(b).

Additionally, electrical circuits in the form of voltage dividers are used so that the variable resistance of the sensors can be converted to change in voltage. The referent voltage of this circuit is 5 V and the dividing resistor has the equal resistance as the nominal resistance of the corresponding sensor. The resulting voltage of these dividers can be derived from:

$$AD_{n-1} = \frac{R_n}{R_n * RS_n} * 5[V] \qquad (1)$$

Where: AD_{n-1}- output voltage to analog input n-1; R_n - nominal resistance of sensor n; RS_n- current (measured) resistance of sensor.

In Fig. 2 the end product of the prototype is shown, with all the components mounted properly on top of the glove.

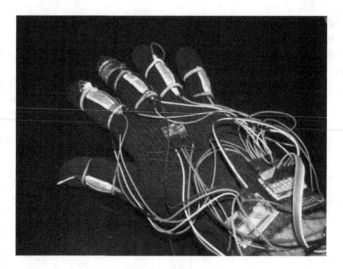

Fig. 2. Complete hardware design

4   Software Implementation

The use of a Arduino microcontroller implies that the programming of it will be done in the Arduino software, which is based on the programming language C. This project also uses a USB connection to communicate with a PC. The microcontroller is used to gather the information from all sensors, gyroscope and contacts, and real time signal processing of the signals from the sensors. The rest of the algorithm including signal filtering and processing, calibration, angle calculation and letter recognition runs on a PC using the program Processing, which incorporates a programming language based on Java.

Naturally, the output signal from the flex sensors is unstable mainly because of its construction. In order to ease the hardware components, real time signal processing is done by the Arduino. The primary raw signal gathered by the microcontroller through ADC contains oscillations and some imminent saturations, as illustrated in Fig. 3(a). In order to stabilize the signals and cut-off the oscillations, two filters are used. The first one is a mean value filter, which computes the current value output as the mean value of the last n readings [5]. And the second filter is a modified low pass filter. Low pass filters are commonly used for canceling out minor oscillations [6]. This filter is based on differential behavior, or every differential (change) that is bigger than a particular value is not modified, but everything that is smaller than that value goes through a cube filter. This "cubed" filter allows the lowest values to be almost completely suppressed, but as that value rises they are less or not at all suppressed. This filter follows the following equation:

$$\begin{cases} y(dx) = \frac{(dx)^3}{n^2}, |dx| < n \\ y(dx) = dx, |dx| > n \end{cases} \tag{2}$$

Where: y - output; dx - differential of the last and current reading (dx = x[i]-x[i-1]); n - cut off value.

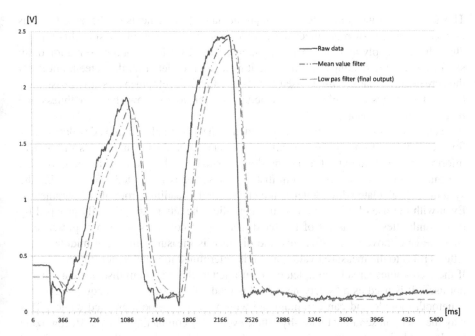

Fig. 3. (a) Raw data directly read from a sensor; (b) Mean value filter applied to raw data; (c) Low pass filter applied for finite processed signal

The finite output signal, shown in Fig. 3(c), is presented after filtering has lost the oscillations and saturations. Because of the nature of the sensors, a calibration procedure is of great essence. This will give the computer insight on the operating range of the sensors and can maximize the precision by knowing the estimated highest and lowest expected values. For this to happen a calibration procedure must be done by the user. After this procedure, the stabilized signal that was previously mentioned can be converted to values that are easier to work with depending on the later use of the system. Through measurements and experiments it was concluded that the joint of the thumb goes approximately from 0° to 90°, but the other fingers can go from 0° to 110°. Some of the letters have very similar readings, so they need to be grouped and internally divided. For example, the letters "U" and "V" use adduction and abduction which something that is not sensed by the flex sensors. For this purpose there is a normally open contact between the index and middle finger in order to sense this movement. If they touch it is "U", if not it is "V". Otherwise, they are completely the same. There are some other letters which can be labeled as similar such as "L" and "G", but aside from all the same readings, they differ by the plain in which the hand sits. This is sensed by the gyroscope and the letters are distinguished. The letters "J" and "Z" have the positioning of the hand just like "I" and "D" respectively, but both include movement with the hand which is picked up by the accelerometer.

In order to ease the coding and memory use, instead of fuzzy logic, the principle for rule giving here was developed by defining the rules of recognition by hand. This means the acceptable range for each parameter is already initially defined in the code. Every rule includes dependency between the parameters which ensures flexibility.

This secondary zone is included so that all the natural movements by the hand (such as twitches or minor swings) affect the outcome as little as possible. Using this type of algorithm and applying to a generated window with realistic visual representation of all sensor data. If the readings match a rule it results with a letter on the screen, but if not the screen stays blank. This is used for research and development, as it is possible to handle the ranges and rules for each letter, as well as to show the smoothness and precision of the sensors.

The previous mode is computer dependent. The second algorithm is developed only for the Arduino, to make the system stand alone. This algorithm entrusts the user to inform the system to expect letters by doing a small hand gestures with the glove. To use this as an advantage, minimum distance classifier is integrated [7]. With this the system will calculate which letter is the closest to the readings from all 12 parameters. Even with the use of minimum distance classifier, the letters are primarily grouped by their similarities such as tilt of the hand, activity of contact sensors and presence of characteristic movement. After this, the distance is measured from the middle of the letter's rules to the measured values and it is determined to which letter it is the closest. If the read values already completely cover a letter, the minimum distance classifier is not used. It is used as a "safety net". In this mode, the system is also equipped with a Bluetooth module and can communicate with a local Bluetooth enabled device. This way the user can send data letter-by-letter, eventually completing a word. Recognizing whole words is not supported as it would need both hands and their mutual digital coordination. This algorithm can be enriched with some basic artificial intelligence which will contribute with active real time redefining of rules of all letters for better and more precise prediction and recognition of them (Fig. 4).

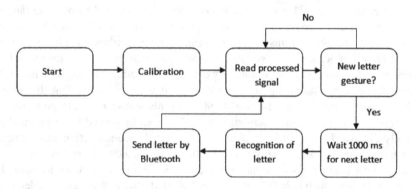

Fig. 4. Flow chart of data acquisition and letter recognition

5 Performance and Accuracy

The performance of this system, as well as its accuracy, is dependent on the letters that are being recognized. Letters such as "M", "N" and "T" are very similar to each other and can cause inconvenience. However, this is not something that happens too often, statistically about 5 % of the time. Similar to the problems of those three letters are "C", "O" and "E". In this case the problem is not only that they are very similar, it is also that the positions of the joints are in the middle of the range, meaning the fingers are not flexed or extended, and oscillations from muscle twitching is almost certainly present. Even though this is mostly surpassed by the given rules or minimum distance classifier, it still is happening at maybe 80%-85% of the time. The other letters in general are carefully divided from each other and when added the minimum distance classifier, the mistakes in decision making are reduced to a minimum.

6 Concluding Remarks

This paper proposes a design tried by users of sign language and has proven effective for converting sign language to text accurately, but also it takes the most out of the handmade sensors by real time signal processing and can with satisfactory precision recreate the movement of fingers for analysis of anthropomorphic hand movements or control of multimedia devices as well as personal computers. The low level approach of coding allows the microcontroller to use as less as possible of its capacity, as well as the construction which is modular and easy to improve. In further research and development the rules can be defined by working with a group of regular users of sign language and teach the system to recognize patterns on itself, through machine learning algorithms such as neural networks.

Acknowledgement. I would like to thank my mentor Prof. Dr. Elizabeta Lazarevska, who has helped and supported me throughout the lengthy period devoted to the realization of this project.

References

1. Pfau, R., Stenbach, M., Woll, B.: Sign Language: An International Handbook. Series: Handbooks of Linguistics and Communication Science (HSK37). De Gruyter Mouton, New York (2012)
2. Haydar, J., Dalal, B., Hussainy, S., El Khansa, L., Fahs, W.: ASL fingerspelling translator glove. IJCSI Int. J. Comput. Sci. Issues 9(6), 254–260 (2012)
3. Kuroda, T., Tabata, Y., Goto, A., Ikuta, H., Murakami, M.: Consumer price data-glove for sign language recognition. In: Proceedings of the 5th International Conference on Disability, Virtual Reality & Associated Technologies, Oxford, UK (2004)
4. Li, K., Chen, I.-M., Yeo, S.H., Lim, C.K.: Development of finger-motion capturing device based on optical linear encoder. Robotics Research Centre, School of Mechanical and Aerospace Engineering, Nanyang Technological Univeristy, Singapore, vol. 48, January 2011
5. Gavrovski, C.: Basics of measuring techniques. Faculty of Electrical Engineering and Information Technologies, Skopje (2011)
6. Kuo, S., Lee, B., Tian, W.: Real-Time Digital Signal Processing: Fundamentals. Implementations and Applications. Wiley, New York (2013)
7. Solomon, C., Breckon, T.: Fundamentals of Digital Image Processing: A Practical Approach with Examples in Matlab. Wiley, Chichester (2011)

Author Index

Printed in the United States
By Bookmasters